The Ne

> 105 THE

Commissioning Editor: Ellen Green
Development Editor: Janice Urquhart
Project Manager: Nancy Arnott
Designer: Erik Bigland
Illustrator: Hardlines; David Banks; Jane Fellows

The Normal Child

Edited by

Martin Bellman MD FRCP FRCPCH DCH

Consultant Paediatrician, Royal Free Hospital, London and Islington Primary Care Trust, London, UK

Ed Peile EdD MB BS FRCP FRCPCH FRCGP DCH DRCOG

Associate Dean (Teaching), Warwick Medical School, University of Warwick, Warwick, UK

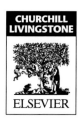

CHURCHILL
LIVINGSTONE

ELSEVIER

EDINBURGH LONDON NEW YORK OXFORD PHILADELPHIA ST LOUIS SYDNEY TORONTO 2006

CHURCHILL
LIVINGSTONE
ELSEVIER

First published 2006

ISBN-10: 0-443-05707-9
ISBN-13: 978-0-443-05707-6
IE ISBN-10: 0-443-05718-4
IE ISBN-13: 978-0-443-05718-2

British Library Cataloguing in Publication Data
A catalogue record for this book is available from the British Library

Library of Congress Cataloging in Publication Data
A catalog record for this book is available from the Library of Congress

Printed and bound by CPI Group (UK) Ltd, Croydon, CR0 4YY

Transferred to Digital Print 2011

Preface

What is a normal child? In our current multiethnic/multicultural society the range is very wide. Global travel is becoming more and more common and the population profile of most countries is constantly changing. Even without immigration, normality is a dynamic concept. Normal standards in the UK for attributes such as growth, educational attainment and social behaviour are not the same now as they were a generation ago and will be different again in another 10 years' time.

Is it then possible to write a textbook on the 'normal child'? Some fundamental facts do not change, such as anatomy and physiology. Prenatal and postnatal human development is also remarkably constant and deviations from the normal patterns are fortunately rare. Relevant information on these subjects is included in chapters that cover genetics, embryology and the senses. Most of the other chapters cover more changing fields as they are significantly influenced by environmental factors to a greater degree (e.g. the preterm infant, feeding and growth) or to a lesser degree (e.g. communication, cognition and emotional behaviour, play and motor skills). The chapter on social environment draws together aspects of how the child is impacted on by many different forces in society and how child advocacy may be able to work towards improving circumstances for future generations. The special senses chapter is about how the child experiences the immediate ambient environment with a comment on the mothering role. Thus, we hope that this book successfully presents information on the normal child in the first part of the 21st century and that it does not get out of date too rapidly.

The book is intended for all professionals who work with children as a learning aid during training and a reference during their careers. However, we also hope that it will be useful for parents who wish to have more information about normal children. Our aim is to describe the health and development of children in a way which will clarify the boundaries of normality. We accept the dangers inherent in talking about the 'normal child': we might be understood to imply the existence of the 'abnormal child'. Far from it: as our concluding case studies demonstrate, we emphasize that every child has norms and that deviations from the 'standard' patterns are often unclear and controversial.

Written from a health perspective, we hope to illustrate the common boundaries of normality in the typical child, rather than to write yet another book about paediatric disease processes. When we refer to diseases, it is to illustrate what happens when the boundaries of 'normality' are crossed. In this way, a picture builds up of what is typical for a child and what is not.

As we hope that many people who are not from a health background will enjoy this book, in addition to doctors, nurses and allied health professionals, we have tried to limit the use of medical terms. However, an understanding of the child depends on some anatomy, physiology and medical science, so we have included as much as we believe is fundamental to this understanding.

The richness of this book is attributable to the different professional backgrounds of the contributing chapter authors. We have not tried to impose too much 'house style' uniformity in order to allow the freshness of their contributions to impact directly on our readers.

We welcome suggestions as to how future editions may be improved.

M. B.
E. P.

Acknowledgements

Many people have given generous help at various stages of this book. We would like to thank in particular: Frances Howard for commenting on the Genetics and Embryology sections, and Joanna Lawson for commenting on the section on the eye, and Charlotte Schembri for secretarial assistance. At Elsevier, Ellen Green offered patient encouragement from the first conception of the book through its early development, and Janice Urquhart and Nancy Arnott have given continuing editorial support. Much of the burden of this endeavour has been borne by our families. We deeply appreciate their support, and we also thank those who have supported the time taken out by our chapter authors.

Contributors

Martin Bellman MD FRCP FRCPCH DCH
Consultant Paediatrician, Royal Free Hospital,
London and Islington Primary Care Trust, London,
UK

Jill Brownson MCSP
Paediatric Physiotherapy Service Manager, St Mary's
Hospital, London, UK

Deborah Christie BSc PhD DipClinPsych
Consultant Clinical Psychologist and Honorary
Senior Lecturer, Head of Paediatric and Adolescent
Psychology, University College London Hospital,
London, UK

Rachel Crowther MB BChir MSc MFPH
Consultant in Public Health Medicine, South East
Public Health Observatory, UK

Margaret Francis RGN RSCN HV DipHSW
Paediatric Liaison Health Visitor, Paediatric Liaison
Health Visitor, Hemel Hempstead Hospital, Dacorum
PCT, Hemel Hempstead Hospital, Hertfordshire, UK

Angela Huertas-Ceballos MD MSc
Consultant Neonatologist, Elizabeth Garret Anderson
Hospital, University College London Hospital, UK

Juliet Jamieson MRCSLT
Specialist Speech and Language Therapist
Child Development Centre, Stevenage, Hertfordshire
and Department of Human Communication Science,
University College London

Nigel Kennedy MB BS FRCP FRCPCH DCH DRCOG
General Practitioner, Aylesbury; Hospital
Practitioner, Paediatrics, Stoke Mandeville Hospital,
Aylesbury, UK

Helen Pegg RGN RHV BSc
Health Visitor, North Derbyshire, UK

Ed Peile EdD MB BS FRCP FRCPCH FRCGP DCH DRCOG
Associate Dean (Teaching), Warwick Medical School,
University of Warwick, Warwick, UK

Sally Scott-Roberts MEd DipCOT ILTM
Lecturer, Occupational Therapy Department, School
of Health Care Studies, Cardiff University, UK

Lyn Westcott MSc BSc DipCOT ILTM
Senior Lecturer, Occupational Therapy Dept, School
of Health Care Studies, Cardiff University, Cardiff,
UK

Contents

List of abbreviations   x

1. **Genetics**   1
   M. Bellman

2. **Embryology**   9
   M. Bellman

3. **The Preterm Infant**   19
   A. Huertas-Ceballos

4. **Growth**   29
   E. Peile

5. **Feeding**   47
   M. Francis, J. Jamieson

6. **Sleep**   61
   H. Pegg

7. **Cognitive, emotional and behavioural development**   73
   D. Christie

8. **Speech and communication**   83
   J. Jamieson

9. **Play**   103
   S. Scott-Roberts, L. Westcott

10. **Motor skills, gait and coordination**   117
    J. Brownson

11. **Special senses: vision, hearing and skills integration**   129
    M. Bellman

12. **Social environment**   149
    R. Crowther

13. **Boundaries of normal in health**   177
    N. Kennedy

14. **Postscript: two case studies**   193
    M. Bellman, E. Peile

Appendix 1
   Tables of normal neurodevelopmental data   195
   M. Bellman, E. Peile

Appendix 2
   Immunization   199
   M. Bellman, E. Peile

Appendix 3
   Sexualized behaviour   201
   M. Bellman, E. Peile

Index   203

List of abbreviations

AA	arachidonic acid	LAD	language acquisition device
ACA	acquired childhood aphasia	LCPs	long chain polyunsaturated fatty acids
ADD	attention deficit disorder	LH	luteinizing hormone
ADHD	attention deficit hyperactivity disorder	MRI	magnetic resonance imaging
AOM	acute otitis media	NREM	non-rapid eye movement
AS	Asperger's syndrome	NICU	neonatal intensive care unit
ASD	autistic spectrum disorder	OAE	oto-acoustic emission
CANS	central auditory nervous system	OME	otitis media with effusion
CAP	central auditory processing	OSA	obstructive sleep apnoea
CDS	child directed speech	OSD	obsessive compulsive disorder
CLD	chronic lung disease	PCR	polymerase chain reaction
CSF	cerebrospinal fluid	PE	physical education
CTG	cardiotocography	RAST	radio-allergo-sorbent test
DHA	docosahexaenoic acid	RDS	respiratory distress syndrome
DNA	deoxyribonucleic acid	REM	rapid eye movement
EEG	electroencephalogram	ROP	retinopathy of prematurity
ENT	ear, nose and throat	RNA	ribonucleic acid
EMG	electromyogram	SCN	suprachiasmatic nucleus
EOG	electro-oculogram	SLI	specific language impairment
FSH	follicle stimulating hormone	SIDS	sudden infant death syndrome
GBS	Group B streptococci	SNiP	single nucleotide polymorphisms
GH-IGF	growth hormone insulin-like growth factor	SOM	secretory otitis media
GORD	gastro-oesophageal reflux disease	SWS	slow-wave sleep
hGC	human chorionic gonadotrophin	TB	tuberculosis
HIV	human immunodeficiency virus	TENS	transcutaneous electronic nerve stimulation
HPL	human placental lactogen	URTI	upper respiratory tract infection
ICP	intrauterine, childhood and puberty	UTI	urinary tract infection
IGF-2	intrauterine growth factor-2	2D	2 dimensional
IUGR	intrauterine growth restriction	3D	3 dimensional

1 Genetics

M. Bellman

▼ OVERVIEW

A person's health and personality are determined by a mixture of genetic endowments from parents (nature) and environmental influences (nurture). The number of human characteristics and diseases that have a recognized genetic basis is steadily increasing.

This chapter will cover basic information about the scientific foundations of genetics, the methods of investigation and the ways in which genetic traits are transmitted from parent to offspring. Some examples of genetic disease are given to illustrate the pathways of inheritance.

INTRODUCTION

The father of genetics was Gregor Mendel who described autosomal inheritance in 1865 following his famous meticulous research on garden peas. In 1902 Garrod introduced the term 'inborn error of metabolism' for alkaptonuria, which he recognized as being transmitted by autosomal recessive inheritance. Interest in clinical genetics grew in the first half of the 20th century and genetic counselling clinics were established in the UK from 1946.

Genetics is one of the most rapidly advancing areas of medical technology and it is likely that soon there will be a complete map of the genes that will open up the way for identifying the locations of genes that determine individual characteristics, including abnormalities that cause a wide range of human illness. As these are identified, methods for diagnosis of potentially affected individuals will become easier and screening of the normal population will become feasible, notwithstanding ethical considerations.

MOLECULAR STRUCTURE (Fig. 1.1)

All genetic information is encoded in DNA molecules contained in chromosomes in every cell. In 1962 Wilkins, Crick and Watson won a Nobel prize for describing the DNA double helix made up of parallel chains of nucleotide sugars. The backbone of DNA and RNA molecules is made up of spiral chains of sugar units (deoxyribose and ribose respectively) linked by phosphate units. A nitrogenous base is attached to each sugar-phosphate group to form a nucleotide. These bases are purines (adenosine [A] and guanine [G]) or pyramidines (cytosine [C] and thymine [T] or uracil [U]). The order of the bases is crucial as it determines the genetic code. The bases

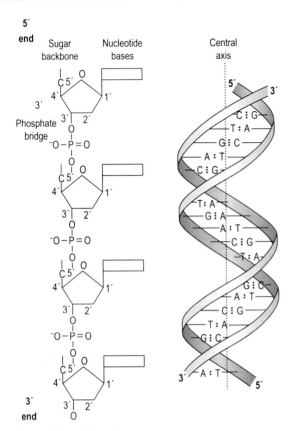

5′
end

Sugar backbone

Nucleotide bases

Central axis

Phosphate bridge

Figure 1.1 Molecular structure

3′
end

are joined by hydrogen bonds, which can split and rejoin to allow separation and replication of the chains. The nucleotide bases on one strand attach to the complementary strand in specific pairs (C–G or A–T) so maintaining the genetic code during replication.

Chromosomes

Normal human cells contain 22 pairs of autosomes and one pair of sex chromosomes. Somatic cells have a diploid complement (46) of which one member of each pair comes from each parent. Gametes are haploid (23): female ova X/X, male sperm X/Y.

Somatic cells multiply by mitosis in which each chromosome replicates into two daughter cells with identical diploid complementary genetic material. Gametes replicate by meiosis when the chromosome number is halved to create a haploid cell. There is random crossing over of genetic material so that each

gamete contains a different selection of chromosomal DNA. Thus, when an ovum is fertilized by a sperm, the resulting chromatid will contain a DNA selection derived from each parent, which will be different to a subsequent chromatid from the same parents.

The human genome

The genetic code is passed on by transcription of the nucleotide basis sequences to messenger RNA and translation to proteins. The DNA double helix unwinds and an RNA molecule is generated as an exact copy of one of the DNA strands. The genetic code is made up of groups of three nucleotide bases (codons), which specify one of the 20 amino acids. Occasionally, this process goes wrong and there is a mutation resulting in an error in the production of a protein. Abnormalities may occur during mitosis or meiosis spontaneously or following exposure to a toxic environmental agent such as ionizing radiation or chemicals.

INHERITANCE

Mendelian inheritance (Fig 1.7)

The laws of Mendelian inheritance remain unchanged since first described 150 years ago and still describe accurately several thousand single-gene disorders. Genetic characteristics (phenotype) are determined by paired alleles, of which one is derived from each parent. The genetic make-up (genotype) can be represented by Punnett's square (Fig. 1.2), which shows the various genetic combinations that can result from gene segregation during meiosis and combination during fertilization.

Autosomal inheritance

A characteristic is dominant if it is manifested when it is determined by only one of the alleles in the pair. In Punnett's square, if the allele A is dominant, then the offspring with the genotype in cells 1 and 3 will exhibit the characteristic. Thus, there is a 50% (1 in 2) chance of it being passed to the next generation. Children who inherit the other allele (a) will neither

Mother's gametes

A   a

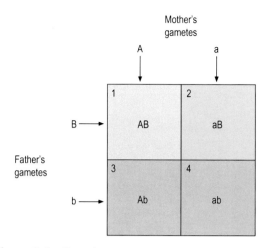

Father's gametes

B ⟶

b ⟶

	1	2
B ⟶	AB	aB
b ⟶	Ab	ab

Figure 1.2 Punnet's square

have the characteristic nor pass it on to their offspring.

Autosomal dominance (Fig. 1.3) There are three features that indicate autosomal-dominant inheritance:

1. Males and females are affected in equal proportions.
2. It occurs in successive generations.
3. Transmission occurs irrespective of gender.

Some important disorders are transmitted by autosomal-dominant inheritance, including achondroplasia, osteogenesis imperfecta, spherocytosis, neurofibromatosis and Huntington's

chorea. However, there may be considerable variability in the severity of the disorder between affected individuals because of reduced penetrance or variable expressivity. Occasionally, a person with a dominant genotype appears normal because the allele has not been expressed, but still has a 50% risk of passing the allele to a child in whom it may penetrate and cause disease.

Autosomal recession (Fig. 1.4) A characteristic that is transmitted by autosomal-recessive inheritance is manifested only when both alleles in the chromosome pair carry the determining gene (homozygous) and is not shown if the relevant gene is present on only one of the alleles in the pair of chromosomes (heterozygous). New mutations for recessive alleles are rare and it is usually assumed that the parents of a child with a recessively inherited characteristic must be heterozygous for the allele and are carriers of the characteristic. In Punnett's square, if the alleles a and b are both determinants of the same recessive characteristic, then children with the genotype in cell 4 will be homozygous for the characteristic and manifest it, children with genotypes in cells 2 and 3 will be heterozygous carriers and children in cell 1 will not have a determinant allele and will not show or carry the characteristic.

Thus, offspring of two carriers of an autosomal recessively inherited characteristic have a 25% chance of manifesting the characteristic, a 50% chance of carrying it and a 25% chance of not inheriting the determinant allele. Affected and carrier individuals

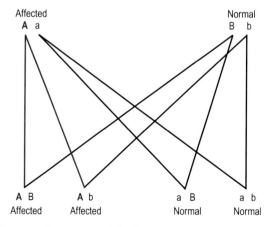

Affected   Normal
A a   B b

A B	A b	a B	a b
Affected	Affected	Normal	Normal

Figure 1.3 Autosomal dominance

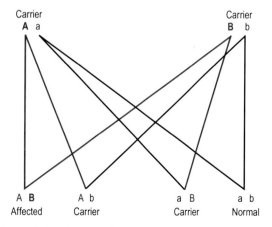

Carrier   Carrier
A a   B b

A B	A b	a B	a b
Affected	Carrier	Carrier	Normal

Figure 1.4 Autosomal recession

of recessively inherited traits are in the same 'horizontal' generation and without gene analysis, family trees cannot be traced.

There are three features that suggest autosomal recessive inheritance:

1. Males and females are affected in equal proportions.
2. Only a single sibship in one generation is affected.
3. The parents are consanguineous.

There are many autosomal-recessive disorders and they tend to be severe and relatively common in a population. The most prevalent worldwide are haemoglobinopathies, such as sickle-cell anaemia and thalassaemia, with a carrier rate in certain populations of approximately 1 in 10. In northern Europe the commonest is cystic fibrosis, with a carrier rate of 1 in 25 and an incidence of 1 in 2500 births. Other important autosomal-recessive disorders include congenital adrenal hyperplasia, mucopolysaccharidosis, spinal muscular atrophy, Tay–Sachs disease and many inborn errors of metabolism, such as galactosaemia, homocystinuria and phenylketonuria.

Sex-linked inheritance

A characteristic is sex-linked if it is carried on either of the sex chromosomes (X or Y). In practice X-linked genes are more important.

X-linked-recessive inheritance (Fig. 1.5) In this type of inheritance pattern the characteristic phenotype is only shown in males who are hemizygous for the allele (**XY**) and in homozygous females (**XX**) the defective trait is balanced out by the equivalent normal allele on the other X chromosome. However, these female carriers have a 50% chance of passing the characteristic phenotype to their sons and the carrier state to their daughters. An affected male will pass the allele to 100% of his daughters (obligate carriers), but his sons will inherit the Y chromosome and be normal.

There are three features that indicate X-linked-recessive inheritance:

1. The trait is virtually always restricted to males.
2. It occurs only in the sons of carrier females.
3. It does not occur in the sons of affected males, but may occur in their grandsons via their obligate carrier daughters.

Important examples of X-linked recessive disorders are Duchenne muscular dystrophy, red–green colour blindness, fragile-X learning disability and haemophilia. Occasionally, heterozygous carrier females can exhibit a modified form of the phenotype, for example in ocular albinism or, if the gene is frequent in the population, a female may be homozygous and have the disorder, for example colour blindness.

X-linked-dominant inheritance (Fig. 1.6) This is similar to autosomal dominant inheritance when the affected allele is on the **X** chromosome. Thus, the

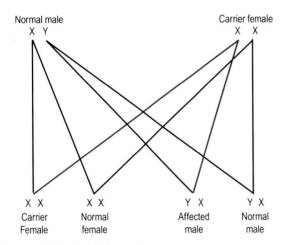

Figure 1.5 X-linked recession

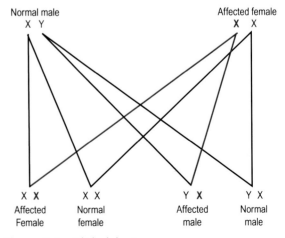

Figure 1.6 X-linked dominance

characteristic phenotype is shown by heterozygous females as well as hemizygous males who have the abnormal allele on their single **X** chromosome. Genotypically, the inheritance pattern is similar to the sex-linked-recessive state but, because the affected **X** chromosome dominates, the phenotype is shown by 50% of an affected female's sons and daughters and 100% of an affected male's daughters.

There are three features that indicate X-linked-dominant inheritance:

1. Both sexes are affected, but females are more frequent.
2. Females are often less severely affected than males.
3. Females transmit the trait to both their sons and daughters, but males transmit only to their daughters.

This type of inheritance is rare and examples of X-linked-dominant disorders are vitamin-D-resistant rickets and incontinentia pigmenti.

Non-Mendelian inheritance

Genomic imprinting

Sometimes an identical genotypic state is expressed as a variable phenotype depending on which parent the genotype is derived from. The imprint occurs in gametogenesis and affects only one generation. It may occur in any number of chromosomes and cause abnormalities of the placenta and fetus or it can affect part of an individual chromosome or gene. An important example is deletion of a specific region (q11–13) of chromosome 15, which results in Prader–Willi syndrome if it is inherited from the father or Angelman syndrome if inherited from the mother.

Uniparental disomy

As a rule, one member of each pair of chromosomes is inherited from each parent. However, on rare occasions both homologues in the pair are derived from one parent. This occurs because of a non-dysjunction error in meiosis when a pair of chromosomes does not divide so that one daughter cell has one extra chromosome and the other has one

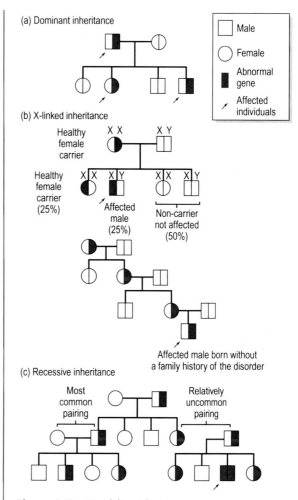

Figure 1.7 Mendelian inheritance

less. On fertilization by the former gamete, the conceptus will be trisomic, but in order to achieve a normal disomic state one chromosome is deleted (trisomy rescue) and if that is the one from the other parent's gamete then the fetus is left with the two inherited from the abnormal gamete, that is uniparental disomy. This mechanism may be the cause of an affected child being born to a carrier parent with an autosomal recessive condition when the other parent is normal. It has been implicated in Beckwith–Wiederman syndrome, in which there are two paternally derived copies of locus 11p15 and no maternal copies, and in some cases of Prader–Willi syndrome and Angelmann's syndrome when there are two identical copies of 15q11–13 derived either from the father or mother respectively.

Mitochondrial inheritance

In addition to the cell nucleus, DNA is contained in the cytoplasm in the mitochondria. As spermatozoa consist exclusively of nuclear material, the entire mitochondrial DNA in a zygote is derived from the cytoplasm of the ovum. This DNA is involved in coding for energy production by oxidative phosphorylation and production of ATP and, therefore, systems with a high demand for aerobic energy such as brain, muscle and the eye can be affected by defective mitochondrial DNA. Disorders that affect both sexes, but are transmitted only through the mother by this mechanism, include Leber's optic atrophy and several types of neuromuscular disease with ragged red fibres.

MOSAICISM

When there is more than one cell line in an individual they are referred to as being mosaic. It is due to an error during mitosis that occurs in a zygote at any time after fertilization. It starts in a single cell and is then transmitted to future generations. The time after fertilization of the initial event determines the proportions of the two cell lines

Mosaicism is the normal situation in females as only one of the two X chromosomes is active in each cell. According to the Lyon hypothesis this happens because the second X chromosome becomes inactive early in embryogenesis. Female carriers of an X-linked disorder are usually asymptomatic because many of the active X chromosomes have a normal allele. However, if the proportion of normal X chromosomes that are inactivated is high enough, they may exhibit symptoms of the characteristic caused by the abnormal gene on the other X chromosome. Females with an X-linked-dominant disorder will have a variable phenotype dependent on the proportion of active chromosomes that carry the mutant gene.

Mosaicism is not infrequent and occurs in some important disorders such as achondroplasia, neurofibromatosis, osteogenesis imperfecta and Turner's (XO/XX) and Down's (trisomy/disomy 21)

syndromes when the phenotype is less severe than in the full condition. It may also be restricted to gonadal cells, for example, in the mothers of children with X-linked-recessive disorders, such as Duchenne's muscular dystrophy or haemophilia, when normal screening investigations on somatic cells are negative.

CHROMOSOMAL IMBALANCE

The number of chromosomes may be abnormal (aneuploidy) due to non-disjunction in the early phases of mitosis. When chromosomes divide unequally, the resulting daughter cells will contain more or less of the chromosomes fragments. The commonest example is Down's syndrome due to the presence of an additional chromosome (trisomy 21). Some cases of Down's syndrome are due to translocation in a parent's chromosome structure when there is abnormal breakage of chromosomes and reconstitution by reciprocal exchange so that the overall chromosome complement is functionally normal (balanced translocation). However, in meiosis the balance is disturbed and one gamete gets an extra chromosome 21. Thus, this parent has an ongoing increased risk of producing children with Down's syndrome.

CHROMOSOME ANALYSIS

Chromosomes can be gathered from any cell, but lymphocytes are the easiest and usual source. They can be seen by light microscopy after staining. The karyotype is determined by banding, identifying and counting each of the 23 chromosomes in a number of cells. Specific gene abnormalities can be found by using fluorescent-labelled probes that will combine with a specific genetic target and show up under ultraviolet light (FISH test).

DNA ANALYSIS

DNA sequencing/cloning

The DNA molecules can be cleaved into specific sequences by restriction enzymes obtained from bacteria. These sequences are combined with a vector and cultured with host DNA material to produce multiple copies of identical DNA sequences (clones). Because of their high specificity, labelled DNA probes can be made to identify their complementary sequences.

Polymerase chain reaction (PCR)

By identifying the DNA adjacent to a specific sequence, complementary oligonucleotide primers can be used to vastly amplify minute amounts of DNA so that it can be identified by conventional techniques. This technology is rapid (a few hours) and can be used very successfully for forensic purposes as well as antenatal diagnosis from small amounts of material taken by chorionic villus sampling or amniocentesis. Amplified DNA sequences can be analyzed by techniques such as Southern blotting to produce a restriction map of DNA structure. Specific genes can be identified and DNA material examined for the presence of particular sequences. Thus, genes can be detected in an asymptomatic person or to identify carriers.

The Human Genome Project

In 1990 two teams in the USA and the UK began to sequence DNA with the aim of mapping the whole human genome. In 2001 a draft of the complete sequence was published, 4 years ahead of schedule, spurred on by competition between the teams.

The genome contains 30–40 000 genes, which is considerably fewer than expected, as worms have 18 000 and some plants 26 000. However, the total number of base pairs in these genomes is approximately 100 million, whereas humans have around 3 billion. There is considerable variability in the density of genes on different chromosomes. Genes seemed to cluster on certain chromosomes, e.g. 19, whereas others, such as 13, 18 and 21 have few genes.

While the genome map is a revelation, it is merely the equivalent of an anatomical diagram. The second stage of the project, which is to define function of the genes, is perhaps of more practical importance. Only about 1.5% of the genome is made up of exons, which are necessary for protein coding and 24% is responsible for introns, which are non-coding sections of the DNA molecule. Much of the remainder consists of repeat sequences that have no apparent function. Functions found for some of the codes include production of transcription factors and enzymes.

A challenging task is to investigate human variation. Only about 0.1% of the genome is different between individuals, whereas 99.9% is identical. Most of the variation is in single nucleotide polymorphisms (SNiPs). The next stage is to produce an accurate SNiP map and identify susceptibility loci for certain disorders. This may be facilitated by work on animal models, such as the mouse and zebra fish, which have considerable similarities to the human genome and disease patterns. Definition of susceptibility loci will eventually allow the identification or specific genes. Many disorders caused by abnormalities on single genes with simple Mendelian inheritance have already been mapped. The next step is to identify susceptibility genes for multifactorially determined disorders such as asthma, cancer, diabetes, epilepsy and behavioural disorders, which are much more common.

Further reading

Kingston HM 2002 ABC of Clinical Genetics, 3rd edn. BMJ Books, London
Read A, Strachan T 2003 Human Molecular Genetics, 3rd edn. Garland Science, Oxford

Websites

http://www.hgmp.mrc.ac.uk/omim/ (catalogue of genetic disorders)
http://www.ebi.ac.uk (databases and information on molecular biology and genetics)

2 Embryology

M. Bellman

▼ OVERVIEW

Embryology is the study of prenatal development. Fetal life starts at the moment of conception and lasts until the time of delivery. In humans the programmed duration of the fetal development period is usually 283 days from the first day of the last menstrual period to term delivery. During that time the embryo undergoes the most amazing changes as the cells divide and differentiate into all the tissues of the human body. The order and manner of this developmental process is highly programmed and the normal sequence of events is invariable. The study of the pattern of fetal development provides a unique perspective on normal and abnormal anatomy that leads to understanding of how congenital anomalies happen and why insults at certain times during gestation cause specific damage to organs and structures developing at that time.

The normal pattern of human fetal development will be described in this chapter with basic information on the formation of some important body systems and structures. At relevant points references are made to some common anomalies that occur when embryogenesis goes wrong.

INTRODUCTION

It is important to know the basics of embryology in order to understand the origin and relationships of anatomical structures and the causes of some congenital anomalies.

Life commences at fertilization when a single sperm penetrates a single oocyte. The precise timing of this awesome event is usually unknown, so the age of the fetus is calculated from the first day of the last menstrual period, which is sometimes also uncertain. Thus, the gestational age is 2 weeks more than the fertilization age.

The oocyte is the female gamete, which divides by meiosis to contain a haploid number of chromosomes (23,X). Similarly, the sperm is the male gamete, which has also undergone meiotic division to become haploid (23, X or Y). The oocyte passes from the ovary and develops into the corpus luteum, which enters the adjacent Fallopian tube where it is fertilized by one of the approximately 300 million sperms that were deposited in the vagina, of which 1% entered the cervix and progressed through the uterus to the Fallopian tube. Immediately on penetration, a chemical barrier is formed to prevent other sperms from penetrating the same oocyte and the second meiotic division of the oocyte is triggered. The zygote results from the combination of the haploid oocyte and sperm that forms the diploid blastomere. This undergoes cleavage by mitosis to maintain a diploid complement of chromosomes and becomes the morula, which contains 16–20 cells, and then the blastocyte, which implants into the uterine wall that has been ripened by several hormones and enzymes secreted after ovulation and fertilization. The sex of the fetus is determined by the type of sex chromosome carried by the sperm so that the diploid sex chromosome is XX (female) or XY (male).

ANTENATAL TIME COURSE (Fig. 2.1)

After implantation, the blastocyte grows rapidly by successive mitotic division and the cells differentiate into the embryoblast, which forms the embryo, and the blastocyst cavity surrounded by the trophoblast. The syncytiotrophoblast invades the endometrium and the embryo is firmly embedded in the uterine wall by 12 days after fertilization. Human chorionic gonadotrophin (hGC) is produced to maintain the corpus luteum. hGC can be detected by immunoassay in vitro, which is the basis for pregnancy testing.

EARLY FETAL DEVELOPMENT (Fig. 2.2)

Two weeks after fertilization, the embryonic disc develops in the embryoblast, which, at first, has two layers and then, by gastrulation, becomes trilaminar. Initially, the cells of the embryo are totipotent and can develop into any part of the body, but after differentiation into three distinct germ layers, the cells become specialized and are destined to develop in specific ways. Age 3 weeks the primitive streak develops at the caudal end of the embryo and extends cranially. Epiblastic cells form the three germ layers that give rise to all the tissues and organs of the body.

Up to 50% of fetuses are aborted, often because of major malformations. Many are shed with the next menstrual period and the mother does not know she was pregnant. Approximately 15% of recognized pregnancies end as spontaneous abortions and threatened abortion occurs in about 25% of pregnancies, of which approximately half can be saved by medical intervention.

Germ layers (Fig 2-3)

The three germ layers develop into ectoderm, mesoderm and endoderm, which form specialized body parts.

Ectoderm

Neuroectoderm The neural plate develops cranial to the primitive streak and by 18 days the notochord, flanked by the neural folds can be seen. The folds start to join early in the 4th week to form the neural tube that is completely closed over by 28–29 days. This develops into the central nervous system and some cells left outside the tube give rise to the neural crest, which forms the autonomic nervous system.

Surface ectoderm Ectoderm cells generate all external tissues including skin, hair and nails as well as some other structures.

Mesoderm

Cells from the deep surface of the embryonic disc form the mesenchyme, which gives rise to the mesoderm. This develops into 38 paired somites on each lateral side of the neural groove and within these the intraembryonic coelom forms in the 3rd week. The coelom is a cavity that divides the mesoderm into a parietal layer and a visceral layer. During the 2nd month the coelom divides into pericardial, pleural and peritoneal cavities.

Endoderm

Some cells from the primitive streak are displaced deep to the mesoderm and form the intraembryonic endoderm, which gives rise to all the epithelial linings and structures of internal organs.

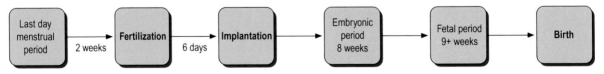

Figure 2.1   Antenatal time course

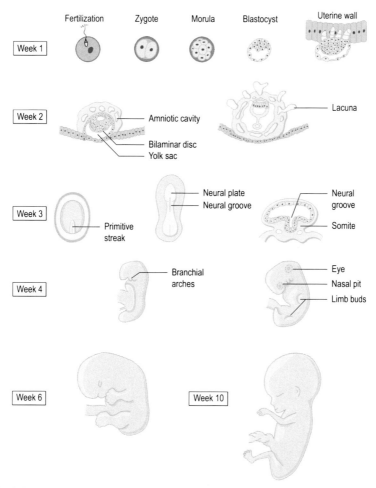

Figure 2.2   Early fetal development

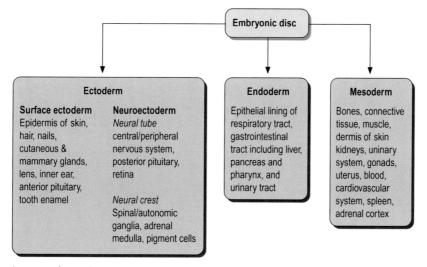

Figure 2.3   Development of germ layers

Nervous system

Central nervous system

The cells of the nervous system are derived from the neural plate that appears in the 3rd week. The neural folds are initially nourished from surrounding amniotic fluid, but after closure to form the neural tube, nourishment depends on blood circulation. The neural tube begins to close in the 4th week in the middle of its axis and extends rostrally to form the brain and caudally to form the spinal cord. The cranial opening closes on the 25/26th day and the caudal end on the 27/28th day. The lumen of the neural tube becomes the ventricular system of the brain and the central canal of the spinal cord.

Three brain vesicles (forebrain, midbrain and hindbrain) form rapidly in the 4th week and divide further in the 5th week to form five vesicles that fold over in the midbrain and hindbrain areas (Fig. 2.4).

Hindbrain The caudal end of the hindbrain (myelencephalon) forms the medulla and the neuroblast cells become organized into the efferent and afferent nerve bundles contiguous with the spinal cord. The cranial part of the hindbrain (metencephalon) becomes the pons, cerebellum and brainstem.

Midbrain The midbrain (mesencephalon) enlarges and the nerve fibres growing between the cerebrum and the brain stem form the cerebral peduncles.

Forebrain In the 4th week two optic vesicles form on the lateral sides of the anterior forebrain (telencephalon) and at the posterior end (diencephalon) two cerebral vesicles develop into the cerebral hemispheres. Within the diencephalon neuroblasts rapidly differentiate and become organized into the epithalamus, thalamus and hypothalamus. The neural tube lumen forms the third ventricle in the forebrain with the paired lateral ventricles within the two cerebral hemispheres that expand over the rest of the brain and eventually meet in the midline. Fissures separate the hemispheres into the frontal, parietal and temporal lobes and the ventricles change in shape so that the lateral ventricles become like paired mirror image 'C' shapes joined by the third ventricle. Nerve fibres grow rapidly and are organized into thick bundles that connect the cortex to the midbrain via the internal capsule and the hemispheres to each other via the corpus callosum.

The pituitary gland consists of a posterior lobe (neurohypophysis) that grows down from neuroectoderm of the diencephalon and an anterior lobe (adenohypophysis) that is an upgrowth from ectoderm of the stomodeum.

The growth of the brain follows a highly structured course. Some parts move relative to others and migrate along pre-programmed routes. Abnormal development may happen and result in failure of growth or incorrect position. Blockage to the cerebrospinal fluid (CSF) system results in hydrocephalus, which will damage cerebral matter if the intracranial pressure increases and is not relieved by release of CSF. Defective closure of the neural tube will cause spina bifida, which may be associated with hydrocephalus.

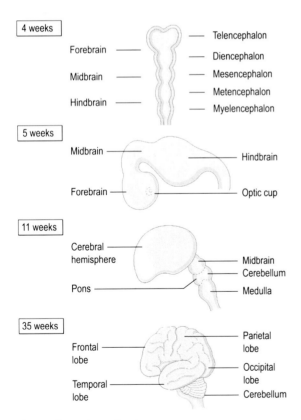

Figure 2.4 Brain development

Peripheral nervous system

The cells of the peripheral nervous system develop from the neural crest and form the nerve ganglia and cranial, spinal and visceral nerves. All sensory nerves derive from the neural crest and motor nerves originate from the basal plates of the brainstem (cranial nerves) and spinal cord (spinal nerves).

Twelve pairs of cranial nerves form in the 5th–6th week. The hypoglossal nerve (XII) grows rostrally to provide the motor innervation to the tongue. The motor nerves to the eyes (III, IV and VI) also go rostrally. Cranial nerves V (trigeminal), VII (facial), IX (glossopharyngeal) and X (vagus) innervate the structures that develop from the embryonic arches. The trigeminal nerve (first arch) has three large divisions (ophthalmic, maxillary and mandibular) and incorporates sensory fibres to the skin of the face and mucous membrane of the nose and mouth. The facial nerve (second arch) supplies motor fibres to the muscles of facial expression and a small branch takes sensory fibres by a tortuous route through the middle ear to taste buds in the anterior two-thirds of the tongue. The glossopharyngeal nerve (third arch) contains efferent (motor) fibres to the salivary glands and sensory fibres including taste to the tongue. The vagus nerve (fourth and sixth arches) supplies visceral efferent and afferent fibres to several organs including the heart and gut and motor fibres to the larynx and pharynx. The accessory nerve (XI) is formed from a cranial root that arises from the vagus nerve in the medulla to supply the muscles of the soft palate and larynx and a spinal root arising from the cervical spinal cord to supply the sternomastoid and trapezius muscles.

There are three special sensory cranial nerves. The olfactory nerve (I) transmits the sense of smell from the nasopharynx through the cribriform plate of the ethmoid bone to the olfactory bulb in the forebrain. The retina is formed as an outgrowth from the forebrain, hence the optic nerve (II) is actually a tract of brain fibres that connect directly to the visual cortex via the optic chiasma where the fibres cross over. The vestibulocochlear nerve (VIII) contains the vestibular nerve, which transmits the sense of balance from the semicircular canals, and the cochlear nerve, which transmits hearing sensation from the cochlea.

CARDIOVASCULAR SYSTEM

By 3 weeks the embryo is too big to get sufficient nourishment by absorption from amniotic fluid and angioblastic tissue from the mesenchyme forms blood vessels and the heart, which starts to contract at the end of the 3rd week. By 4 weeks blood is circulating and the sinus venosus receives oxygenated blood from the placenta through the umbilical veins and deoxygenated blood from the yolk sac via the vitelline veins and from the embryo body via the cardinal veins. This mixed blood enters the atrium and passes through the atrioventricular canal to the primitive ventricle where it is pumped to the bulbus cordis, truncus arteriosus and via the aortic arches to the dorsal aorta, which supplies the embryo, yolk sac and placenta. Paired umbilical arteries carry mixed, poorly oxygenated blood from the caudal ends of the embryonic circulation back to the placenta.

Initially, the cardinal veins empty into the sinus venosus and at 7 weeks the ductus venosus develops, which shunts oxygenated blood from the placenta through the liver to the inferior vena cava and into the heart. At the same time the two dorsal aortae fuse to form a single aorta.

By 4 weeks the heart cavity becomes divided into a primitive atrium and ventricle and during the 4th week endocardial cushions grow out from the heart wall between the atrium and the ventricle and fuse to divide the atrioventricular canal into a right and left half. The atrium is divided by the septum primum, which grows down from the roof of the primitive atrium and fuses with the endocardial cushions. The septum primum is crescent shaped and the hole in the middle is the foramen primum that gets progressively smaller. However, before it closes, the foramen secundum appears in the middle of the septum primum, which is overlapped at 6 weeks by the septum secundum that grows down from the top of the atrium. A valved opening (foramen ovale) is left between the atria that allows one-way passage of partially oxygenated blood from the inferior vena cava to pass from the right to left atrium and thence to the embryo body. The primitive ventricle is divided by the interventricular septum, which grows up from the apex of the ventricle and fuses with the endocardial cushions in week 7. Simultaneously, the outlet of the common ventricle (bulbus cordis and truncus arteriosus) is divided by a midline septum so that the left ventricle connects to the aorta and the right to the pulmonary trunk.

Fetal circulation (Fig. 2.5)

The fetus receives oxygenated blood from the placenta via the umbilical vein, which either enters the liver circulation or goes through the ductus venosus into the inferior vena cava and then into the right atrium. Most of the blood stream passes through the foramen ovale to the left atrium and mixes with a small amount of deoxygenated blood from the pulmonary veins. It then passes into the left ventricle and is pumped into the ascending aorta and thence to the heart, head, neck and upper limbs. The small amount of oxygenated blood left in the right atrium, mixed with deoxygenated blood from the superior vena cava passes into the right ventricle, to the pulmonary trunk and then most goes through the ductus arteriosus into the descending aorta. This supplies the lower trunk, viscera and lower limbs

and the umbilical arteries, which return blood to the placenta for reoxygenation.

Neonatal circulation

When breathing commences after birth, the pulmonary vascular resistance falls and blood flow increases. Pressure in the right atrium falls below that in the left and the foramen ovale closes so that the only outlet of the atria is into their respective ventricle. The ductus venosus closes and the ductus ateriosus and the umbilical arteries constrict. These changes start as soon as the first breath is taken, but may take several days to complete.

Many things may go wrong with the complex development of the cardiovascular system such as *failure of normal division*, for example common atrium or ventricle, persistent truncus arteriosus; *failure of fusion*, for example atrial or ventricular septal defect; *failure of normal growth*, for example valve abnormality, hypoplastic ventricle, coarctation of the aorta and *failure of neonatal change*, for example patent ductus arteriosus.

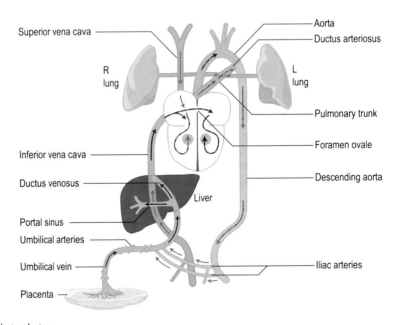

Figure 2.5 Fetal circulation

THE ABDOMEN

Digestive system

During the 4th week the primitive gut develops from the yolk sac and can be differentiated into three sections that give rise to specific structures.

Foregut

The pharynx and accessory structures such as the tongue, tonsils, salivary glands and pharyngeal pouches derive from the foregut. The upper respiratory system develops from the first and second pharyngeal pouches and the lower respiratory system forms from the laryngotracheal diverticulum, which is a side-growth from the floor of the primitive pharynx caudal to the fourth pharyngeal pouch. The rostral end of the diverticulum is separated from the oesophageal section of the pharynx by the tracheo-oesophageal septum to become the larynx and the distal end enlarges to form a lung bud that bifurcates at 34 days to develop into the bronchi and lungs.

The oesophagus elongates rapidly with the growth of the mediastinum and connects the pharynx to the stomach, which appears as a dilatation of the foregut during the 4th week. In approximately 1 in 3000 births, there is an abnormality of development of the tracheo-oesophageal septum resulting in oesophageal atresia usually associated with a tracheo-oesophageal fistula.

As the stomach enlarges it rotates clockwise to lie almost horizontally across the abdomen. Simultaneously, the duodenum forms as a 'C' shaped structure from the lower foregut and the upper midgut. At this junction the common bile duct opens, which grows outwards and produces a liver, gall bladder and pancreatic bud. The liver enlarges rapidly between weeks 5 and 10, when it occupies most of the abdominal cavity.

Midgut

Derivatives of the midgut are most of the duodenum, the small intestine (jejunum and ileum) and most of the large intestine (caecum, appendix, ascending colon and approximately half of the transverse colon). As the midgut loop elongates it cannot be accommodated within the embryonic abdomen and herniates into the umbilical cord and communicates with the yolk sac via the yolk stalk. The loop rotates anticlockwise through approximately 90° before returning to the abdomen during the 10th week, when it rotates an additional 180° anticlockwise. As the midgut grows the epithelial lining proliferates so rapidly that the lumen is occluded and later recanalizes. If this does not happen efficiently, stenosis or atresia occurs, particularly in the duodenum. Several other developmental abnormalities of the midgut may occur, including omphalocele when the intestines fail to return to the abdomen, umbilical hernia when a small section of the intestine protrudes through an imcompletely closed umbilicus after returning to the abdomen, gastroschisis when the intestines and viscera herniate through a defect in the abdominal wall and abnormalities of rotation, such as non-rotation and volvulus.

Hindgut

Derivatives of the hindgut are the distal half of the transverse colon, the descending and sigmoid colon, the rectum, the proximal part of the anal canal and the epithelium of the bladder and urethra. At first the caudal part of the hindgut terminates in the cloaca, which is divided by the urorectal septum into the rectum and urogenital sinus. The rectum and upper two-thirds of the anal canal fuse with the lower anal canal, which is derived from ectoderm of the proctodeum. Abnormal development of the urorectal septum may result in anal agenesis, imperforate anus and fistula. Failure of innervation of the colon causes Hirschsprung's disease.

Urogenital system

Urinary system

The first functioning kidneys are the mesonephroi (plural of mesonephros), which develop in the 4th week and excrete urine into the urogenital sinus. In the 5th week the permanent kidneys (metanephroi) appear and start to function around 9 weeks. Urine is excreted into the amniotic fluid, which the fetus drinks, and waste products are eliminated through the placenta into the maternal circulation.

The metanephroi consist of two parts: the metanephric diverticulum (ureteric bud), which develops into the ureter, renal pelvis, calices and collecting tubules, and the metanephric mesoderm, which produces the metanephric vesicles, nephrons and glomeruli. The fetal kidneys are divided into lobes that coalesce during fetal and early postnatal life, but rarely persist. At first the kidneys are located close to each other in the pelvis and gradually move superiorly and laterally, so that by the 9th week they are in the adult position. Congenital abnormalities of the kidneys include renal agenesis, which may be asymptomatic if unilateral, when it is often associated with a single umbilical artery, or fatal if it is bilateral, when it is often associated with other abnormalities; oligohydramnios; abnormal rotation or position (ectopic); fusion (horseshoe kidney) and polycystic disease.

The bladder is derived from the vesical section of the urogenital sinus and the distal part of the mesonephric ducts, which forms the trigone. It is continuous with the urachus, which is the persisting vestigial remnant of the allantois that connects the urogenital sinus to the umbilicus and may abnormally remain patent.

Genital system

During the 4th week spherical sex germ cells appear near the allantois and migrate along the hindgut to the gonadal ridges medial to the mesonephroi. In the 6th week primary sex cords grow into the mesenchyme and develop into undifferentiated gonads with an internal medulla and an outer cortex. If the fertilizing sperm contained a sex-determining region in a gene on the short arm of the Y chromosome, the medulla develops into a testis under the influence of the testis-determining factor and the cortex regresses. In the absence of a Y chromosome, the medulla regresses and the undifferentiated gonad becomes an ovary. The fetal testes produce an androgen testosterone that results in the formation of the male sex structures. If this does not occur, female differentiation takes place even in the absence of ovaries.

Male genitalia Seminiferous tubules form in the medulla of the gonad to form the rete testis, which is encased in the tunic albuginea. The tubules are separated by mesenchyme, which contains the interstitial cells of Leydig that produce testosterone at 8 weeks. The testis separates from the mesonephros and is suspended by the mesorchium. Other hormones important for male development are human chorionic gonadotrophin (hGC) and Müllerian inhibiting factor. The mesonephric duct, which drained urine from the mesonephric kidneys, forms the epididymis, vas deferens and ejaculatory duct.

Up to the 7th week there is an undifferentiated genital tubercle at the rostral end of the cloacal membrane that develops a phallus. Under the influence of testosterone, the phallus becomes a penis and urogenital folds develop on each side of its ventral surface. These fold over and fuse to form the urethra. Laterally, on each side, labioscrotal swellings grow towards the midline and fuse to form the scrotum. At the end of the penis the glans forms and a layer of epithelium separates to form the prepuce, which remains adherent to the glans.

The testes develop in the lower abdomen, but gradually 'descend' due to the relative separation of the rostral and caudal (pelvic) parts of the abdomen. At 28 weeks the testis passes through the inguinal canal and, usually, by 32 weeks enters the scrotum. Thus, it is normal for the testes to be undescended in premature babies and even in term infants it may not reach the scrotum until several weeks after birth.

Female genitalia The ovaries are visible from the 10th week. Cortical cords form from the cortex of the primitive gonad into the medulla, which then regresses. The cords form primordial follicles containing an oogonium and these multiply by mitosis to produce around 2 million germ cells by the end of the prenatal period. These will enlarge and become primary oocytes and no more oogonia are formed after birth. The ovary is surrounded by the tunica albuginea, separates from the mesonephros and is suspended by the mesovarium.

In the absence of testosterone, the undifferentiated phallus develops into the clitoris. The urogenital folds fuse only at the ends, and in the middle they become the labia minora. The labioscrotal folds enlarge and become the labia majora. The uterus develops from the paramesonephric ducts and the vagina from the mesenchyme around the urogenital sinus. The vagina is separated from the urogenital sinus by the hymen until late pregnancy.

The commonest abnormality of the genitalia is due to congenital adrenal hyperplasia, when there are excessive androgens resulting from a metabolic enzyme deficiency. This will cause masculinization of a female fetus. Diagnosis and treatment is urgent because of the systemic effects of abnormal cortisol production.

SPECIFIC STRUCTURES

Face (Fig. 2.6)

The origin of the mouth appears in the middle of the cranial prominence of the embryo as the stomodeum

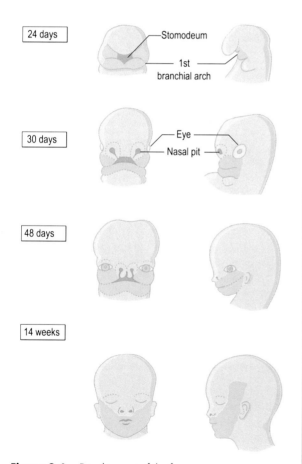

Figure 2.6   Development of the face

in the 3rd week. Ectodermal cells from the neural crest accumulate on either side of the stomodeum to form paired pharyngeal arches that develop into the connective tissues of the face. The nasal placodes develop in the 4th week, followed by the optic vesicles, which arise from the forebrain. At the end of the 5th week the external ears are visible and in the 6th to 7th week the nasolacrimal duct develops to connect the nose and the eye, although it only becomes patent after birth. Between the 7th and 10th weeks the lateralized nasal prominences move medially and merge and the nose is separated from the mouth around which lips form. Failure of this process results in cleft lip. By the 10th week the face has a clearly human form.

Palate

In the 6th week the primary palate begins to develop in the anterior midline from the maxilla and the secondary palate develops as lateral palatine processes on each side of the tongue. These grow towards the midline during the 7th and 8th weeks and the tongue moves inferiorly, so that the palatine processes fuse above it in the midline and with the primary palate and the nasal septum, which has been growing down concurrently. Cleft palate results from failure of fusion of the palatal processes. It may be part of the first arch syndrome and associated with a small mandible (Pierre Robin sequence) or maxillary hypoplasia and abnormalities of the eyes and ears (Treacher Collins' syndrome).

Eye

In the 4th week bilateral optic sulci appear in the neural folds. These grow laterally to become optic vesicles connected to the forebrain by optic stalks. When the vesicles meet the ectoderm the surface folds over to enclose a lens vesicle. Simultaneously, the optic vesicle invaginates to form the optic cup. The wall of this becomes the retina which is composed of a pigmentary layer nearer the ectoderm through which light will have to pass to reach a neural layer nearer the brain. The retina is connected to the brain by ganglion cells, which grow in the optic stalk to form the optic nerve. This continues to myelinate after birth while visual function develops.

While the lens vesicle enlarges and forms specialized transparent cells, it is vascular and supplied by the hyaloid artery, which degenerates before birth. The ciliary body and iris are derived from the optic cup and maldevelopment may result in a coloboma. Occasionally, the lens is opaque due to genetic, infective or metabolic causes and blindness results unless the abnormality is diagnosed quickly and the lens removed.

Ear

Internal ear

Early in the 4th week bilateral otic placodes appear in the ectoderm of the hindbrain and invaginate to form otic vesicles. These develop into the vestibular organ consisting of the endolymphatic duct, semicircular canals, utricle and saccule and the hearing organ comprising the cochlear duct and cochlea (spiral organ of Corti). The inner ear is full-sized by 22 weeks and does not grow further.

Middle ear

The tubotympanic cavity develops from the first pharyngeal pouch. The proximal part becomes the Eustachian tube and the distal section expands to become the tympanic cavity containing the ossicles and the mastoid antrum. The middle ear continues to grow in size throughout childhood.

External ear

The tympanic membrane has two layers: the inner is derived from the endoderm of the tubotympanic recess and the outer from surface ectoderm. The external auditory meatus develops from the first pharyngeal groove and is a solid meatal plug until late pregnancy. It is short at birth and lengthens during the first 9 years of life. The pinna (auricle) arises from mesenchyme of the first pharyngeal groove, which is known as the seven 'hillocks of His'. If they fail to fuse, a pit results, if one is left out, a tag forms. As the mandible grows the pinnae move up to eye level and continue growing during childhood.

Deafness may result from abnormalities of the cochlea (sensorineural) or middle ear (conductive), which may be associated with developmental anomalies of the outer ear, such as pre-auricular pits and abnormal pinnae.

The ears develop at the same time as the kidneys so associated defects are often seen in both systems.

Further reading

Larson WJ 2001 Human Embryology, 3rd edn. Churchill Livingstone, New York

Moore KL, Persaud PVN 2003 Before We Were Born: Essentials of Embryology and Birth Defects. Saunders, Philadelphia

---

Websites

http://embryology.med.unsw.edu.au (educational resource developed for learning concepts in embryological development)

3

The Preterm infant

A. Huertas-Ceballos

▼ OVERVIEW

With advancing neonatal technology and expertise, it is now common to see survivors of preterm birth in normal nurseries and schools. Ten years ago it was rare that an infant born below 30 weeks' gestation would achieve a normal outcome. Now babies born at 24 weeks' gestation have a significant chance of leading a normal life; others will be severely disabled and more will have moderate degrees of disability, but be able to function in a normal mainstream environment. It used to be thought that a fetus under 24 weeks of gestation was non-viable, but that has steadily reduced and who knows where science will go?

This chapter covers background information, definitions and factors relevant to preterm infants. There is a description of services to help them and some common problems seen in 'normal' preterm-born children. The concluding section gives information on prognosis and outcome.

INTRODUCTION

There have been dramatic improvements in the results of neonatal care over the past 30 years and now premature babies are surviving against all odds at earlier gestations than ever before. Infants of more than 34 weeks are no longer the difficult ones. The literature and experience of neonatologists all over the world is more focused on the very preterm (less than 28 weeks). As survival improves and mechanisms of disease are understood, the aim is to have a more protective and preventive approach. Therapies and diagnostic procedures are constantly under revision. The literature, however, lacks good and robust evidence for most of them. This chapter aims to provide a general idea of the 'normal preterm infant' and what to expect when faced with a preterm delivery.

DEFINITION

Worldwide, it is well accepted that a normal pregnancy lasts from 37 to 41 weeks. Therefore, preterm infants are babies that are born before 37 weeks' gestation. Very preterm babies are delivered at less than 32 weeks and the extremely premature are babies of less than 28 weeks. Current legislation in the UK states that an unborn of less than 24 weeks is still considered as a fetus. However, babies of less than 23 weeks are delivered and are surviving. Babies of less than 22 weeks' gestation are still considered below the limits of viability and neither science nor clinical expertise has overcome the enormous difficulties of treating these babies.

Premature does not always means small. In fact, premature babies could either be appropriate for gestational age if their weight increment is between 2 s.d. either side of the mean, large for gestation if it

Table 3.1 Definitions of terms used in neonatology

Neonate	Infant below 28 days old
Term baby	Gestational age between 37 and 41 weeks at birth
Premature baby	Gestational age of less than 37 weeks at birth
Extremely premature baby	Gestational age of less than 28 weeks at birth
Small for gestational age	Birth weight less than 2 standard deviations
Large for gestational age	Birth weight more than 2 standard deviations
Appropriate for gestational age	Birth weight ± 2 standard deviations of mean
Low birth weight	Infants of 2500 g or less
Very low birth weight	Infants of 1500 g or less
Extremely low birth weight	Infants of 1000 g or less
Intrauterine growth restriction	Small for dates due to intrauterine starvation
Stillbirth	Fetal death after 24 weeks' gestation
Abortion	Fetal death and expulsion before 24 weeks' gestation

of an abortion. Increasingly, antenatal scans rather than the last menstrual period date are used to estimate gestational age. Therefore, it is advisable that pregnant women have an ultrasound measurement of crown–rump length at 7–11 weeks' gestation and/or biparietal diameter at 14–20 weeks' gestation.

In the USA the rate of preterm delivery is between 5 and 12%. Extreme premature births are between 1% and 1.5%. For low birth weight the incidence in the UK is around 6% and one-third of these are small for dates.

CAUSES OF PRETERM DELIVERY

About one-third of premature births occur for no apparent reason. Major causes remain antepartum haemorrhage and premature rupture of membranes. Although in many preterm deliveries a definite cause can not be found, it is possible to identify several factors that are generally associated with preterm labour and delivery. Obstetricians and midwives have long used this information to identify 'at-risk' women and to design interventions that prevent or reduce the occurrence of fetal and neonatal complications. It is equally important for neonatologists in order to anticipate the baby's immediate needs and make appropriate preparations for resuscitation and initial care (Fig. 3.1, Table 3.2).

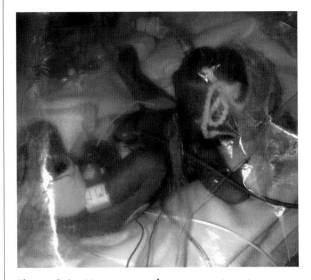

Figure 3.1 Very preterm infant receiving intensive care

falls above 2 s.d. or small if it is below 2 s.d. (see Table 3.1) The term intrauterine growth restriction (IUGR) is reserved for those fetuses that experience progressive growth restriction. These babies must be approached in a different way to pure preterm babies (even if they are small for dates) as the implications of in-utero starvation are quite different.

With improvements in neonatal care, preterm deliveries have increased in number considerably. Attempting to find a figure for rate is difficult. The apparent rise in the incidence of preterm birth over time might reflect changes in clinical practice and also changes in UK legislation with a lowering of the gestational age from 28 to 24 weeks for the definition

Table 3.2 Risk factors associated with preterm delivery		
Maternal history	**Pregnancy**	**Fetal**
Chronic disease	Inadequate weight gain	Fetal anomalies
Diabetes	Acute maternal illness	Infections
Renal disease	Pregnancy induced hypertension	
Cardiovascular disease	Urinary tract infection	
Respiratory disease	Chorioamnionitis, vaginal infection	
Underweight before pregnancy	Antepartum haemorrhage	
Reproductive tract anomalies	Isoimmunization	
Smoking	Premature rupture of membranes	
Age extremes (below 18 and above 40)	Multiple gestation	
Previous preterm labour	Polyhydramnios	
Low socioeconomic status	Retained intrauterine device	

ASSESSMENT OF FETAL WELLBEING

Not long ago the ability to assess fetal wellbeing was provided by simple auscultation of the fetal heart. Nowadays obstetric care has dramatically improved and there are a number of methods that can be used to measure the fetal status and to provide an approximation of its wellbeing.

History

First and foremost, the maternal medical history provides the background for a risk assessment and indirectly of the fetal health. Maternal condition and previous diseases, habits, and health status added to any complications during previous or the current pregnancy would identify the risks to a woman of having a preterm delivery.

At each antenatal visit, clinical assessment of fetal movements, fetal heart rate, symphyseal–fundal height measurement and liquor volume is done.

Fetal movements

Fetal motor activity reflects the fetal condition in utero and the simple 'kick-count' of fetal movement is a low-tech, low-cost screening tool. In the USA a decrease in or absence of fetal movements is relied upon by obstetricians as one of the most sensitive tests that would lead to emergency investigations because of the high risk of fetal death. In the UK a similar method, the Cardiff 'count to ten' failed to show overall benefit. However, reduced fetal movements should always alert the midwife and would normally lead to further investigations.

Other common methods available include cardiotocography (CTG) and ultrasonography to measure fetal growth velocity, amniotic fluid volume, and fetal Dopplers. Some units may consider the use of biophysical profile scoring that includes 30 min observation on fetal breathing, movement, tone, CTG and amniotic fluid volume.

Fetal heart rate

CTG is a test used to assess the integrity of the fetal autonomic nervous system. The fetal heart rate is under the dual influences of the sympathetic and parasympathetic nervous systems. By approximately 28 weeks' gestation, 85% of fetuses will demonstrate fetal heart rate accelerations in response to fetal movements. Interpretation of the CTG depends upon the gestation of pregnancy.

Ultrasound measurements

In pregnancies at risk of growth restriction, routine practice is to estimate the fetal growth by serial antenatal scans measuring the circumferences of the head and the abdomen. A fall in the growth velocity of the abdominal circumference is a marker of growth restriction.

Fetal blood flow

In addition the assessment of the maternal uterine arterial Dopplers at 24 weeks' gestation can be used in high-risk pregnancies to predict the risk of IUGR or stillbirth.

Doppler flow provides assessment of the fetal arterial and venous systems. Umbilical arterial blood flow becomes abnormal when there is placental insufficiency. Its usefulness is that absence of end-diastolic flow may appear days before conventional antenatal tests become abnormal leading to further investigations, which would include Doppler of the middle cerebral artery and fetal heart rate.

INTERVENTIONS TO PREVENT PRETERM DELIVERY

Several medical approaches have been used with the aim of, either preventing preterm labour and delivery, or preventing respiratory distress syndrome in the preterm baby. In any case, arrangement for transfer to a perinatal centre with neonatal intensive care unit (NICU) facilities is desirable.

Specific conditions may need different treatments (i.e. pregnancy-induced hypertension or gestational diabetes). For uncomplicated pregnancies that present with preterm labour, there is no evidence to support the contention that bed-rest and monitoring of contractions prevent preterm delivery. Interventions including education about smoking cessation, etc., have been shown to be beneficial.

The only role for tocolytic medication is to allow transfer of the woman to an appropriate unit where she would get antenatal steroids (see interventions to reduce the risk of complications in the baby).

Cerclage or cervical suture is only considered for women with a history suggestive of cervical incompetence (painless miscarriage in the second trimester).

INTERVENTIONS TO REDUCE THE RISK OF COMPLICATIONS IN THE BABY

A single dose of antenatal steroids reduces the risk of death, respiratory distress syndrome and intraventricular haemorrhage in the preterm infant. The current recommendation is to give it to women between 24 and 34 weeks' gestation who are at risk of preterm delivery within the next 7 days. Beclomethasone is preferred to dexamethasone because of less long-term side effects on the baby. There is no robust evidence to support repeated courses of steroids.

Group B streptococci (GBS) are a common inhabitant of the gastrointestinal and genitourinary tract. Colonization rate ranges from 15 to 40%. The newborn becomes colonized when passing through the birth canal. Symptomatic infection is usually systemic and severe. Women who are known carriers of GBS or who have had a previous infant with invasive GBS infection should receive intrapartum antibiotics (IV penicillin). This intervention has decreased the incidence of systemic infection in babies by more than 70%.

THE DECISION ON DELIVERY

About 15% to 25% of preterm infants are electively delivered because of fetal complications during pregnancy like maternal hypertension and intrauterine growth restriction. The decision to deliver these babies is taken by balancing the risks of preterm birth for the infant against the consequence of continuing the pregnancy for the mother and the fetus.

PERINATAL AND NEONATAL SERVICES: REGIONALIZATION

In the UK the neonatal mortality rate for very low birth weight infants (less than 1500 g) fell from 50% in 1975 to less than 20% in 1995 thanks to major improvements in standards of care. It is currently advised that preterm deliveries are planned in advance and that these women are transferred to an appropriate centre for monitoring and birth arrangements.

The UK provides a neonatal service with nationwide coverage through regionalization, which is the process of resource allocation or service delivery based on geographical boundaries. Each region has various units to provide different levels of care from special to intensive care. The aim is to ensure that the population in the region has local access to facilities that can at least provide special care. Hospitals that can give only special care should arrange for preterm babies to be delivered elsewhere. These hospitals, however, must ensure that adequate equipment and appropriately trained staff are available in case of unexpected delivery of a preterm baby.

In 1998 the British Association of Perinatal Medicine defined the standards of centres where babies are delivered (Table 3.3).

Transitional care units

Transitional care units are well recognized for the care of the mother and baby and are ideal for the management of preterm babies of more than 34 weeks. These units are designed to encourage bonding and attachment and to provide support especially with breast feeding. The staff includes midwives and neonatal nurses with a special interest in breast feeding. Services also include phototherapy for babies with jaundice and monitoring for hypoglycaemia.

Transport

Well planned in-utero transfer is the best way of transfer for a premature baby. Outcomes of extremely premature babies are significantly better when transferred in-utero to a tertiary or perinatal centre than when transferred ex-utero.

When a premature baby needs transfer, however, referral criteria are established and the transport service gives high-risk patients timely access to the appropriate services without interrupting their care. It provides an adequately trained service for transport of preterm babies from one centre to another. The ideal team is configured in a centralized neonatal transport team or in the Level 3 unit and is also responsible for the wellbeing of babies from tertiary centres that are returning to their local hospitals.

THE PRETERM BABY AT DELIVERY

Ideally, preterm delivery should be anticipated and planned in advance so that the neonatal unit can

Table 3.3	Perinatal and neonatal levels of care	
Level 1	Special care	Such a unit is essentially midwifery led, but with the safeguard of recourse to medical assistance (obstetrician, GP, anaesthetist or paediatrician) should unexpected complications arise. It is particularly suitable for women without obvious risk factors who wish to have a labour with minimum technological intervention. The emphasis of these units is on support for breast feeding
Level 2	High dependency	Based in district general hospitals and with short-term neonatal intensive care capability
Emphasis on babies that require continuous monitoring, supplemental oxygen and parenteral nutrition
Level 3	Intensive care	Generally based in tertiary perinatal centres where fetal-medicine units services are available
Adequately trained staff in labour ward and in the neonatal unit with all the facilities for full intensive care and availability of surgery and cardiology
The higher survival rate for premature babies is related to them being delivered in these units
Ideally, preterm deliveries of less than 28 weeks or babies of less than 1000 g should be transferred in utero and delivered in these centres

prepare and the neonatal team is available. There is not enough evidence to evaluate the use of a policy for elective Caesarean delivery for small babies. When a preterm delivery happens unexpectedly or in a non-tertiary centre, however, staff trained in neonatal resuscitation should be present at delivery. Once the baby is delivered, a rapid assessment will reveal an approximate gestational age and the condition at birth. General condition at birth, although not proven to be predictive of outcome, is an excellent indicator for subsequent management and should be documented. Apgar score (Table 3.4) should also be recorded, but also efforts should be made to describe the baby's condition and responsiveness.

Maternal, pregnancy, perinatal and fetal risk factors should always be taken into consideration when planning the management of the preterm baby. In terms of resuscitation, however, most babies of less than 30 weeks will have similar treatment, i.e. placement inside a polyethylene bag, surfactant at delivery and admission to intensive care for supportive ventilation and parenteral nutrition. On the other hand, most babies of more than 35 weeks will be fit and well enough to be nursed in a transitional care unit with their mothers. Babies between 30 and 34 weeks would probably need admission to a Level 1 or 2 unit for tube feeding.

INITIAL MANAGEMENT

Management depends on gestational age and condition at birth as well as the risk factors already mentioned. Parents are counselled and it is generally agreed that most babies will be in hospital until their expected delivery date. Therapies administered through the admission are diverse according to the baby's condition. Temperature stability is paramount and a radiant heater should be available at delivery and closed incubators or steam units should be available. There is good evidence that babies of less than 30 weeks should be placed inside a polyethylene bag to effectively maintain temperature. Environment plays an enormous role and developmental care is important to keep the baby as comfortable as possible. Therefore, light should be controlled, loud noise should be avoided, gentle touch is encouraged and minimal handling is desirable.

COMMON PROBLEMS OF PRETERM BABIES

Energy requirements and feeding

Energy requirement for preterm infants is 110–120 kcal/kg/day. The best source for provision of these requirements is breast milk from the baby's mother. However, the ability to suck, swallow and breathe in a coordinated fashion is not achieved until 34–36 weeks' gestation. Therefore, expressed breast milk is provided by orogastric or nasogastric tube initially while the baby learns to breast feed. Bottles or formula feeds should not be promoted as they are deleterious for the learning process.

Table 3.4 Apgar scores			
Sign	Score		
	0	1	2
Heart rate	Absent	Under 100 beats per minute	Over 100 beats per minute
Respiratory effort	Absent	Slow (irregular)	Good crying
Muscle tone	Limp	Some flexion of extremities	Active motion
Reflex irritability	No response	Grimace	Cough or sneeze
Colour	Blue, pale	Pink body, blue extremities	All pink

Gastro-oesophageal reflux

Preterm infants frequently have gastro-oesophageal reflux and an immature gag reflex, which increases the risk of aspiration of feed. Some of these babies will need anti-reflux medication and expert advice by a speech and language therapist with experience in feeding problems. There is no evidence that feed thickeners are effective.

Temperature instability

Preterm babies have a decreased ability to maintain body temperature and are susceptible to heat and fluid loss especially immediately after delivery and in the first few days of life. Heat loss in the preterm neonate is accelerated because of a high ratio of surface area to body mass, reduced insulation of subcutaneous tissue and water loss through the immature skin. Hypothermia is associated with increased mortality and morbidity. Kangaroo mother care with skin-to-skin contact between mother and baby as soon as the latter is stable enough, is an extremely valuable experience for parents and it is claimed that it is useful in controlling the baby's temperature.

Respiratory distress syndrome (RDS)

Babies under 28 weeks of gestation have pulmonary immaturity due to surfactant deficiency, non-compliant lungs and an extremely flexible chest wall. In addition, metabolic acidosis due to hypothermia or infection reduces surfactant production. There is very good evidence that exogenous surfactant given as soon as possible after delivery, via an endotracheal tube in babies of less than 30 weeks is associated with a 40% reduction in neonatal mortality from RDS.

Hypoglycaemia

Hypoglycaemia is very common in preterm infants as they have minimal energy reserves, higher metabolic rate, and limited fat and glycogen reserves if IUGR. Monitoring the blood glucose is particularly important in very and extremely preterm babies (Fig. 3.1). More mature infants may show signs such as lethargy and poor feeding that could be associated with hypoglycaemia.

Immature brain

Very preterm babies have immature cerebral vasculature and fragile white matter predisposing them to intraventricular haemorrhage and ischaemia. Reducing the incidence of cerebral damage in preterm infants has become the objective of perinatal medicine. The main risk factors associated with cerebral palsy are preterm birth, multiple pregnancy, intrauterine infection, hypoxaemia, hypocapnia, and haemodynamic disorders.

Ductus arteriosus

The ductus arteriosus normally obliterates soon after birth in a term baby, however, sometimes it remains patent maintaining a constant blood flow from the systemic circulation into the pulmonary circulation compromising the pulmonary gas exchange. If symptomatic it is usually medically or surgically closed.

Infections

Preterm babies are prone to infections because of an immature immune system. Local infections can rapidly become systemic and the mortality rate is high (40% more than babies without infection). This has led to the common practice of giving intravenous broad-spectrum antibiotics when risk factors for sepsis are identified. As the newborn, and especially the premature baby, is unable to localize the infection, a full septic screen (chest and abdomen X-rays and cultures of cerebrospinal fluid, urine and blood) is mandatory. Necrotizing enterocolitis is the most commonly acquired gastrointestinal emergency in the newborn infant; it most often affects preterm infants with an incidence of 10% in babies of birth weight less than 1500 g.

Apnoea

Apnoea of prematurity is a very common condition presented mostly by very preterm babies. It is usually secondary to an immature brain-stem response to

CO_2, but several causes are associated as well. Temperature instability, gastro-oesophageal reflux, hypoxaemia, infection, hypoglycaemia, intracranial haemorrhage, medication, or seizures are associated risk factors.

Jaundice

Hyperbilirubinaemia is a benign condition for most babies and is due to limitations in the metabolism and clearance of bilirubin from the plasma. All newborn infants, whether term or premature, exhibit a rise in the serum concentration of unconjugated bilirubin in the first few days of life and 50% of term and 80% of premature become jaundiced. Some risk factors like Rh incompatibility, birth trauma, infection, polycythaemia, or poor feeding may lead to high levels of bilirubin with the potential for neurotoxic effects and permanent brain damage or kernicterus. Clinical examination is not a reliable measurement of the level of serum bilirubin. Therefore, if risk factors are present, the level of bilirubin should be measured in a blood sample (if in hospital) or with a transcutaneous bilirubinometer (if at home) and early phototherapy started if required. Very high levels might require exchange transfusion.

Some babies have prolonged jaundice (>10 days). The commonest reason is breast milk jaundice when most of the hyperbilirubinaemia is unconjugated. Mothers can be reassured that it usually resolves by approximately 6 weeks, but may continue for 3 months. The jaundice disappears if breast feeding is discontinued, but this should only be advised in exceptional circumstances.

OUTCOMES

As more and more extremely low birth weight infants survive, demands for information about their long-term prognosis increase. Most of the disabilities like cerebral palsy, hearing loss, visual impairment, and educational and behavioural problems occur in the extremely preterm babies. The survival rate has increased, but the disability rate, especially cerebral palsy has not changed. Most of the studies around the world show similar results.

A study from the UK and Ireland (EPICure) evaluated the outcomes of babies born at 25 weeks' gestation or less in 1995 and found that, overall, 39% survived and that 49% of survivors, had no disability when developmentally assessed at 30 months corrected age (Costeloe et al. 2000, Wood et al. 2000). They were, however, smaller when compared to the population means (Wood 2003). The same group studied the survivors at 6 years of age and found that most of them had moderate-to-severe disabilities (Marlow 2005).

An American study followed up 59% (126 of 213) of children born at less than 29 weeks' gestation and found that at primary-school age 31% had no physical or educational impairment, 15% had cerebral palsy, 19% had cognitive problems and 32% had special needs and behavioural problems. At secondary-school age 41% had no physical or educational impairment, the cerebral palsy rate remained unchanged and 29% had special needs. Neonatal intraventricular haemorrhage and low socioeconomic status were the strongest predictors of adverse outcome (D'Angio 2002).

Other studies have shown that preterm babies achieve lower mean scores in tests of coordination, cognitive and language skills. However, when measures of quality of life were explored in ex-premature teenage children, there was no difference between them and controls.

FOLLOW-UP

Retinopathy of prematurity (ROP)

Extremely premature babies exposed to high concentrations of oxygen and sudden changes in oxygenation are prone to develop abnormal proliferation of retinal vessels, and require regular ophthalmologic reviews during the first year to monitor the degree of retinal involvement. The grading of ROP is from 1 to 3. Grade 1 usually recovers with time but can progress to grade 2 or 3. Grade 3 means retinal detachment and requires urgent laser therapy.

Hearing

Because of prematurity and aminoglycoside medication hearing should be monitored and hearing tests (OAE or AABR) are performed in every preterm baby born at less than 32 weeks' gestation.

Chronic lung disease (CLD)

CLD is defined as oxygen dependency in a baby at 36 weeks corrected age, or at 28 days from delivery. CLD is the result of oxygen therapy and assisted ventilation. Lungs become non-compliant and very difficult to ventilate. In the later stages cystic appearances and areas of scars are seen and gas exchange is impaired. Babies are institutionalized for long periods of time and sometimes discharged home with oxygen. Diverse treatments have been empirically used in an attempt to reduce the consequences of CLD; however, none are very effective. Steroids are no longer recommended, because they have been associated with cerebral palsy. Babies with CLD are more prone to asthma, chest infections and feeding problems. A protocol should be in place to monitor these babies, including immunizations against influenzae and pneumococcal infection; teaching of parents on smoking cessation; the correct use of inhalers for their babies, and treatment of associated feeding problems or gastro-oesophageal reflux.

Neurodevelopment

The neurodevelopment follow-up programme is a screening process provided for the very preterm graduates from neonatal units that begins on admission. The babies are assessed at regular intervals in order to determine the presence of physical, mental or emotional limitations. It involves an assessment of the parents of the baby and the environment where he/she is developing. It attempts to provide a comprehensive service by listening, examining and assessing at the same time as using anticipatory guidance. Early signs of deficiencies in normal development are identified and the baby is referred to the appropriate team for more specific therapy.

During their stay in the neonatal unit, babies should have regular head circumference measurement, and regular transfontanelle ultrasound scans for monitoring brain growth and development and for screening for brain damage. An MRI scan at term-corrected age is a valuable prognostic tool of further infant neurodevelopment.

The neurodevelopment follow-up should be a continuous process that starts in the neonatal unit and continues through infancy, school age and adolescence.

Counselling

Parents of a preterm baby are likely to be in desperate need of support. Few anticipate the possibility of having a preterm baby and antenatal courses do not cover this issue as a possible outcome for the pregnancy. When counselling a couple it is important to note the gestational age at which the baby was delivered as outcomes vary according to gestational age. Although parents are keen for knowledge, their understanding may be limited by the overwhelming amount of information they get, mostly from the Internet. Both obstetricians and paediatricians acknowledge the importance of fully informing the parents and their attitude is an important factor in parents' expectations. It is important to emphasize that once the baby is born other factors will immediately take place that might change the predictions.

References

D'Angio C 2002 Longitudinal 15-year follow-up of children born at less than 29 weeks' gestation after introduction of surfactant therapy into a region: neurologic, cognitive and educational outcomes. Pediatrics 110: 1094–1102

Costeloe K, Hennessy E, Gibson AT et al 2000 The EPICure Study: outcomes to discharge from hospital born infants born at the threshold of viability. Pediatrics 106(4): 659–671

Marlow N, Wolke D, Bracewell MA, Samara M, EPICure study group 2005 Neurologic and developmental disability at six years of age after extreme preterm birth. New England Journal of Medicine 352: 9–19

Wood N, Marlow N, Costeloe K, Gibson AT, Wilkinson AR 2000 Neurological and developmental disability after extremely preterm birth. New England Journal of Medicine 343(6): 378–384

Wood NS, Costeloe K, Gibson AT, Hennessy EM, Marlow N, Wilkinson AR, the EPICure study group 2003 The EPICure study: growth and associated problems in children born at 25 weeks of gestational age or less. Archives of Diseases in Children; Fetal Neonatal Edition 88(6):F492–500

Further reading

ABC of preterm birth 2004 BMJ monthly reviews from 18 September 2004 to 11 Dec 2004

Rennie J, Roberton N 1999 Textbook of Neonatology, 3rd edn. Churchill Livingstone, Edinburgh

4 Growth

E. Peile

▼ OVERVIEW

This chapter will describe the processes of growth in the normal child, looking at three stages: *Intrauterine*, *Childhood* and *Puberty* – the so-called ICP model of growth. At each stage the main determinants of growth will be highlighted.

Differential growth of the normal child's body components is illustrated before hormonal, genetic, and environmental factors are described in more detail. Nutrition, although of crucial importance to the growth process, will not be examined here, as it is covered in Chapter 5.

Finally, measurement of growth will be considered. Conditions causing pathological growth, and short or large stature will not be covered.

INTRODUCTION

Human growth starts when a sperm fertilizes an egg. It is much more difficult to define when growth ends, although mature adult size is usually reached around the mid-to-late teens. Some human tissues and organs (such as the male prostate gland) continue growing until death in old age. Birth is just one point in this continuum; this is important because the child's environment changes so drastically with transformations in the way nutrients are delivered.

Puberty likewise is an important stage for growth, less on account of the obvious 'growth spurt', than because puberty signals the beginning of the end of the previously relentless increase in body size. A later onset of puberty allows more growing time before the growth plates in long bones fuse. If children of similar pubertal size and growth patterns are compared, those with later puberties will grow taller.

GROWTH IN THE UTERUS

Growth will never be as fast again as it is in the 40-week period of gestation, during which time the human fetus repeatedly doubles in size, undergoing some 42 cycles of cell division before birth, against an estimated further five cycles from birth to adulthood. The size of a baby at birth is determined by the length of gestation time, by the size of the mother, and by the placental nutrient supply. Maternal regulation of fetal growth is believed to act by means of a biological constraint on growth, rather than by any accelerator. There is a direct relationship between the mother's own birth weight and her baby's birth weight, but no such relationship exists for fathers. Of course, obstetricians are concerned about small mothers carrying large babies, lest the size of the passage through the pelvis be too small for the fetal head to traverse.

Maternal smoking affects fetal growth, whereas socio-economic factors exert their effect on birth weight by increasing the risk of pre-term delivery.

Length of gestation is clearly an important predictor of birth size as premature delivery cuts short this most rapid growth phase.

Thus, if labour commences early for whatever reason, a smaller infant is born than would have been expected had labour proceeded to term. Term, defined as the period between 37 and 42 weeks of gestation, shows a marked slowing of intrauterine growth, and babies remaining in-utero after this time often actually achieve less growth in the perinatal period than their counterparts who were delivered earlier.

Of course, for some babies premature birth arises out of an intrauterine condition that, by its very nature, slows growth. Such babies are termed small-for-dates, by comparison with normally growing babies delivered 'pre-term'. The small-for-dates baby may have an early birth because the intrauterine condition triggers an early onset of labour, or because of intervention by the obstetrician, who has been carefully monitoring growth as an indicator of fetal wellbeing.

By about 10 weeks into the gestation, ultrasound measurements become reliable to the extent that the fetus can be tracked on a perinatal centile chart. Babies born a long time pre-term very seldom catch up the growth lost in utero, and may remain smaller than predicted by mid-parental height. Those small-for-dates babies whose intrauterine growth delay is detected early may experience considerable catch-up if they are skillfully nurtured as neonates. Those that have suffered marked or prolonged intrauterine growth retardation may remain affected by this blight on their growth long term.

Rapid growth in infancy has been associated with risk factors for cardiovascular disease in later life; however 'catch-up growth' confers demonstrable benefits on the baby born after intrauterine growth retardation. Catch-up growth, which is predicted by factors relating to the intrauterine restraint of fetal growth, may still result in obesity as children who showed catch-up growth between 0 and 2 years are fatter and have more central fat distribution at 5 years than other children.

Intrauterine nutrition is a key determinant of a baby's growth. Placental function is much more important than the mother's nutrient intake, though this is important as related to her state of health. Babies born to mothers with undetected or poorly controlled diabetes may be large for dates, but they are disadvantaged in the perinatal period. Placental function is a key determinant of the main growth factors of the infant, which are intrauterine growth factor-2 (IGF-2), human placental lactogen (HPL) and insulin.

GROWTH AND OBESITY: A RELATIONSHIP THAT STARTS BEFORE BIRTH

Reduced fetal growth leads to insulin resistance and associated disorders: raised blood pressure, high-serum triglyceride and low-serum, high-density, lipoprotein cholesterol concentrations. The highest values of these coronary risk factors occur in people who were small at birth and become obese. Intrauterine conditions that affect prenatal growth and postnatal growth both affect the risk of development of childhood diabetes in the same way: a poor growth decreases and an excess growth increases the risk.

One-third of obese UK children and adolescents of different ethnicities have the insulin resistance syndrome. Because being overweight is associated with various risk factors even among young children, it is possible that the successful prevention and treatment of obesity in childhood could reduce the adult incidence of cardiovascular disease. Obesity is discussed further in Chapter 5. By adolescence, body weight is on track for adult weight, and it is suggested that emphasizing and supporting physical activity in adolescence is one of the most helpful strategies (Kvaavik et al 2003).

BIRTH AS AN INTERRUPTION IN GROWTH

Growth in the period shortly after birth is conventionally measured in terms of weight rather than length. It is quite normal for the newborn infant to lose up to 10% of body weight in the first 4 days of life, but birth weight is normally regained by the 10th day. The interruption in growth is attributable to the change in circulation from fetal to neonatal, with the accompanying fluid shifts exacerbated by the trauma of delivery.

As the infant acclimatizes to life outside the womb, feeding becomes established and weight gain is typically around 180–200 g per week in the full-term infant, reducing to around 140–160 g per week in the second 3 months of life. Neonatal illness will, of course, affect growth temporarily.

INFANT AND TODDLER GROWTH

The normal child gets on with the business of growing in the weeks after delivery, when growth may be monitored both in terms of weight and supine length. Normal weight gain in the second year of life is around 2.5 kg for the average weight infant. Feeding difficulties are not uncommon at this time (see Chapter 5) and can have a pronounced temporary effect on weight, as can intercurrent illness. It needs to be remembered that fluid depletion can have a profound effect on the infant's weight and moderate dehydration can be reflected as 10% weight loss. Likewise measurements need to be carefully interpreted when the infant is so small, as there is a marked difference in weight depending on whether the infant has defecated or not.

Parents will need no reminder of the speed with which children outgrow their clothes in the first 2 years of life. Although growth is not as rapid as it was before birth, the average birth weight infant can expect to double birth weight by around 5 months of age, and treble it by 15 months of age. Thankfully, for most children this rapid growth is accompanied by increasing independent mobility so that parents need to do less moving and handling as the infant passes the 10 kg weight of a medium-sized suitcase (Figs 4.1a, b).

Once out of the immediate neonatal period, genetic determinants of size begin to exert more influence. Thus, while birth weight reflects principally the state of transplacental nutrition, the 2-year-old is established on a growth trajectory principally determined by parental size. During the first 2 years it is not uncommon to see some healthy normal babies gradually crossing centile lines. The infant of small parents who thrived in utero may change from growing along the 90th centile to growing under the 25th centile, whereas with catch-up growth a baby who was born on the 10th centile as a result of mild intrauterine growth retardation could, by the age of 2 years, be progressing along the 75th centiles for height and weight.

There is an old adage that you can double the height of the 2-year-old to predict adult height. Because the normal child usually grows predictably along a centile line from this time, it can be seen from the centile charts that this approximation is not without some factual basis.

DIFFERENTIAL GROWTH IN CHILDHOOD

Growth is not a uniform process in all body tissues. The head of the newborn infant makes up almost one-third of total size compared with the adult proportion of approximately 1:7. It is obvious that there is a differential in the growth of different tissues.

Another example of differential tissue growth velocity is the lymphoid tissue in normal tonsils. Because there is a disproportionate rate of growth in relation to the rest of the oropharynx, the tonsils of a 6-year-old can appear to be very big. As tonsillar growth slows down at this age, by the time the child is postpubertal, the tonsils will appear to be 'normal' size again. Earlier demonstration of this simple physiological fact by longitudinal observation of normal children might have saved countless unnecessary tonsillectomies.

In terms of the overall size of the child and of the eventual adult, the most important component is the growth of bones, particularly the long bones that determine limb length. Skeletal maturation is used as an indicator of growth progress. By X-raying the hand and wrist, skeletal maturation can be estimated from radiological norms of epiphyseal state, and compared to chronological age. Bone age behind chronological age indicates that there is more growing time left, and augurs a taller adult height than would be predicted from present height for age.

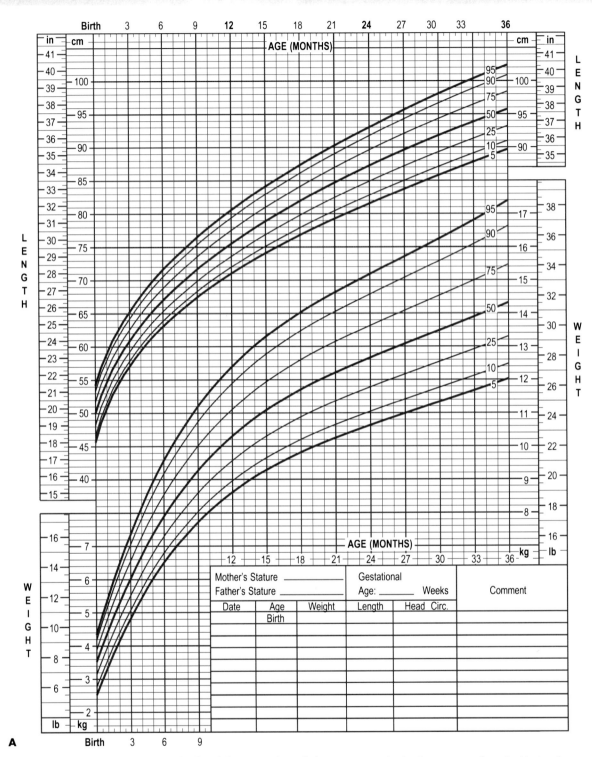

Figure 4.1 (a) Boys: birth–36 months, length-for-age and weight-for-age percentiles (with permission from the National Center for Health Statistics)

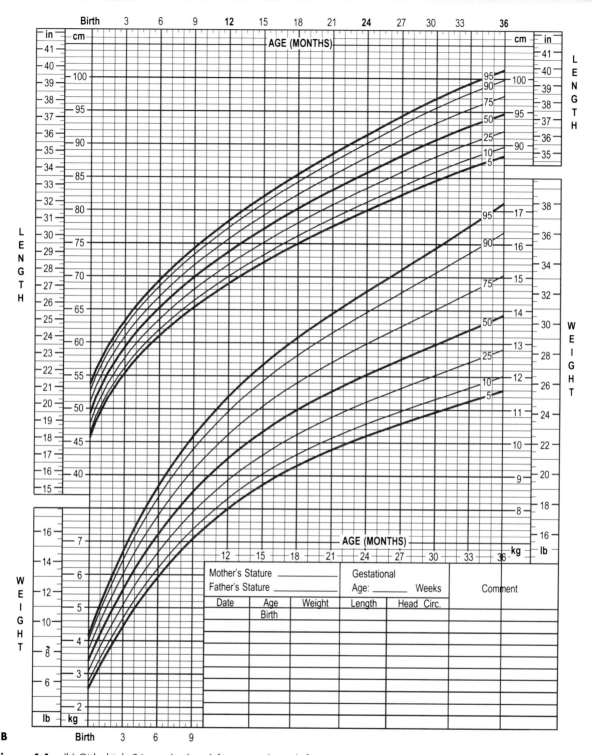

Figure 4.1 (b) Girls: birth–36 months, length-for-age and weight-for-age percentiles (with permission from the National Center for Health Statistics)

Conversely, advanced bone age indicates that growing time will be reduced.

Growth hormone is an important determinant of bone age. When small children are given growth hormone, not only does their height increase, but also the progression of bone age appears to be normal at least over the 1st year of treatment in pre-puberty.

Head size attracts particular attention in infancy (Figs 4.2a, b). The occipitofrontal circumference of the skull is measured soon after birth, not only to ensure that the baby does not have microcephaly, reflecting poor brain growth in utero, but also to establish a baseline for the 1st year of life. Until the bones of the skull fuse with closure of the anterior and posterior fontanelles (the baby's 'soft spots') a skull that enlarges faster than normal may be a warning sign of a dangerous increase in intracranial pressure requiring neurosurgical attention. Most large heads turn out to be familial, and merely indicate that the child will require a large hat size in later life!

PUBERTY

Skeletal growth

In many children's minds puberty is the time when growth is most noticeable; over a very short time period the child's body assumes adult proportions. The long bones are expanding rapidly, causing growth trajectories to kick upwards (see Figs 4.3a, b and Figs 4.4a, b), but this period is short lived, as bone growth slows rapidly after the initial pubertal growth spurt with the closure of the epiphyseal plates. Thus, it is puberty that signals the tailing off of a child's growth. By the time a girl has her first period (menarche) she has completed two-thirds of her pubertal growth spurt, and is unlikely to grow more than another 3–5 cm. Similarly for boys, later onset of puberty prolongs the growing time and leads to greater eventual height. Homeostatic mechanisms appear to be in play here as there is a tendency for smaller children to have later puberty and taller children to be earlier, moderating the population height towards the mean. The situation where this does not hold true is for children who were already small (under 5th centile) at age 7 years. These children are likely to stay small, and age of puberty has little effect on their growth progress (Jefferis 2002).

Girls usually start their adolescent growth spurt about 2 years before boys. The first acceleration is in the long bones of the legs, followed by pelvic bone and vertebral growth in the trunk occurring before the shoulders and chest broaden out. Both increasing density of the bony skeleton and an increase in bulk of muscle and fat contribute to adolescent weight gain.

In the adolescent growth spurt gender differences are accentuated. Whereas the shape of the prepubescent boy differs little from that of a prepubescent girl, in puberty girls not only develop breasts, but their hips broaden more and their soft tissue development has a higher ratio of fat to muscle. Boys broaden out more at the shoulders, and develop their neck musculature. The average male will lose body fat during adolescence.

Other cardiovascular and respiratory changes emphasize the gender differences in organ growth. As puberty advances, the male heart and lungs grow larger and consequent differences in blood pressure, heart rate, and tidal volume of air intake account for some of the differences in stamina between adult men and women.

Secondary sexual changes

A further important example of differential growth is that of the primary sex organs, or gonads, accompanied by the development of secondary sexual characteristics at the time of puberty.

Relatively early in puberty, as the penis grows, boys begin to experience spontaneous erections and shortly afterwards spontaneous ejaculation is evidence of spermarche as the male testes produce sperm cells along with semen from the prostate gland.

In girls, menarche (the first menstrual period) signals that the ovaries are releasing mature ova into the Fallopian tubes and that endometrial shedding is occurring in response to the cyclical hormonal changes.

Both oestrogens and androgens are present in males and females, but in different amounts. In boys the large quantities of the androgen testosterone

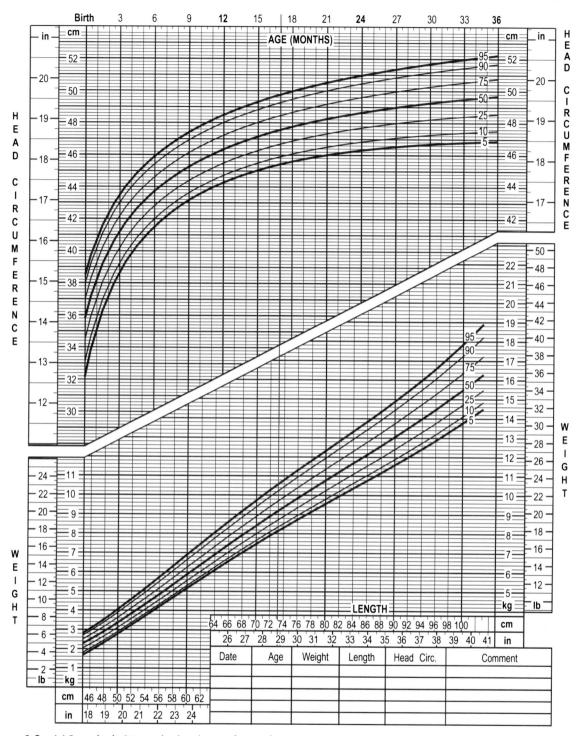

Figure 4.2 (a) Boys: birth–36 months, head circumference-for-age and weight-for-length percentiles (with permission from the National Center for Health Statistics)

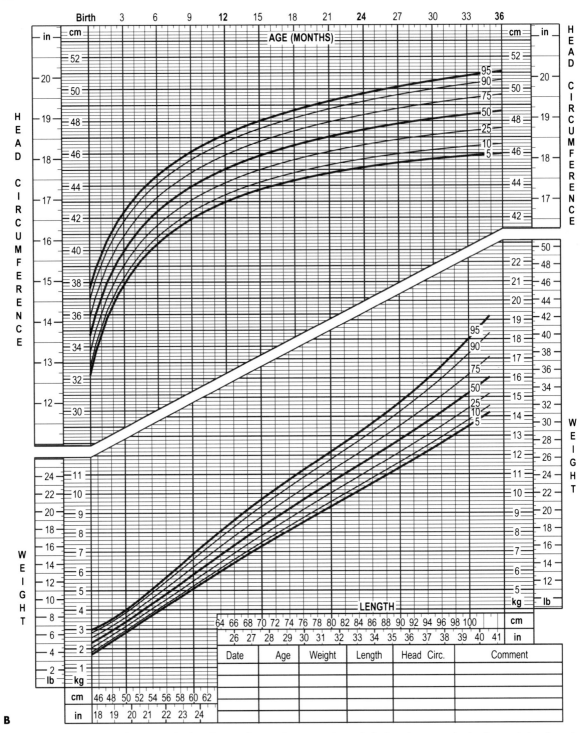

Figure 4.2 (b) Girls: birth–36 months, head circumference-for-age and weight-for-length percentiles (with permission from the National Center for Health Statistics)

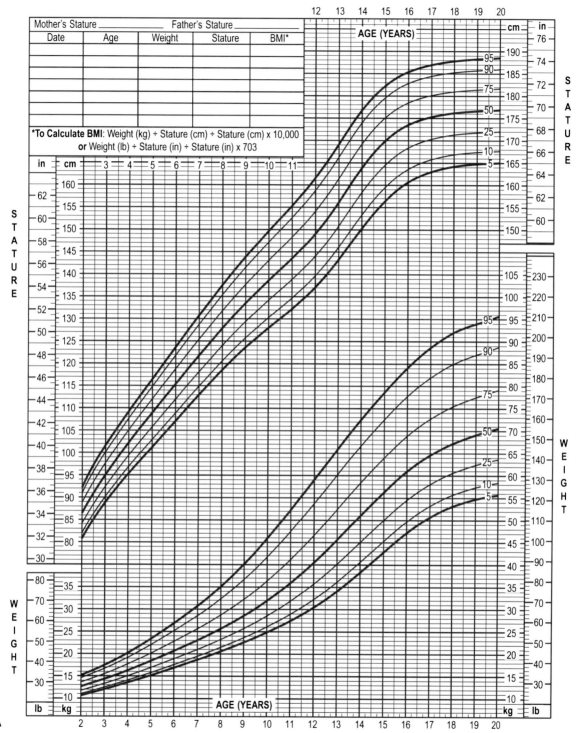

Figure 4.3 (a) Boys: 2–20 years, stature-for-age and weight-for-age percentiles (with permission from the National Center for Health Statistics)

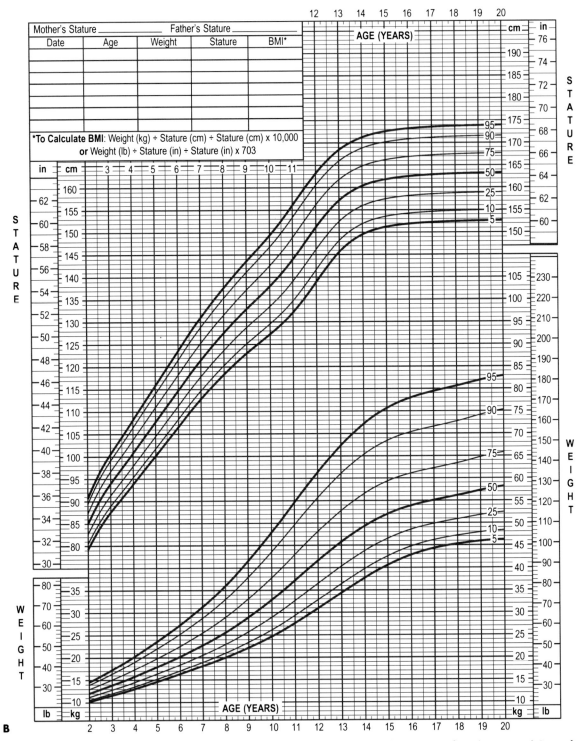

Figure 4.3 (b) Girls: 2–20 years, stature-for-age and weight-for-age percentiles (with permission from the National Center for Health Statistics)

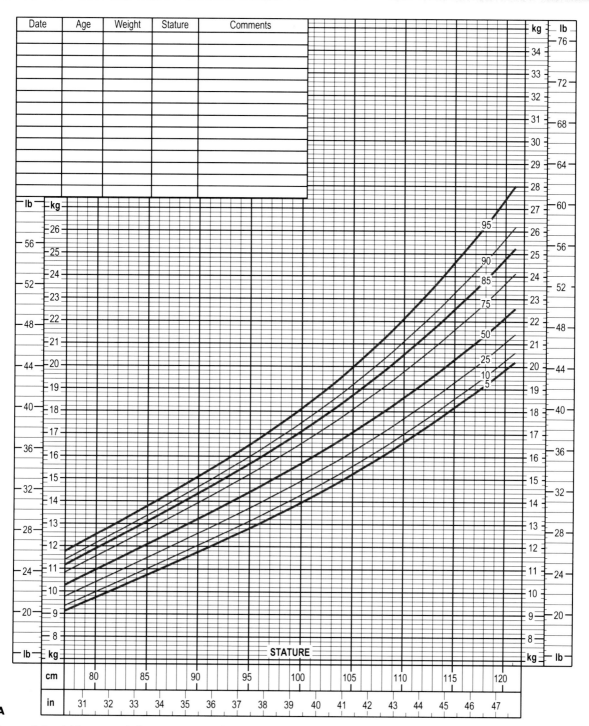

Figure 4.4 (a) Boys: weight-for-stature percentiles (with permission from the National Center for Health Statistics)

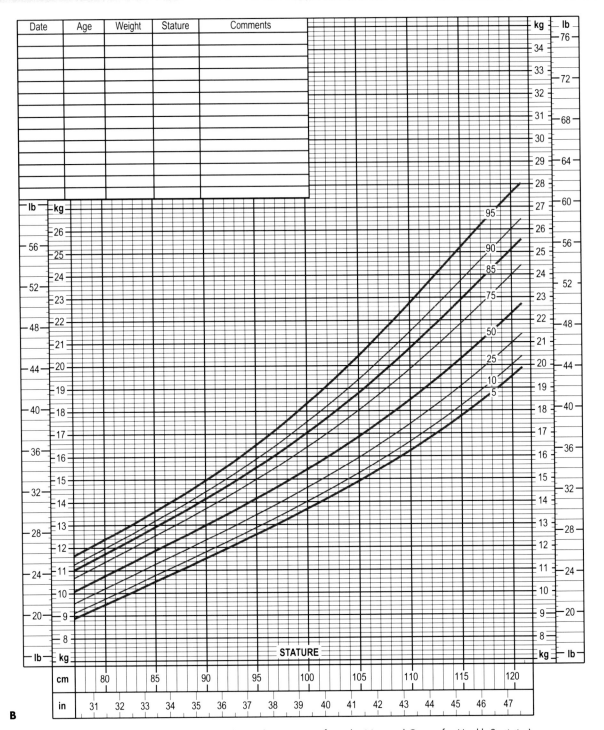

Figure 4.4 (b) Girls: weight-for-stature percentiles (with permission from the National Center for Health Statistics)

B

released by the testes contribute to muscle growth, body and facial hair, and other male sex characteristics. Testosterone also contributes to gains in body size.

In girls ovarian oestrogen release is important for maturation of breasts, uterus and vagina, and contributes to the body assuming feminine proportions. Regulation of the menstrual cycle depends not only on oestrogens, but also on progestogens from the corpus luteum and the pituitary gonadotrophins luteinizing hormone (LH) and follicle stimulating hormone (FSH) all of which interact in a feedback cycle.

Like boys, girls' pubertal growth spurts are also affected by androgens. In girls the main source of androgen production is the adrenal glands, and these adrenal androgens are also largely responsible for growth of axillary and pubic hair.

The approximate timings of some of these changes are summarized in Table 4.1.

Table 4.1	Age ranges for pubertal changes	
Typical age range in girls	Features of puberty	Typical age range in boys
9½–14½ years	Main pubertal growth spurt (around 18–24 months accelerated growth)	10½–16 years
	Testes start to enlarge	10–13 years
8–13 years	Thelarche (breasts start to grow)	
8–14 years	Pubic hair grows. Underarm hair develops around 2 years later along with facial hair in boys, at about the same time as the sweat glands develop	10–15 years
	Penis develops and voice breaks	11–14½ years
10–16½ years	Menarche (first period)	

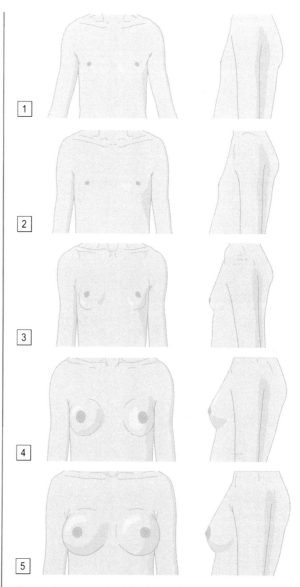

Figure 4.5 Standards for breast development (after Tanner)

Breast changes

The commonly accepted classification of Tanner and Whitehouse enables growth specialists to determine the pubertal stage of breast development (Fig. 4.5). The stages are:

- B1: preadolescent – elevation of papilla only
- B2: breast bud stage – elevation of breast and papilla as small mound. Areolar diameter enlarged over stage B1

- B3: breast and areola both enlarged and elevated more than in stage B2, but with no separation of their contours
- B4: the areola and papilla form a secondary mound projecting above the contour of the breast
- B5: mature stage – papilla only projects, with the areola recessed to the general contour of the breast.

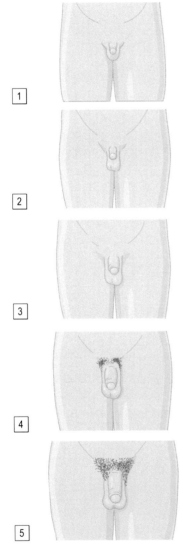

Figure 4.6 Standards for genital development (after Tanner)

Penis and testis development

Likewise, Tanner and Whitehouse defined the standards for assessing pubertal development of the penis, scrotal sac and testes in boys (Fig. 4.6). The stages are as follows:

- G1: preadolescent – testes, scrotum and penis are about the same size and shape as in early childhood
- G2: scrotum slightly enlarged, with reddening of the skin and changes in texture. Little or no enlargement of the penis at this stage
- G3: penis slightly enlarged, at first mainly in length. Scrotum further enlarged than in stage G2
- G4: penis further enlarged with growth in breadth and development of glans. Further enlargement of scrotum and darkening of scrotal skin
- G5: genitalia adult in size and shape.

Development of pubic and body hair

Again the Tanner and Whitehouse stages are used as shown in Figure 4.7. The stages for boys and girls are as follows:

- PH1: preadolescent – the vellus over the pubes is not further developed than that over the abdominal wall, i.e. no pubic hair
- PH2: sparse growth of long, slightly pigmented downy hair, straight or slightly curled, chiefly at the base of the penis or along the labia
- PH3: considerably darker, coarser and more curled. The hair spreads sparsely over the junction of the pubes
- PH4: hair now adult in type, but area covered is still considerably smaller than in adults. No spread to medial surface of thighs
- PH5: adult in quantity and type with distribution of the horizontal (or classically 'feminine' pattern). Spread to medial surface of thighs, but not up the linea alba
- PH6: spread upwards along the linea alba (the typical male escutcheon).

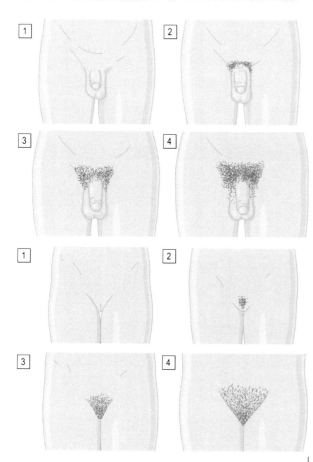

Figure 4.7 Standards for pubic hair development in boys and girls (after Tanner)

The biological clock

We have seen how puberty can be defined in terms of the stage of development of the breasts in girls and penis and testes in boys, along with the development of body hair in both sexes. Pubertal stage 1 is the prepubertal stage. As the adolescent proceeds through puberty the most accurate description is one of the component stages (for example breast stage 3; pubic hair stage 2) but sometimes an approximation of global stage is given (for example puberty stage 3). The sequence is usually fairly uniform in line with the ranges indicated in Table 4.1, but sometimes there is some variation in the synchrony as in premature thelarche, which is one form of precocious puberty.

Precocious puberty is usually defined as sexual development before the age of 8 years in girls or

10 years in boys. This happens four times more commonly in girls than boys and, although generally an innocent happening (sometimes familial, sometimes unexplained), it always requires investigation, as in some 15% of cases a serious cause, for example adrenal or gonadal tumour, will be found.

Full-blown precocious puberty, as might be expected, accelerates and then halts growth before the child has reached normal adult height with girls typically reaching a height of around 152 cm and boys about 5 cm taller. But, interestingly, girls with premature thelarche grow significantly taller than normal controls of the same age, suggesting that premature thelarche is an incomplete form of precocious sexual development probably due to derangement in the maturation of the hypothalamo-pituitary-gonadal axis, which results in a higher than normal FSH secretion.

Hormonal regulation

Hormonal changes precede physical changes in male puberty. As puberty approaches, levels of inhibin B, FSH, LH, testosterone and oestradiol levels increase significantly between stages 1 and 2 of puberty. Inhibin B, which in boys is thought to be produced mainly by the Sertoli cells of the testis, is probably a key initiator of puberty. Its production is stimulated by testosterone from the Leydig cells of the testis. Inhibin B has a complex feedback relationship with FSH, the level of which continues to increase between stages 2 and 3 of puberty before levelling off and slightly decreasing at pubertal stage 5. From stage 2 of puberty the inhibin B level remains relatively constant, whereas levels of serum LH, testosterone, and estradiol increase progressively throughout puberty. By the end of puberty the closed loop feedback regulation system, operating in adult men, has been established.

The finding that mature levels of inhibin B are achieved early in puberty may explain the observation that spermarche also is achieved early in puberty and may occur when the testes have grown only slightly and with little or no pubic hair development.

Inhibin B, which in girls is produced by granulosa cells in the ovary, is again believed to be important in the initial stages of puberty, with levels rising between stage 1 and stage 2. It has been suggested that the interaction between inhibin B and FSH may be critical for follicle development. Serum levels of FSH and inhibin B and FSH peak earlier in puberty than those of LH and oestradiol, which continue to rise throughout puberty until the adult female cyclical pattern is established.

GROWTH AS A MARKER OF WELLBEING

'My, how you've grown', is the refrain of proud grandparents, indicating growth as a marker of successful nurturing. Height has an association with social class (upper socioeconomic groupings tending to be taller), with reproductive success in men and women, and to economic success in Western cultures, so it is no wonder that growth is prized. What is also true is that good physical and emotional health is a prerequisite for satisfactory growth. In the same way as physical illness of many kinds can detrimentally affect growth, so emotional deprivation is a well-known cause of failure to thrive. Indeed, growth charts are often produced in court as evidence of emotional deprivation when it can be seen that a particular environment has a marked effect on growth rate.

Brain growth and cognitive development are emotive subjects. To what extent does brain growth reflect a child's overall growth pattern, and how does growth affect IQ?

Across the range of normal birth weights, weight at birth is associated with later cognitive development. School attainment is related to birth weight and, independently, to social class, which has a more pronounced effect on school attainment (Jefferis et al 2002). There is also evidence that IQ tends to be higher in those who were heavier at birth or who grew taller in childhood and adolescence, and it appears that brain growth during infancy and early childhood is more important than growth during fetal life in determining cognitive function (Gale et al 2004).

In a large study, boys who grew slowly during infancy had poor educational achievements and lower incomes than those who grew more rapidly,

irrespective of the social class into which they were born. It has been suggested that biological processes linked to slow infant growth may lead to lifelong impairment of cognitive function.

Two points should be emphasized here. Growth is not a constant velocity process. If growth is measured accurately it can be seen that the trajectory is often rather 'staircase' like, with periods of upward movement followed by flat periods of barely measurable growth. The second point is that all poor growth is not symptomatic of physical, social or emotional problems. There is a condition of constitutional growth delay, evidenced by delay in the bone age, which occurs in the normal child and can run in families. This condition resolves spontaneously, when a subsequent growth spurt, typically coming 1 or 2 years later than normal, enables the child to reach normal adult height a little later than their peers.

DRIVERS OF GROWTH

Nutritional state is perhaps the most important variable predicting growth in infancy, although it appears that levels of growth hormone–insulin-like growth factor (GH–IGF) are also important. As childhood progresses, this, and other hormonal controllers assume greater importance. Around puberty, the sex hormones both amplify growth hormone secretion and increase tissue responsiveness to GH–IGF.

Growth hormone, which is released in pulses, is a key determinant of health and wellbeing, from childhood well into adult life (it is thought to play no role in fetal growth). It is a metabolic regulator, crucial to fat metabolism, and important for bone metabolism.

In children and young adults, it appears that the early night-time period when deep sleep occurs, is an important time in the daily secretion of growth hormone (Fig. 4.8).

There are also significant changes in the amount of growth hormone secretion that correspond with age. Growth hormone secretion peaks early in the pubertal growth spurt and thereafter falls to adult levels, which are much lower than those in childhood.

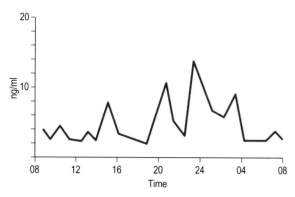

Figure 4.8 *Diurnal variation in growth hormone (with permission from the National Center for Health Statistics)*

MEASUREMENT OF GROWTH

Measuring growth is a preoccupation of parents, health visitors and paediatricians alike. Both weight and linear measurements are important reflections of size, and they can be combined in the body mass index. Measuring techniques need to change as childhood advances. The fetus is measured ultrasonically in its curled up state; infants are weighed and also measured lying flat on a measuring mat; whereas, from 2 to 3 years of age, a child's longitudinal growth can be measured in terms of erect height.

Reference standards for the original crown–rump measurements used in antenatal ultrasound measurements were derived from measurements of aborted fetuses and live-born infants covering the range of 8 to 44 weeks' gestation, and correction factors were applied for parity, race, socioeconomic status and fetal sex. It is now commonplace for ultrasonographers to predict birth weight on the basis of their measurement computations.

It is worth remembering that changes in the process of measurement affect the accuracy with which we can measure children. Specialists in growth measurement (auxologists) have developed charts that facilitate predictions of future growth and eventual size, the most important determinants of which are the measured rates of growth to date.

Very small errors of measurement can affect predictions drastically. Few child health nurses would claim to measure to an accuracy of less than ±3 mm, but think about how much even such a small error can affect predictions. If a child is measured and re-measured after 6 months, and if the first measurement is 3 mm out in one direction, and the second is 3 mm out in the other direction, then that is a 6 mm error. Compare this child to another who has been measured with errors in the opposite direction, and one child may be deemed to have grown 12 mm more than the other when, in fact, their growth has been the same. When the expected growth for both children over the 6-month period was 20 mm, a 12 mm difference is enormous. Measurement errors are reduced by means of accurate equipment, trained measurers and attention to detail both in measuring and plotting on charts. The impact of errors of measurement is reduced by repeated measurements over prolonged periods of time.

One of the most important pieces of information for the child worried about being too small or too tall is a prediction of eventual adult height. This is facilitated by charts that take account of the genetic contribution of parents' height. Mid-parental centile charts are available, but an acceptable approximation for boys is to add 7 cm to the mother's height and to then calculate the midpoint between this and father's height. For girls the procedure is to deduct 7 cm from father's height and the calculated mid-parental height is then the midpoint between this and mother's height. Using the mid-parental height, it is then possible to predict that the child's eventual height has a 96% chance of ending up within 2 s.d. of the mid-parental height.

An even more rough-and-ready piece of reassurance for the short boy is the observation that he has a 93% chance of growing taller than his mother.

CONCLUSION

Growing pains are largely fictitious, invented to explain otherwise unexplained limb pains in childhood. Growth is normally a painless process, physically and emotionally. Emotional pain around growth or the lack of it can often be allayed by a sensitive explanation of the natural processes at play. Growth is an important marker of health and wellbeing, but careful interpretation is needed. Each normal child must be seen in his or her genetic, environmental, and nutritional context.

References

Gale CR, O'Callaghan FJ, Godfrey KM et al 2004 Critical periods of brain growth and cognitive function in children. Brain 127: 321–329

Jefferis BJMH, Power C, Hertzman C 2002 Birth weight, childhood socio-economic environment, and cognitive development in the 1958 British birth cohort study. British Medical Journal 325: 305–308

Kvaavik E, Tell GS, Klepp K-I 2003 Predictors and tracking of body mass index from adolescence into adulthood. Archives of Pediatric and Adolescent Medicine 157: 1212–1218

Tanner JM, Whitehouse RH 1976 Clinical longitudinal standards for height, weight, height velocity, weight velocity, and stages of puberty. Archives of Diseases in Childhood 51: 170–179

Further reading

Gardosi J, Chang A, Kalyan B, Sahota D, Symonds EM 1992 Customized antenatal growth charts. The Lancet 339: 283–287

5

Feeding

M. Francis, J. Jamieson

▼ OVERVIEW

Feeding children a nutritionally adequate diet for the first few years of their life is of great importance. The primary objective is to achieve optimum growth and development, with a second objective of developing and maintaining good food habits.

The intention of this chapter is to lead the reader from the first few days of breast/formula feeding through to the introduction of solid foods and then the ongoing development for a good diet, nutrition and eating habits. Along the way some of the more common problems that may occur will be discussed.

BREAST OR BOTTLE?

Preparation for feeding a baby begins during pregnancy. The breasts start preparing for making milk as soon as conception takes place. The nipples develop prominent little spots, the opening of tiny glands called Montgomery's tubercles. These secrete an oily substance that keeps the nipples soft. Inside the breast the fatty tissue is replaced by the milk-producing and storing cells.

The mother must be allowed to choose what is right for her and not to be made to feel guilty if artificial feeding is the chosen decision. She should feel relaxed and enjoy the baby whatever her decision.

BREAST FEEDING

The World Health Organization (WHO) recommends that 'breast is best' as it is uniquely designed to meet the baby's every need and its properties can never be accurately reproduced in formula milks. The act of breast feeding provides a close bond between mother and child. Breast feeding offers the newborn the best nutrition to provide nourishment and protection during a vulnerable period of life. It offers an appropriate balance and concentration of nutrients in a digestible form with enzymes being provided to aid digestion. There are no rules to breast feeding. Successful breast feeding depends on two hormones (Table 5.1).

Colostrum

In the first few days after birth a breast fluid called colostrum is produced in small quantities suitable for the baby learning to suckle. Colostrum is high in protein and helps babies to resist infection. It also acts

Table 5.1	Breast-feeding hormones
Prolactin	Milk-producing hormone that is released from the anterior pituitary gland after delivery of the placenta and membranes. This produces milk in the acini (milk-producing cells) in the breast
Oxytocin	Hormone released from the posterior pituitary gland, in response to the baby suckling. It causes the myoepithelial cells around the acini cells to contract, enabling the manufactured and stored milk to be released. The milk then drains into the ampullae or reservoir that lies behind the nipple and milk is then removed by the baby suckling. This process is known as the 'let down' reflex

Table 5.2	Some important nutrient components for formula feeds
Long chain polyunsaturated fatty acids (LCPs)	A special group of fats, which are essential components of all cell membranes and play an important role particularly in the development of new cells in the nervous system, brain and eyes Two of particular note are arachidonic acid (AA) and docosahexaenoic acid (DHA)
Nucleotides	Amino acid components for growth and development involved in immunity and also important for infant manufacture of LCPs
Beta-carotene	Antioxidant that helps in the development of the immune system, skin and body tissue
Selenium	Essential trace mineral and a key antioxidant for balanced nutrition It is essential for the normal functioning of the immune system and thyroid gland

as a laxative and so helps the baby pass meconium and is important in avoiding the development of jaundice. Colostrum is rich in protein, immunoglobulins, vitamins, anti-infective agents such as lactoferrin and lysozyme, living cells and minerals.

After 3 days mature breast milk develops and is a constantly changing food that adjusts to the age and needs of the baby. Each mother produces the perfect food for her baby. Early suckling straight after delivery influences the success and duration of breast feeding and should be encouraged if possible. The very action of sucking not only fills the baby's stomach, but it sends an impulse to the mother's pituitary gland, which then produces oxytocin. This then releases the milk stored in the storage cells deep in the breast. A further message is then sent to the brain telling the breast to replace the milk that the baby has used.

ARTIFICIAL FEEDING

Cow's milk has to be specially adapted for human consumption to contain the necessary basic nutrients. Modified cow's milk can attempt to copy breast milk, but this is made more difficult as all the properties contained in breast milk are still unknown. However, more and more research into the field of infant nutrition increases the awareness of the importance of certain nutrients, such as those listed in Table 5.2. Many of the available brands of manufactured infant formulae will now contain all or some of these. Table 5.3 compares human milk, cow's milk and formula.

ADVANTAGES OF BREAST FEEDING

In 2003 the UK Department of Health revised its infant feeding guidelines and recommended breastfeeding exclusively for the first 6 months, but ideally throughout the first year. It should be reduced following the introduction of weaning.

Composition of breast milk is never constant: the amount of protein, fat, sugar (lactose) and other components change. At the beginning of the feed *fore-milk* is produced, high in volume, low in fat and,

Table 5.3   Comparison of milks: human, cow's and formula

	Breast milk	Cow's milk	Formula milk
Protein	Needed for growth. This is quickly digested; it breaks down into casein and whey but is largely whey. It has no lactoglobulin. Only 1% of breast milk is protein as babies are meant to grow slowly and feed often	Levels are three times higher and are of a different type and less digestible. Can cause allergic reaction in some babies. Protein needs to be diluted to a safe level. This dilutes the calories	Lactose is added to provide extra calories
Fat	For energy and growth. Easily deposited with very little waste. A higher concentration of long chain fatty acids, which is thought to be important for the growth of the brain and nervous system	Less easily absorbed and of a different type. Essential long chain fatty acids are not naturally present	Essential long chain fatty acids are not naturally present, and manufacturers are trying to add them
Carbohydrate	Important source of energy and very important for brain growth. Produced in the form of lactose	Lactose content one third less than human breast milk	Added to cow's milk as lactose (milk and sugar) to make up to the same energy value and amount in breast milk
Vitamins	Adequate maternal diet provides all necessary vitamins	Small amounts and less available	Not present in the right amount and some vitamins are destroyed by processing and then have to be added after
Minerals	The iron content is low, but 20 times more easily absorbed. Other minerals are present in the right balance	Three times more sodium, potassium, calcium and chloride are present and six times more phosphorous. Iron and zinc are less well absorbed	Iron added. Other minerals adjusted to approximate levels of breast milk
Water	It contains all the water a baby requires	The water content cannot be changed to suit the needs of the baby so additional water needs to be given	The water content cannot be changed to suit the needs of the baby so additional water needs to be given

therefore, satisfying thirst. The second part of the feed (*hind-milk*) is low in quantity, but richer in calories and satisfies hunger.

Protection from infection is provided by maternally derived antibodies in breast milk and by iron-binding protein that, in the baby's gut, helps to protect from illnesses such as necrotizing enterocolitis and gastroenteritis. Formula-fed babies are five times more likely to develop these. A breast-fed baby is also five times less likely than a formula-fed baby to develop urinary tract infections. If breast feeding is exclusive for longer than the first 6 months it has been found to reduce the number of ear infections including otitis media. If a supplementary formula feed is introduced this risk is increased.

Breast feeding studies have also shown protection against breathing problems such as bronchitis, bronchiolitis and pneumonia (Villalpando & Hamosh 1998, Oddy 2003) and these effects can be long term. Babies breast fed for the first 2 months of life are also less likely to develop insulin-dependent diabetes as juveniles, coeliac disease, inflammatory bowel disease and some childhood cancers (Davis 2001). There is also evidence that breast feeding may promote an optimal lipid profile and thus protect against atherosclerotic disease in adult life (Golding et al 1997).

It is now generally accepted that breast feeding can help to reduce the risk and severity of allergic diseases, such as eczema and rhinitis (Gdalevich 2001, Kuli et al 2002). Because atopic babies' immune systems can react adversely to cow's milk protein (lactoglobulin) by producing allergic symptoms, it is usually recommended that breast feeding continues for the first 6 months.

Breast feeding is also beneficial to the mother, reducing the risk of ovarian cancer and pre-menopausal breast cancer. It helps to prevent osteoporosis, increasing the strength of bones in later life. It also gives a faster return to the pre-pregnancy figure.

BREAST FEEDING IN SPECIAL CIRCUMSTANCES

Prematurity

Breast milk is extremely beneficial for premature babies as it is more easily digested. It contains an enzyme called lipase, which helps the baby digest fat more efficiently. This is significant as fat is an important source of energy for a premature baby's growth. Studies have shown that giving premature babies breast milk reduces the chances of illness and death considerably. The optimal growth of the brain is dependent on the baby receiving essential fatty acids through the milk and this is important for visual development. The protective element of breast milk is even more important for premature babies. The immune system of the pre-term infant is not fully mature and using breast milk encourages protection from potentially life-threatening conditions such as necrotizing enterocolitis (NEC), meningitis and viral infections. Infants of 30–36 weeks gestation who are fed formula are 20 times more likely to get NEC.

The birth of a premature baby is, however, often a time of crisis and emotional turmoil and much effort is needed to establish and maintain a supply of breast milk. Some babies may be too weak to suck at the breast or if they go to the breast they are easily exhausted. For those babies who have not established a sucking reflex, feeds of expressed breast milk may be given via a nasogastric tube. Breast feeding can then be gradually introduced as the baby becomes stronger.

Special needs

Breast feeding should be encouraged whenever possible for a baby born with recognized special needs, as it will enhance bonding of mother and child, and can help the mother to feel that she is playing some part when there is increased medical intervention.

Three of the most common special needs are Down's syndrome, cleft palate and heart problems, but with professional help and maternal determination breast feeding can be achieved.

Multiple births

Breast feeding of twins does at first seem insurmountable, but with some planning can be achieved. Feeding both together is the ideal solution, but this can prove difficult for the first time mother. Good support and positive management in the early days will be required as feeding is a major task during the day. Careful positioning of the babies using supportive cushions or pillows is important. It is essential that mother and twins are comfortable.

HIV and AIDS

The increasing prevalence of human immunodeficiency virus and AIDS has fuelled the debate about whether or not infected HIV mothers should breast feed and risk passing on the infection to the baby. At present, there is still no known cure and breast feeding should be discouraged. The most usual way for a baby to be infected is by the mother passing it to the unborn fetus during pregnancy, but it can be passed by blood or breast milk. However, in developing countries the balance of risks is different and breast feeding may be the preferred option.

Most of the children in the UK who acquire HIV infection do so as a result of transmission from their mothers either before or during the birth or afterwards through breast feeding. The risk of transmission can be greatly reduced by antiretroviral therapy, elective Caesarean section and avoidance of breast feeding. These interventions together reduce the risk of mother-to-child transmission from 15–25% to less than 5%.

PROBLEMS WITH EARLY FEEDING

Mastitis and maternal medication

Mastitis usually results from the ineffective emptying of the mother's breast, resulting in stasis of milk causing inflammation of the breast tissue, and sometimes infection and even abscess formation. It is important for the mother that breast feeding continues from both breasts, allowing the milk to flow thereby helping to resolve the mastitis. Feeding from the affected side first can aid the let down reflex to help the mother stop experiencing discomfort, and even in the presence of breast infection, the milk is not harmful to the baby. If antibiotics are used to treat the mother, consideration must be given to the baby's safety. Drugs and medicines enter breast milk in variable concentrations, and prescribers must always refer to the literature to ascertain if a temporary pause in breast feeding is needed while a mother is on medication.

Possetting

Most babies at some time will bring back some milk feed. Possetting is the name given to the small amount of feed that is often seen at the corner of the mouth; a dribble of milk. The baby will otherwise be thriving.

Oesophageal reflux

This is the most common cause of vomiting in babies under 6 months and is caused by the incompetence of the sphincter at the top of the stomach. Acid refluxing into the oesophagus, which lacks the protective lining of the stomach, is painful. Excessive and persistent crying after a feed can, therefore, give a clue that oesophageal reflux is happening. Ten per cent of term babies and 33% of premature babies will be affected by reflux, which is often accompanied by a failure to gain weight.

In order to relieve this distressing condition, it is worth remembering that babies spend a lot of their time in the prone position and these babies often find comfort in being nursed more upright, for example in a recliner chair, and being handled gently without squeezing after feeds. Specially designed infant formulas or food thickeners may be tried. Medication may be needed for a short while, but the subsequent introduction of solids often alleviates the intense symptoms.

Colic

Infantile colic describes the excessive crying in healthy and thriving babies. It usually starts in the early weeks of life with paroxysmal episodes of screaming, drawing up of the legs and refusing to be comforted. Examination reveals no physical abnormality. It occurs in 20% of babies. There is no recognized aetiology for the condition, but theories include:

1. It may be a problem with the gut. The crying is the result of painful contractions due to an allergy to cow's milk, lactose intolerance or excessive gas.
2. It may be a behavioural problem, problems with parent–infant interaction.

3. It may be merely the extreme end of normal crying.

Whatever the cause, periods of being unsettled and excessive crying can often cause parents much anxiety. Everything that they try to pacify with appears not to work and this can lead to feelings of inadequacy. There may be a case in the most severe for removing cow's milk protein from the diet, but the majority of unsettled babies settle by 4 months, although this is of small comfort when a parent is experiencing the worst.

Pyloric stenosis

This is a condition where the muscle surrounding the outlet at the end of the stomach hypertrophies, narrowing the lumen. Five times as many boys as girls will present with a history of persistent projectile vomiting together with a loss of weight. Diagnosis is made by feeling a lump in the abdomen over the pylorus that softens and hardens during feeding and observation of vigorous muscle contractions attempting to force food through the obstructed pylorus (visible peristalsis). It can be corrected by a simple operation – pyloromyotomy (Ramstedt procedure). Untreated pyloric stenosis is life threatening as it causes dehydration and metabolic disturbance (hypochloraemic alkalosis).

WEANING

The first year of life is a period of rapid growth and development. Breast or bottle feeding exclusively for the first 6 months provides vital sources of fat, protein and calcium for the baby and is the only food that a baby can digest.

Weaning, the introduction of solid foods, should be an enjoyable time of learning and exploration for both mother and baby (Table 5.4). Solids should be introduced from 6 months old as additional iron and other nutrients need to be provided by foods other than milk. If weaning is delayed beyond 6 months there may also be problems with introducing lumpy foods, as there appears to be a 'window of opportunity' in babies' development as regards

Table 5.4 Signs that a baby is ready for weaning

Baby not sleeping through the night, having previously done so
Unsettled after a feed where previously had been content
Demanding more frequent feeds
Diminishing weight gain

chewing and masticating. As well as solid food, breast milk or formula milk must be continued, until the introduction of cow's milk after 1 year of age.

For successful weaning, the extrusion reflex should have disappeared thus allowing the tongue not to push the food out.

Taking food from a spoon instead of sucking, then moving it to the back of the mouth and swallowing is a hard concept for a baby. Some babies will be happy to accept liquids, but reject smooth solids because it does not have the continuous flow of a liquid when presented on a spoon. Some children may experience oral hypersensitivity and may find it difficult to tolerate the wide variety of smells, tastes and texture of the new food offered. Weaning needs to be taken slowly and at first one new taste at a time should be introduced.

Composition of weaning foods

Fruit and vegetable mashes using single components like carrot, parsnip, potato, banana, cooked eating apple or pear make ideal first foods. Baby rice made up with breast milk, formula milk or water can be given.

Presenting the immature gut with some allergens too early can lead to problems. It is for this reason that that any cereal containing gluten is best eliminated from the diet until after 6 months of age. Other foods to be avoided are nuts and seeds including ground nuts, peanut butter and other nut spreads. Eggs, fish and shellfish and citrus foods should also be avoided.

As babies are unable to adequately regulate their sodium balance, it is essential that no salt is added to home cooked foods, and added sugar is also discouraged.

Milk is still an important part of the diet in the weaning period, but gradually the amount will decrease as a second and third solid meal is introduced. Water can also be used to substitute a milk feed.

Progression from mashes to lumps

After 6 months the texture of food gradually changes from mashed to lumpier foods over the next 6 months. Variety is still really important and meat, fish and cheese can be given. Parents worry about babies going onto chewy foods because they are anxious about them choking. The most effective way of teaching a child to chew is to give foods that require chewing. Babies are active and growing, but only have small stomachs and, therefore, need to eat regularly and to include high calorie foods.

Full-fat cow's milk can be used to mix foods, but should not be used as a drink until 1 year. This is because a baby still needs a good supply of nutrients and iron. For breast-fed babies after the age of 6 months, mothers may need to consider taking a vitamin supplement. Follow-on milks advertised from 6 months are not needed as long as the baby has food rich in iron such as breakfast cereals, green vegetables and other iron-rich foods, such as baked beans and, therefore, they should not need the extra iron in follow-on milk.

It is advisable to give a combination of family food as well as manufactured variety for several reasons including cost and the difficulty of introducing family food if the baby has only had jars or packets from the beginning. A balance of home cooked and commercial foods is often an alternative that offers more flexibility. Together with lumpier foods, finger foods can be introduced to encourage self-feeding and chewing practice that also allows development of speech muscles. It is important to let a baby try even though there will be a mess guaranteed!

After 6 months a lidded beaker may be given for tap water to replace a milk feed. By the age of 12 months a baby would be having about 20 fluid ounces (500 ml) of milk that includes cheese, yoghurt and any milk used to mix with food.

It is important that children experiment with food and learn to feed themselves. Getting messy is all part of the fun as children need to know what food feels like. This encourages them to become more independent and more adept at eating food. Family mealtimes are an important learning environment.

Vegetarian weaning

There are many types of vegetarian diets ranging from those of vegans, who avoid all foods of animal origin, to people who just eliminate meat from their diet.

If a baby is going to have a vegetarian diet it is essential that care is taken in making sure they get all the nutrients and energy they need to grow and develop. Vegetarian diets can tend to be bulky and lower in calories than a diet including meats, therefore, care needs to be taken to include foods that have little or no fibre, such as eggs, milk and cheese, so as to provide the baby with sufficient calories before they are full. It is essential to make sure that the diet has plenty of protein, vitamin A, calcium and zinc. Iron is often lacking in a vegetarian diet, although it is present in many vegetables and pulses, such as beans, lentils and chickpeas, and some of these should be eaten every day. Absorption is helped by eating foods rich in vitamin C.

Very restrictive diets, such as Rastafarian or strict macrobiotic diets, are not recommended at the weaning stage as they risk many deficiencies that could prove seriously harmful to the baby's health.

Balancing the diet

Poor nutrition can adversely affect the child's growth, development and health and it is now recognized that it may be a contributing factor to an increased risk of illness in adult life. It is important to recognize that children's food requirements are different from those of adults. Children require a lot more energy and also more fat in their diet as they are growing and developing at a rapid rate. The metabolic rate of a child is quite different from that of adults.

The essential elements of a healthy diet are carbohydrates (including fibre, starches and sugars), fats (including essential fatty acids), proteins, vitamins, minerals and water. In the UK many people are aware of the reasons for 'Healthy Eating', but the recommended healthy eating diets for adults should not be inflicted on children, as they could actually harm a child. A growing child needs plenty of protein and higher levels of sugar and carbohydrate than an adult. The UK Department of Health recommends that children should not be given semi-skimmed or skimmed milk under the age of two years and even after then only if their diet is varied and full. Added fibre or high-fibre cereals especially bran can compromise a child's vitamin intake because of poor absorption in the bowel. A child needs natural sugars rather than the chemical sugars found in many low-calorie food products. However, this does not mean the child should have unlimited access to sweets and biscuits! Many sugary foods are higher in calories, but low in other nutrients, which increases the risk of getting fat without providing any of the fuel that the body needs to function. It is important to help children avoid wanting all food sweetened, as acquiring a 'sweet tooth' may impair their diet in later life.

As previously mentioned, the young child has inadequate mechanisms for regulating sodium balance, and as children grow older, the average diet contains more than enough salt. Added salt is discouraged as excess salt intake can contribute to hypertension and heart disease in later life.

Recent studies of school age children have found insufficient iron and zinc to be common problems. Iron is found in meat, green vegetables and pulses as well as fortified breakfast cereals. Zinc is found in

Table 5.5   Dietary components and their characteristics

Milk and milk products	Protein for body building and repair Calcium for teeth and bones Some essential B vitamins
Meat, fish, eggs and pulses	Protein for body building and repair especially muscle and tissue Some of these are rich in iron, needed for blood formation Some are especially rich in vitamin D for strong bones For vegetarians, pulses can provide protein, iron and vitamins
Bread and cereals	High-energy foods especially if wholegrain products are used Contain some vitamins and minerals Fibre makes the bowel work properly and reduces problems with constipation
Fruit and vegetables	Vitamin A is important for eyesight, health of skin, hair and nails. It can also build resistance to infection Carotene, converted to vitamin A, is a substance found in carrots, tomato and all green and some yellow vegetables Vitamin C in normal quantities is important for resistance to infection and for tissue repair and normal growth; it is found in citrus fruit, berries, green leafy vegetables but will often be destroyed by cooking
Fats and oils	Some source of dietary fat is needed to enable production of body fat essential for metabolism, thermoregulation, and insulation of vital organs Some fats also contain fat soluble vitamins A, D and E Fat can either be saturated, monosaturated or polyunsaturated Eating too much saturated fat, usually from red meat sources may be linked to heart disorders; however, red meat is a good source of iron and zinc and should not be cut from the diet altogether Polyunsaturated fats should replace saturated fats and can be found in poultry, fish, rabbit, oily fish and oils from plant sources

cheese, eggs and bread as well as fruit and vegetables.

Types of food are divided into five groups each providing the required daily nutrients and it is accepted that a daily diet should be a little taken from each of the groups shown in Table 5.5.

OBESITY

Obesity is often defined as a condition of abnormal or excessive fat accumulation in adipose tissue to the extent that health may be affected. Adipose tissue is a normal and essential constituent of the body, providing a reserve of energy, which can be mobilized as metabolic demands are required.

The preferred and recommended method for assessing classification of body weight is calculation of body mass index (BMI), i.e. weight in kilograms over height in metres squared. This is sometimes also referred to as the 'Quetelet Index' named after the Belgian Astronomer who observed that in normal individuals there is a more or less constant ratio between weight to the square of height:

$$BMI = weight (kg)/height (m)^2$$

Figures 5.1a and b show BMI charts for boys and girls.

Childhood obesity can simply be defined as weight above the 97th centile compared to the normal height or more than 20% above the mean weight. Weight compared to height centile is a simple way of making sure that a child is not overweight. Most parents worry about their child becoming overweight. In today's society the incidence of childhood obesity is growing. Parents who have a tendency to being overweight themselves often do not want their child to progress the same way or conversely do not recognize the problem at all.

A child who is overweight is known to take in more energy from food than is needed so that extra energy is stored as fat. It is thought to greatly increase the risk of heart disease, strokes and diabetes in adult life. It is, therefore, important to do something earlier rather than later when a pattern of eating too much and being fat is established and can be very hard to change. The pre-school years are often easier times to adjust the child's eating habits. Good eating habits lessen the risk of a problem and increase the likelihood of good health. A child of seven who is overweight has almost a 50% chance of being overweight in adulthood. It is now recognized that this can also have an adverse effect on self-esteem and academic progress.

Changes need to be introduced slowly as resistance is less likely and these changes can benefit all family members. Eating should be adjusted to three mealtimes. Sitting down as a family with everyone having the same food in the same amount is good practice. Continual nibbling in between meals of crisps or sweets will deter the appetite at mealtimes so exchanging these for fruit or vegetables is better. Provide plenty of opportunity for exercise and outdoor activities. Always, remind all family members what the objective is so that they can offer support and encouragement.

Obesity runs in families; whether this is a genetic tendency or poor eating habits is unknown. Parents may also overfeed children to compensate for the feeling of inadequacy in some other aspect of their relationship with the child. Food may also be used as the only means of comforting the child, extra milk during the night, extra snacks while the parent is involved elsewhere in the house.

Professional help may be considered, keeping a simple food diary and talking to a health visitor can help. A referral to a paediatric dietician may be indicated for severe problems.

FOOD INTOLERANCE

Allergy and intolerance

An allergy implies that the body's immune system is involved in producing antibodies to the food in order to fight against it. Reactions can range from itchy blisters, skin rashes, vomiting and diarrhoea to breathing problems, swelling of the lips and even loss of consciousness or death. These symptoms can occur within a few minutes or 2–3 hrs later. The more severe the allergy then the smaller the amount of allergen required to trigger the reaction.

Intolerance is a reaction of the body to a food or foods that differs from an allergy in that the immune system is not involved. Most signs of intolerance are noted within 24–48 h of foods being introduced. The baby or child appears to reject the food by becoming

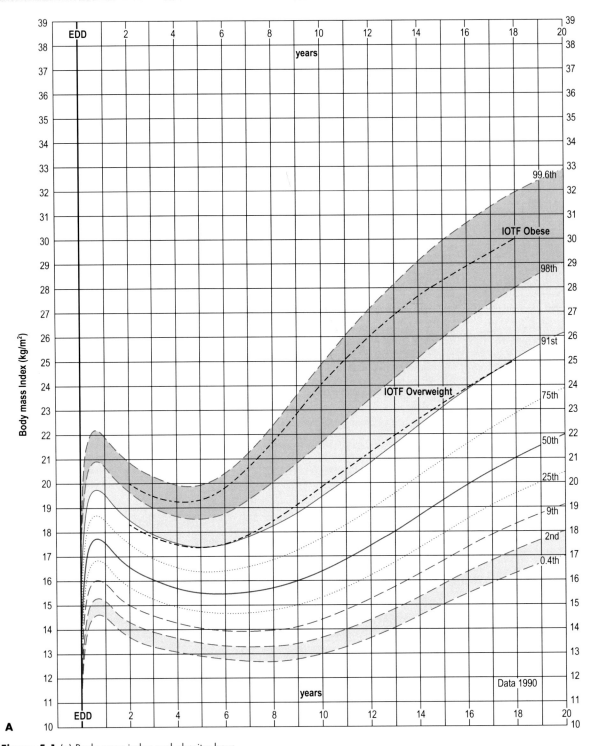

Figure 5.1 (a) Body mass index and obesity: boys

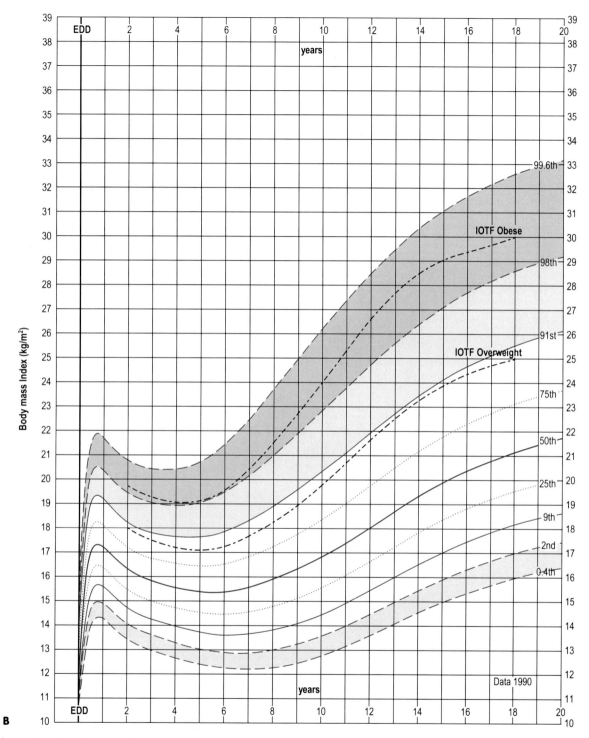

Figure 5.1 (b) Body mass index and obesity: girls

sick. Common foods include nuts, citrus foods, eggs, strawberries and shellfish, but these are also potential allergens.

Peanut allergy

Nuts, especially peanuts, can be the trigger for one of the most severe allergic reactions, anaphylactic shock, which is potentially life threatening. Emergency medical help is needed for children who experience swelling of lips and face after contact with nuts, and once this allergy has been reported, the child's carers can be equipped with epinephrine (adrenaline) injectors, which should always be carried, and the family needs to be vigilant about hidden sources of nuts in foods.

Cow's milk intolerance

This is an allergic reaction to one of the proteins found in cow's milk. It often presents as failure to thrive demonstrated by weight loss, diarrhoea, blood in stools and vomiting, but can also give abdominal pains, eczema and lactose intolerance. These babies need to be referred to a paediatrician for investigation. A milk-free diet including solids is started and generally not reduced until the age of 2 years. Parents may require dietetic advice. Most children appear to grow out of this and are eventually able to take milk products in some form later in life.

Lactose intolerance

Lactose is the sugar in milk. Inability to digest this sugar often occurs after gastroenteritis, but is generally temporary and can be aided by the introduction of milk-free formula under the direction of a paediatrician.

Gluten intolerance

Wheat, barley and oats and their products contain gluten and can produce symptoms similar to lactose intolerance. It is advised that gluten-free products should be given to all infants before the age of 6 months. Chronic gluten intolerance (celiac disease) requires investigation by a paediatrician and proper dietary management.

BEHAVIOURAL EATING PROBLEMS

Food wars and food refusal

Most children go through a period of food refusal at some time in their first 5 years. It is often the first sign of them asserting their independence and being able to manipulate mealtimes. All children go through periods of eating very little or refusing certain foods. It usually starts in the 2nd year and will often have disappeared by the time the child gets to school. This is extremely disconcerting and stressful for parents. Food wars are very common in family life, but always counterproductive, and the parents are always the losers. Parental attitudes towards food have a real influence on children's eating habits. Recognizing the reality of food as only a small part of everyday life may help to diffuse the situation of difficult mealtimes. It is important that the parent keeps calm and that no pressure is put on the child to get them to eat food offered. It should not become confrontational, though most children seem to enjoy testing their parents' patience. Parents may need help in becoming disengaged from the eating process and allowing the child their independence.

Mealtimes should be fun, a social activity for all the family. Forcing a child to eat achieves nothing. The effective strategy is to encourage parents to allow the child to be independent and to encourage self-feeding. Smaller portions and also letting the child help with the food preparation are all strategies that may help to defuse a difficult situation. Praise should be encouraged for the occasional mouthful eaten. The child will not starve and often just keeping a simple food diary for a few days will help to convince that this is so. The child will eat when hungry.

INFANT NUTRITION IN DEVELOPING COUNTRIES

It is now recognized that nutritional improvement, economic growth and developmental trends in a society are interrelated. Adequate nutrition is closely related to good health, physical and mental development and the state of wellbeing of individuals and populations. Economic development is now recognized as necessary for the sustaining of improvements in nutrition. However, this may be difficult to achieve and such interim measures as nutrition programmes may be required. With the current increasing economic crisis (developing world debt, famine and war) this is becoming more evident. The effectiveness of such programmes depends on how well it can reach those individuals it intends to reach and how well the research on their needs has been conducted. The programmes must also be affordable and sustainable for the authorities involved after the outside help has been withdrawn. Good leadership and training of locals is vital to carry many programmes forward. Large-scale nutrition programmes in Botswana, Costa Rica, India, Tanzania and Zimbabwe are well documented and include measures such as drought relief, self awareness and reliance, community mobilization, health education, including immunization programmes, and, of course, infant nutrition.

Breast feeding

Even in countries where poverty prevails, mothers that are reasonably well nourished can produce sufficient milk to meet all the nutritional requirements for their babies for 6 months. In times of famine and other such economic difficulties a mother may not be able to produce adequate milk to nourish the baby. There has been a trend for mothers to continue with sole breast feeding beyond 6 months and this can increase the undernourished status of the baby together with their growth faltering and increased risk to infection. Addition of supplements can help to improve this both for the mother and the baby.

Artificial feeding

The trend now is to move away from the promotion of artificial feeding and to encourage the promotion of breast feeding, which is the safest option for babies in conditions of poor hygiene. When clean water supplies are not always achievable, the risk of babies acquiring infection in bottle feeds is greatly increased, and the bottle-fed baby lacks the immunoprotection and other advantages afforded by breast milk. It is WHO policy to strongly promote breast feeding and to resist the sometimes aggressive advertising of formula milk by some multinational food companies.

References

Infant Feeding Recommendation. Department of Health, London, UK: May 2003

Davis MK 2001 Breastfeeding and chronic disease in childhood and adolescence. Pediatric Clinics of North America 48: 125–141

Gdalevich M, Mimouni D, David M et al 2001 Breast feeding and the onset of atopic dermatitis in childhood: a systematic review and meta-analysis of prospective studies. Journal of the American Academy of Dermatology 45(4): 520–527

Golding J, Emmett PM, Rogers IS 1997 Does breast feeding have any impact on non-infectious allergic disorders? Early Human Development 49(Suppl): S131–142

Kuli I, Wickman M, Lilja G, Nordvall SL, Pershagen G 2002 Breast feeding and allergic diseases in infants – a prospective birth cohort study. Archives of Disease in Childhood 87: 478–481

Oddy WH, Sly PD, de Klerk NH et al 2003 Breast feeding and a birth cohort study of respiratory morbidity in infancy: a birth cohort study. Archives of Disease in Childhood 88(3): 224–228

Villalpando S, Hamosh M. 1998 Early and late effects of breast feeding: does breast feeding really matter? Biology of the Neonate 74: 177–191

Further reading

Aggett PJ, Bresson J, Haschke F et al 1997 Recommended intakes. Journal of Pediatric Gastroenterology and Nutrition 25: 236–241

Bender A 1997 Introduction to Nutrition and Metabolism, 2nd edn. Taylor & Francis Ltd, London

Websites

www.ukmicentral.nhs.uk/drugpreg (information on breast feeding and drugs taken by mothers)

6 Sleep

H. Pegg

▼ OVERVIEW

The ability to sleep is essential for the normal functioning of all body systems of children and of their carers. Newborn babies are not born with the capacity to sleep through the night; this is acquired through a changing relationship between waking and sleeping as the child matures through childhood and adolescence into adulthood. Until the 1950s it was commonly believed that sleep was a period of inactivity, a negation of waking. There is still much about sleep that is not fully understood, but through a combination of laboratory and observational studies, a body of knowledge now exists that explains the physiology and characteristics of children's sleep. This knowledge underpins advice given to parents who wish to satisfy their own need for good-quality sleep with that of their child's.

NORMAL PHYSIOLOGY OF SLEEP

Sleep is a reversible state of reduced awareness and responsiveness to the environment. It is physiologically distinct from the other states of inactivity such as coma, stupor or hibernation and consists of two types of sleep: non rapid eye movement (NREM) sleep and rapid eye movement (REM) sleep.

Wakefulness is maintained by the release of noradrenaline, dopamine and acetylcholine from the brainstem neurones. In order for sleep to occur, activity in the ascending reticular activating centre has to diminish. NREM sleep depends on activity in the basal forebrain systems while REM sleep depends upon mechanisms in the pons. NREM sleep is also known as slow-wave sleep (SWS) because of the electroencephalogram (EEG) patterns. No single substance is responsible for promoting sleep, although various neuropeptides appear to have specific effects upon sleep regulation.

SLEEP STAGES

From observational and laboratory studies it has been possible to identify four stages of NREM sleep (Table 6.1) and one stage of REM sleep. The laboratory studies have made use of polysomnographic techniques such as EEG to record brain activity, electromyogram (EMG) to record muscle activity, and electro-oculogram (EOG) to record eye movements.

Rapid eye movement sleep

REM sleep is physiologically very different from NREM sleep. Brain metabolism is highest at this

Table 6.1 Stages of non-rapid eye movement (NREM) sleep	
Stage I	Occurs at the onset of sleep or following arousal from another stage of sleep Slow rolling eye movements are seen and muscle activity slows Sudden muscle contractions called 'hypnic myoclonia' cause the child to suddenly jump The child is easily woken at this stage
Stage II	Contains more slow activity and eye movements stop
Stage III	Consists of very slow brain waves called delta waves interspersed with smaller, faster waves The child is very difficult to awaken
Stage IV	The deepest form of sleep when only delta waves are seen on EEG There are no eye movements or muscle activity People awakened from this stage do not adjust immediately and feel groggy and disoriented The combination of stages III and IV is called slow-wave sleep (SWS)

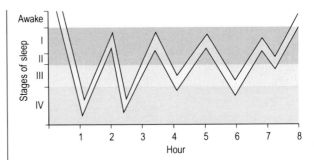

Figure 6.1   Sleep stages and sleep cycles in children

stage. Spontaneous rapid eye movements are seen and EMG activity is virtually absent in the skeletal muscles; there is temporary paralysis. Heart rate, blood pressure, and respiration are all variable, body temperature regulation ceases temporarily, and penile or clitoral tumescence occurs. Most dreaming occurs in REM sleep and when people are awakened from REM sleep they describe dreams in detail.

Intermediate sleep

This sleep state is used to describe the transitional sleep state experienced only by young infants and is a combination of NREM and REM sleep.

Sleep cycles

NREM and REM sleep alternate cyclically throughout the period of sleep and each cycle is repeated several times depending upon the length of the sleep. Adults begin with stage I NREM sleep, moving to stage II,

then to stage III, then to stage IV. Then back up to stage III, stage II then to REM sleep before the cycle restarts. Infants often begin a cycle with a period of REM sleep (Fig. 6.1).

In infants and young children each cycle can be as short as 30 min, whereas in adults cycles last about 90 min. Each sleep cycle is repeated up to seven to eight times per night in young children and about four times in adults. Most of the SWS is seen in the first two cycles. As the individual changes from one sleep stage to another, brief arousals can occur and are normal. A high number of brief arousals occur in certain pathological conditions when there is pain or discomfort.

Circadian and ultradian rhythms

Circadian rhythms are endogenously generated rhythms with a period length of about 24 h. A biological clock in the suprachiasmatic nucleus (SCN) of the hypothalamus in the brain is responsible for the generation of such circadian rhythms as the sleep–wake cycle, daily rhythms in body temperature and day–night rhythms in cortisol and melatonin production. Day–night differences are seen also in the secretion of gonadotrophin, testosterone, growth hormone and thyrotropin.

Signals from the SCN travel to several brain regions including the pineal gland, which responds to the daylight-induced signals by switching off the production of melatonin. The body's level of melatonin increases after darkness causing drowsiness. In recent years, some use has been made of melatonin as a sleep-promoting agent in some children, for example visually-impaired children who lack awareness of daylight.

The tendency to sleep displays an ultradian pattern in which sleepiness is greatest in the early hours of the morning and again in the afternoon. Level of alertness is usually highest in the evening before the onset of sleepiness as bedtime approaches. Individual differences are seen in the timing of this pattern. Some people wake early and tire early (larks), while others are at their best in the evening (owls). Such differences are thought to exist in children from an early age.

THE FUNCTION OF SLEEP

There are many theories about the function of sleep. Most have emphasized the physical and psychological restorative function of sleep and also energy conservation, memory consolidation, discharge of emotions, growth and other biological functions including the maintenance of the immune system.

It has also been suggested that waking and sleeping in the early months of life is an adaptive behaviour to secure frequent feeding and to allow for rapid weight gain and brain growth. Deep sleep in children coincides with the release of growth hormone.

During REM sleep signals travel from the pons at the base of the brain to the cerebral cortex, which is responsible for learning, thinking and organizing information. This may be important for normal brain function in infancy and could explain why infants spend much more time in REM sleep than adults.

Sleep deprivation

Persistent disturbance of sleep causes physical and psychological impairment. If people are deprived of SWS by waking them up each time they get to stage IV NREM sleep they complain of being physically tired. If people are deprived of REM sleep they can get anxious and irritable, and there is some evidence that if a person is deprived of REM sleep for several days, they will have more REM sleep when they do fall asleep.

The adverse effects of chronic sleep deprivation on mood, behaviour and cognitive function both for parents and children can be substantial. In adults sleep deprivation is often accompanied by a strong desire to sleep whereas in children it can have the effect of increasing activity with irritability or tantrums.

NORMAL SLEEP CHARACTERISTICS IN CHILDREN AND ADOLESCENTS

Although there are changes in sleep throughout the whole life span, the most profound changes take place in childhood. Many of the characteristics of adult sleep are present from as early as 6 months of age.

Sleep–wake behaviour

Newborn

The average amount of sleep in 24 h at this age is 16–18 hours and the sleep–wake cycle lasts 3–4 h. At this age there is no discernible difference in behaviour during day or night. Newborns display a higher proportion of REM sleep than NREM sleep and much of their sleep is indeterminate sleep, which does not correspond to either REM sleep or NREM sleep. During REM sleep, bursts of rapid eye movements under closed eyelids are seen and are accompanied by sucking movements, fine twitches, tremors, grimaces and smiles together with intermittent stretching. NREM or quiet sleep is characterized by minimal movement and no movement of the eyeballs.

A sleep cycle can last for 30–70 min and often starts with a period of REM sleep. The high proportion of REM sleep is thought to explain the fragility of sleep in early infancy. In the newborn period, the EEG characteristics of REM and NREM sleep vary by only subtle differences and EMG tone, and respirations are the most useful features in distinguishing sleep stages and wakefulness.

Infants aged 0–1 year

The newborn baby has a 'free-running' circadian cycle of 25 h. By 6 weeks of age, a more well-defined 24-h circadian cycle is beginning to emerge and sleep is consolidated in relation to the light–dark cycle. A priming of the circadian sleep–wake cycle seems to be organized by the feeding cycle.

By 1 month of age, infants' sleeping periods are longer at night, and a sustained wakening begins to occur in the early evening. By 3 months many infants are showing a predictable and stable diurnal distribution of wakefulness and sleep due to a combination of developmental and environmental factors.

By 3 or 4 months, the frequent rapid eye movements seen in the newborn during REM sleep have decreased and occur in bursts separated by periods without ocular activity.

In the first 2–3 months, rhythmic melatonin secretion does not occur, but from 3 months there is a rapid increase until night-time levels peak between 1 and 3 years.

At 6 months EEG recordings show the disappearance of the indeterminate sleep. NREM sleep is now the predominant state. For the first time at around 6 months EEG recordings show the presence of the stage II sleep spindles and K complexes and slow-wave delta activity, which are all seen in adult sleep and there is also a distinction between stage III and stage IV NREM sleep on EEG recordings.

By 6 months of age, a greater percentage of babies will be having a regular longer period of sleep at night. Although some babies still demand night-time feeds at this age, many now sleep up to 10 h without food or drink. However, it is common for night waking to increase after 6 months. The exact reason for this is unclear but it may be linked to the baby's growing awareness at this age of separation from mother on wakening. Teething is often cited as a reason for these increased waking, but there is no evidence to support this. The baby at this age is capable of using self-soothing methods, e.g. finger-sucking to return to sleep and does not always require an adult's presence.

Children aged 1–5 years

At this age, changes are appearing more slowly than in the first year. By 4–5 years of age, children sleep a total of 10–12 h in 24 h, often consolidated into one sleep period. This is largely due to a reduction in the daytime sleep, which is reduced on average from two sleeps at 1 year to one at about 3 years. Daytime sleep has been eliminated by most children at age 5 years.

Between the age of 1 and 5 years the proportion of REM sleep has reduced to 30% of all sleep. Sleep cycles, which have been gradually increasing in length, last an average of 60 min and children usually have 7–10 cycles during each nocturnal sleep period.

By 4–5 years many children are exhibiting a prolongation of the bedtime routine, and experience more delays in falling asleep than when younger. Frequent night-time waking in this age group is reported by 20–30% of parents. Many children have gained daytime bladder control by the age of 2–3, but night-time control is achieved later with approximately 1 in 5 children still enuretic at the age of 5 years.

Children aged 5–10 years

Total sleep time shows a steady decline in this age group. Daytime naps are rare and most children sleep for 95% of the 8–10 h that they are in bed (Fig. 6.2). At this age, most children sleep very deeply and are very alert during the day. The proportion of stage II NREM sleep increases slightly in this group as the amount of stage IV NREM sleep decreases. Stage II sleep now accounts for 40% of the total sleep time. Most REM sleep is now in the latter part of the night.

In this group sleep becomes quieter and body movements decrease in frequency, but are still more frequent than in older children. Boys have been shown to have a greater proportion of deep SWS than girls. Difficulties in initiating and maintaining sleep are reported in about 10–15% of this age-group. Up to 30% of this group will experience temporary night

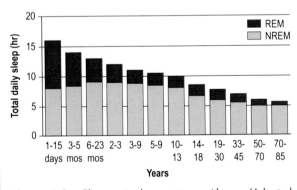

Figure 6.2 Changes in sleep patterns with age. (Adapted with permission from Ferber R, Kryger M (eds) 1995 Principles and practice of sleep medicine in the child. WB Saunders)

disturbance, such as enuresis, sleep talking or walking, or night terrors. The role of anxiety in causing sleep disturbance is more common in this age group as it coincides with starting school and children are more aware of family difficulties than they were at younger ages.

Adolescents aged 11–19 years

After the relatively stable sleep patterns of the preceding age group, adolescence is a time of turbulent sleep behaviour. The amount of REM and NREM sleep is now at the adult level of 25% and 75% respectively. The amount of SWS continues to fall to the adult levels of about 20% of total sleep time. Sleep cycles now last for about 90 min and will continue at that length throughout adulthood.

With the onset of puberty, the sleep requirement is higher than the adult levels, but adolescents often sleep less due to pressures of school and social life. Daytime alertness declines and it is common to take daytime naps, which further distort the already shattered circadian rhythm. The sleep disturbance may be worsened by the consumption of caffeine, alcohol, nicotine and illegal substances. Difficulty getting to sleep is reported by 15% of adolescents. Differences between adults' and children's sleep are summarized in Table 6.2.

OTHER SLEEP CHARACTERISTICS OF INFANTS AND CHILDREN

Respiration

In infants and young children the respiratory rate decreases in all sleep states, but is lowest during

---

Table 6.2   Summary of differences in children's sleep compared with adults

- Longer total sleep time depending on age
- Slow-wave sleep (SWS) prominent in children
- Early reduction in proportion of REM sleep
- Greater number of shorter NREM/REM sleep cycles
- Possible period of SWS before finally waking

---

stage II NREM sleep of the last cycle of the night. Significant breathing irregularities owing to periodic breathing are seen in neonates and persist for several months, but with decreasing frequency. Central apnoeas, lasting 20 s or less, are normal in infancy especially after movement and occur less in REM sleep. Obstructive sleep apnoea (OSA) of short duration is present in about 10% of children, but only 2% of these will experience any sleep disturbance or any daytime symptoms. The most common cause of OSA is enlarged tonsils or adenoids; obesity, passive smoking and the use of sedative medication are predisposing factors. If OSA is causing persistent symptoms of snoring, restless sleep, frequent night waking or daytime somnolence or irritability, sleep studies should be performed and ear, nose and throat (ENT) referral for adenotonsillectomy should be considered.

Cardiovascular control

The heart rate is generally reduced during NREM sleep and further reduced during REM sleep. During REM-related bursts of rapid eye movements, short-lasting tachycardia can be observed. Cardiac output is only slightly reduced during NREM sleep, but further reduced during REM sleep.

Gastrointestinal function

Swallowing and salivary flow are significantly reduced during sleep. The resulting decrease in acid clearance from the oesophagus is most noticeable during REM sleep. In infants, acid reflux reaching the proximal portion of the oesophagus acts as a strong arousal stimulus. This condition, gastro-oesophageal reflux disorder, affects up to 12% of infants.

Body temperature regulation during sleep

Core body temperature follows a stable circadian rhythm. Core temperature falls as the night progresses reaching its lowest point during the early hours of the morning. During REM sleep, it follows environmental temperature, rising and falling in response to the ambient temperature. Although there is an apparent lack of homeostasis during REM sleep, major temperature regulating mechanisms such as sweating and shivering are still active in infants. In both REM and NREM sleep, sweating decreases between 0200 and 0400 h. This cyclic fluctuation is similar to that seen in body temperature and metabolic rate.

Bladder function

The neurological control of bladder function and the ability to be dry during sleep involves the acquisition of control during waking and also the establishment of a circadian rhythm in vasopressin release and the ability to rouse to a full bladder during sleep. Most children acquire the ability to remain dry during daytime naps between 2 and 3 years, and for the majority night-time control is also acquired before the age of 5 years. By the age of 10 years, 3% of children still wet the bed and 1% at 14 years. Enuresis can occur at any stage of sleep. It may be associated with obstructive sleep apnoea and is more common in boys.

REQUIREMENTS FOR ESTABLISHING NORMAL SLEEP BEHAVIOUR

Comfortable environment

Children require a cot or bed in a room designated for sleeping. The cot or bed should be appropriate to their age and stage of development. There should be a minimum of stimulation for the child, so efforts should be made to reduce daylight in summer months, to reduce noise, and to keep toys out of sight when the child is due to sleep. Televisions and computers are not suitable pieces of equipment for a bedroom (at any age).

The room needs to be a comfortable temperature (16–20°C) and the bedding appropriate for that temperature. Young children under about 2 years of age rarely sleep under covers and if the room temperature drops during the night, they need to be dressed in warm suits, but with head exposed. Pillows and duvets are not recommended for infants under 1 year.

Many children share a room with their parents or siblings and in this case it is helpful if the child does not have sight of the companions when falling asleep.

Table 6.3 Sleep and sudden infant death syndrome (SIDS)
Preventative advice on reducing the risk of SIDS in sleep
• Place the baby on its back to sleep • Cut smoking in pregnancy • Do not let anyone smoke in the dwelling • Do not let the baby get too hot • Do not use pillows and duvets • Keep the baby's head uncovered, put the baby's feet at the foot of the cot • If the baby is unwell, seek medical advice immediately • Sleep the baby in a cot in the parents' room for the first 6 months • Parents should avoid falling asleep with the baby on the sofa • Parents should not share the bed with the baby if they are smokers, have been drinking alcohol, take drugs, are obese or excessively tired

In many cultures it is common practice for babies to sleep in the same bed as their parents, called *co-sleeping*. Some parents find that their baby is more content and that both mother and child obtain more sleep when co-sleeping. In recent years there has been some concern that this may increase the risk of the baby suffering a sudden infant death. Current research is not conclusive, but parents are advised not to co-sleep with the baby if they have used tobacco, drugs or alcohol or are obese or overtired. For more details of the full advice for reducing the risk of sudden infant death syndrome see Table 6.3.

Freedom from pain, irritation and anxiety

Many sleep problems in children have originated from a period of illness or discomfort and it is important to address any source of discomfort before it causes a regular disturbance. In young babies common causes of sleeplessness are gastro-oesophageal reflux, infantile colic and middle-ear infection, which can affect children of all ages. After 6 months of age, sleeplessness may be ascribed to teething, but it is unlikely to cause prolonged sleep disturbance and other explanations should be considered. Conditions that cause irritation and discomfort at nights include eczema, asthma and threadworms. These can all contribute to sleep disturbance and will require medical treatment.

Efforts should be made to ensure the child is as free from anxiety as possible. In the infant this can take the form of separation anxiety when the parent leaves the room. In older children it may be anxiety arising from family problems, peer relationships or fears. Some of this anxiety can be easily removed, for example by leaving a light on if the child is afraid of the dark. If the cause of the anxiety is not addressed the child will be reluctant to sleep or may have sleep disturbance.

Learning associations for sleep

From birth most babies fall asleep at the end of a feed and come to associate a feed with going to sleep. These cues to sleep help the child to establish the circadian rhythm of sleeping and waking. Parents can also entrain babies and children to associate other positive conditions with sleep, with the ultimate aim that the child will be able to soothe him- or herself to sleep without the help of another person. Some babies appear to be able to do this with little help; others appear to need more guidance.

It is helpful to the child if there is a regular daytime routine so that the child is able to anticipate when the time for sleep is approaching. A regular bedtime routine that aims to provide an opportunity for the child to 'wind down' from the day's activities and provides a calm period of adult contact will help the child to prepare for sleep. The routine may involve a bath or wash, changing into night-time clothes, and a bedtime story in the bedroom prior to getting into bed. Many children have a period of alertness in the early evening and it is important to allow for this before the bedtime routine.

Many children will also make an association between a particular toy or blanket and sleep and it is important to reserve this just for those times when the child is expected to sleep. Light and dark are also powerful cues to sleep and many children require blackouts in their bedroom to help onset of sleep during light evenings and to prevent early rising in mornings.

Children can also learn negative associations for sleep. The memory of pain or fear from a previous episode of poor sleep can affect the child's ability to sleep as can the presence of negative associations such as the use of the bedroom as a place of punishment.

Daytime routines

A child who feels that their basic needs are not being met during the day may demand that these needs be met during the night.

Newborn babies feed and sleep every 3–4 h throughout the 24-h cycle. By the age of 6 months many babies are able to sleep for 10–12 h and take all their food and drink in the daytime. However, if the baby is not taking sufficient nutrients and calories during the day, then it may reduce his ability to sleep at night and lead to circadian rhythm disturbance. If the child does wake during the night once night-time feeds have stopped, a drink of water may be required and attention paid to correcting the daytime calorie intake. The reintroduction of a feed can start a new habit of feeding at night and should only be recommended if there are concerns about the child's growth.

Children require opportunities for exercising and developing the whole range of skills. If the opportunities for these are denied during the day, they will be less able to relax at the end of the day. Exercise, particularly combined with exposure to daylight, has been shown to help night-time sleep problems. Children also need to experience attention from their carers and sleep disturbance may for some children, be a route to spend more time with their parents or carers.

Gradual separation from parents

From the time of birth, children are experiencing increasing separation from their mother. Some children require little attention between feeds from birth and are content to be placed awake in a cot to fall asleep. Others are very reluctant to fall asleep without being fed, rocked or cuddled, and cry when separated from their mother. Some parents enjoy this feeling of closeness and the dependency of the baby. Others parents find it distressing. By the age of 6 months many babies have learnt to fall asleep without being held, but may still require hearing a familiar voice or touch.

Ability to self-soothe

Some babies have learnt to suck on a dummy, fingers or thumb, to soothe themselves to sleep. Other children find the presence of a favourite toy or blanket provides comfort and the ability to self-soothe. Between 6 and 12 months many of those babies who had learnt to settle on their own may be more difficult to settle. This is due to separation anxiety and is common at this age as the child becomes aware of themselves as a separate person from the mother. Many of these children will also become distressed if the mother leaves the room during the daytime and provided the child is not allowed to become distressed during the daytime and allowed to remain with the mother, the problem is usually short-lived.

Older toddlers and children will also appear to have separation anxiety when their parent tries to leave the room at bedtime. This may be learned behaviour where the child is learning to exercise control over his parents. However, it may also signal a period of insecurity or distress on the part of the child and parents may need some help to handle the situation.

Avoidance of stimulant substances

The use of stimulant substances by children can be deliberate or incidental. Mothers who have a high caffeine intake while breast feeding can pass the stimulant effect to their baby with a noticeable effect on the baby's sleep pattern. Some drugs prescribed to alleviate sleep problems, for example promethazine, can cause sleeplessness as can products containing pseudoephedrine. Some children's sleep pattern can be affected by the ingestion of certain food additives and colourings and certain foods, notably chocolate. Older children may choose to take high-caffeine drinks, nicotine, and illegal drugs, which all have a stimulant effect. The effect of these products is to cause a period when

sleep is difficult followed by a period of excessive sleepiness.

NORMAL VARIATIONS IN CHILDREN'S SLEEP

Most children, even those described by their parents as 'good sleepers' will have an occasional episode when their sleep pattern is disturbed. At any one time it is estimated that as many as 30% of children will be described by their parents as having a sleep problem. Sometimes it is easy to see the cause, such as a family holiday where the routine was different from that at home. For other children there is no obvious reason. Many of these children will resume their previous pattern after a few days, but will repeat the episode at a later stage. This section will describe the most common 'normal variations' and ways in which parents can handle the situation on a short-term basis.

Sleeplessness

This can take the form of:

- reluctance to go to sleep
- waking during the night
- waking early in the morning.

Reluctance to go to sleep (sleep-phase delay)

In a child who has previously had a good routine of falling asleep, there may be an obvious reason, such as illness, discomfort, for example from eczema or there may have been a temporary change in the family. Parents need to ensure that all the requirements for sleep are being met especially the formation and maintenance of positive sleep associations. It is very easy when a child is refusing to go to bed to allow them to come downstairs to watch television. This, unfortunately, has the effect of prolonging the problem as the child is rewarded for their reluctance to comply by being allowed to watch television. Toddlers who still need daytime naps often show reluctance to go to bed in the evening when their nap has been too late in the afternoon.

Naps can be retimed to earlier in the day. If the child does go to sleep late in the evening, he or she should be woken at the usual time the following morning in order to correct the sleep–wake rhythm. In pre-school age children, reluctance to go to bed is very common and it may be that the child does not need to go to sleep as early in the evening as previously. The key to this is whether there is sleepiness during the daytime.

Adolescents often have problems falling asleep and this may be due not only to their lifestyle and the onset of puberty, but also to changes in the timing of melatonin secretion in relation to the sleep-phase delay. Changes to their day and night routine may alleviate the problem, which can require specialist help to correct.

Waking during the night

If a child wakes at night, the behaviour is more likely to be repeated if it is rewarded by a cuddle, drink, feed or attention. After checking that the child is not distressed or in pain, the child should be settled back in the bed and left as soon as possible. Various schedules have been recommended over the years for curing children of this habit; they have ranged from total extinction (leaving the child to cry until morning), to checking the child every few minutes to reassure them that they have not been abandoned. Many parents find it distressing when their child becomes distressed and they may need professional support to follow a behaviour-modification programme that can minimize distress for parent and child.

Waking early in the morning

A child who wakes at 4–5 am is often well-refreshed and unlikely to return to sleep. He or she may have already had enough sleep and it may be that the bedtime needs to be made later in the evening. At 4–5 am the body temperature falls with the room temperature and it may be that the child is not warm enough. Many children who wake early will then be ready for their next nap by 8 am. One explanation for early morning waking is that the final sleep-cycle of the night has become separated from the night sleep. It may be helpful not to let the child have a nap in the early part of the morning, but to try to delay any daytime nap until the average time of 10–11 am.

Older children are sometimes allowed to get up when they awaken, but children should be encouraged to remain in bed until an agreed time and they may fall asleep again. For young children who get up unaccompanied in the early morning, there may be safety concerns to address. Some children have an ultradian rhythm of waking early that identifies them as 'larks' and they will probably also be 'larks' as adults.

Normal sleep at the wrong time

Some children will take their normal sleep requirements at a time that does not fit in with family routines. This is not usually a problem for the young child, although adolescents find it inconvenient when they are late for school. Children may have difficulty falling asleep and then difficulty waking up at the necessary time. Conversely, they may fall asleep early in the evening and wake up in the early morning. By gradually altering the routines, the circadian rhythm can be reset to a more acceptable pattern.

Interruptions during sleep (parasomnias)

A parasomnia is a recurrent episode of behaviour that occurs exclusively or predominantly during or in relation to sleep.

Sleep onset related

A number of phenomena occur in the process of falling asleep and do not have any significance, although they can cause concern. Sudden, single jerks of the limbs or whole body at sleep onset are called 'hypnic myoclonia' or 'sleep starts' and occur at all ages. *Hypnagogic hallucinations* may accompany these sleep starts, but often occur separately. They can be quite frightening and are accompanied by an awareness of the environment in which objects may be seen, heard, felt or tasted. *Sleep paralysis* consists of a brief episode of an inability to move or speak and there is a feeling of not being able to breathe for a few seconds.

Rhythmic movement disorder refers to a group of stereotyped movements, mainly of the upper part of the body, usually occurring at sleep onset, but it can be at the end of the sleep period. In normal children the activity is pleasurable and may be viewed as an aid to getting to sleep or returning to sleep following a waking during the night. Headbanging or head-rolling are the best known forms, often accompanied by rhythmic vocalizations such as humming. Many children exhibit some form of rhythmic movement in their first year of life, but the behaviour almost always stops spontaneously by the age of 3–4 years. Intervention is only necessary if the child is at risk of injury.

Light sleep (NREM stages I and II) related

Bruxism or toothgrinding is the forcible grinding of teeth in a paroxysmal fashion producing a loud grinding sound at night without the child being aware of it. It usually occurs in light sleep and affects up to 50% of children at some time. The child may complain of pain in the face or headache later and, rarely, the teeth may be damaged. There has been very little research into treatment for children, but an individually made soft dental plate may help.

Deep sleep (NREM stages III and IV) related

Disturbances caused by arousal from sleep are called arousal disorders and include confusional arousals, sleep-walking and sleep terrors. These are all very common in childhood. Arousal in this context does not mean that the child wakes up; the arousal is partial usually from deep NREM sleep to another lighter stage of NREM sleep or REM sleep. All three forms have in common a curious combination of features that are suggestive of being simultaneously awake and asleep. Despite seeming alert, there is usually confusion and disorientation, they usually remain asleep during the episode, they are unresponsive to parents' attempts to communicate with them and they have little or no recall of the behaviour.

Confusional arousals occur mainly in infants and toddlers and may begin with movements and moaning, progressing to agitated and confused behaviour with crying, calling out and thrashing about. Each episode usually lasts about 10–15 min before the child calms down spontaneously and returns to restful sleep.

Sleep walking is said to occur in up to 17% of children mainly between 4 and 8 years. Episodes usually last up to 10 min. The child may crawl or walk around his cot or he may calmly walk around the house. He will have his eyes open, but will be unresponsive. Urinating in inappropriate places is common. Accidental injury in sleep-walking is a serious risk and requires installation of stair-gates, locks and fire-guards.

Night terrors are associated with sleep during the night or day. They occur in about 3% of children mainly in later childhood. The parents are usually awoken by the child's scream; the child appears to be terrified with staring eyes, intense sweating, rapid pulse and cries suggesting intense distress. He may rush about frantically and risk of injury is real.

Management of these arousals is mainly by keeping the child safe, and not trying to wake or restrain the child, but to put him or her back to bed when the terror subsides. The general principles of regular sleep routines are important.

REM sleep-related parasomnias

Nightmares are the manifestation of a REM-related sleep disturbance. They occur in the later part of overnight sleep when REM sleep is most abundant and are very common from early childhood in up to 50% of children. The child wakes up frightened and fully alert and relates the fear to a vividly recalled dream. They may be precipitated by illness or stress and are a prominent part of post-traumatic stress disorder. They need no special measures except to comfort the child at the time and to avoid the child seeing disturbing events or videos, especially before going to bed.

Related to all sleep stages

Sleeptalking is common and occurs through all sleep stages. It is usually brief, but can continue for some minutes. It is not of any significance except to those trying to sleep nearby.

PROBLEMATIC SLEEP

As many as 30% of children are reported as having sleep problems and parents often seek professional help in solving these problems.

Children's sleep should be viewed as problematic in any of the following situations:

1. Parents are distressed in any way by their child's sleep.
2. The child is distressed by their own sleep.
3. The child's sleep pattern is interfering with the ability to function normally, e.g. daytime sleepiness after age 5 years, persistent night disturbance, persistent delayed sleep-onset.

Referral options for sleep problems

Primary health care

The parents will often approach primary health care staff such as general practitioners and health visitors about their child's sleep. It is useful for the general practitioner to ensure that the child is not suffering from any medical condition that is impairing the child's sleep and to establish whether there are symptoms of a sleep disorder requiring specialist help, for example narcolepsy or REM sleep behaviour disorder.

For the majority of children, health visitors have the skills and training to work with parents to identify the exact nature of the problem, to establish whether the basic requirements for normal sleep are in place and to suggest ways of modifying the child's behaviour through a gradual programme of change that will not cause undue distress to the child or parents. Some health visitors have established sleep clinics and groups to work with parents both to prevent sleep problems and to address existing problems. Such groups can help to alleviate the isolation and sense of failure felt by some parents when their child is unable to sleep through the night

Medication with sedatives has been used to treat children's sleep problems, but it has been shown only to have short-term use with some children and is not successful in achieving long-term change. Short-term prescription of manufactured melatonin helps some children to achieve a normal wake–sleep cycle.

Secondary health care

Consultant paediatricians will accept referrals from general practitioners who feel that the child has a serious sleep disorder, or that their sleep problem is associated with another medical condition, or where attempts to solve the problem at primary care level have failed.

Child and adolescent mental health teams will accept referrals of children for whom it is believed that the problem is mainly behavioural and where there is willingness to view the matter as a family problem. This referral can be particularly appropriate when it is suspected that the maternal–child attachment is such that is may be contributing to the problem. It has been shown that maternal depression is often present when a child has sleep problems, and it is unknown whether the depression or the sleep problem came first. It may be appropriate to consider treatment for the mother's depression when there is a child with a sleep problem.

Tertiary care Where the first two tiers of care are unsuccessful in treating the problem, a specialized sleep disorders service is indicated. At present, there are few available, although many sleepless parents will travel great distances to solve their child's sleep problems.

Further reading

Ferber R 1985 Solve Your Child's Sleep Problems. Dorling Kindersley, London

Kahn A et al 1996 Normal sleep architecture in infants and children. Journal of Clinical Neurophysiology 13: 184–197

Stores 0 2001 A Clinical Guide to Sleep Disorders in Children and Adolescents. Cambridge University Press, Cambridge

Cognitive, emotional, and behavioural development

D. Christie

▼ OVERVIEW

This chapter will look at child development in terms of *thinking, feeling* and *doing.*

Fundamental concepts of cognition and thinking functions are first considered together with a brief account of how attempts can be made to measure them. Later the normal processes by which a child progresses from total dependency towards independent capacity are reviewed, with particular emphasis on language, memory and attention.

Some common problems of childhood development are examined, as these shed light on the way in which the normal child makes progress on the road to autonomy. One such problem that few children avoid is temper tantrums, and this leads to a discussion of the child's emotional and behavioural development. Again there is mention of some conditions characterizing abnormal emotional and behavioural development, as these serve to delineate the boundaries of normal.

EARLY COGNITION

The word infant comes from the Latin meaning without speech, however, a newborn baby has a very powerful way to communicate its needs to parents. The infant communicates through pre-symbolic sounds like crying in order to indicate primary needs like hunger or physical discomfort. After birth there is a very rapid period of development where the baby starts to smile, achieves head control and the ability to reach and grasp within a few months. Communication in infants up to the first 12 months of life is through gaze, gesture and babbling. Infants learn that they can control their immediate world non-verbally. An infant learns that an action is usually followed by an event (for example if an object is thrown on the floor it will reappear in front of me; if I cry then a familiar face will usually pick me up and cuddle me; if I point to something it will be given to me). This ability to learn contingencies allows an infant to begin to control and influence his or her environment.

During the first 12 months of life children start to differentiate their 'self' from objects. They start to develop a mental representation of an object and become aware that an object is permanent and exists even when it cannot be seen and develop basic short-term memory skills.

By the age of 9–12 months a baby can recognize faces and can distinguish between familiar and non-familiar faces. The ability to learn and remember is available even before birth and provides the building blocks upon which more complex skills, such as reasoning and problem solving, can develop.

Cognition involves developing the ability to handle information in order to solve problems. The information must be selected, represented, stored, retrieved and transformed. Cognitive functions describe the different way the brain obtains information about the environment, which includes physical objects and events, our 'self' and other people. Young children develop internal rules or theories about how these different components are connected and related through categories, rules, skills and procedures. A range of processes allows them to understand the environment and influence it in return. These processes include learning, memory, perception, attention, language, reasoning and problem solving.

Cognitive development is a complex interplay of biological, social and environmental interactions. The ability to develop theories about the world is both helped and constrained by biological endowment, current cognitive competencies, capacity, knowledge and opportunities provided by the environment. The development of these cognitive skills requires the ability to take in and make sense of and use experiences to produce appropriate responses.

The brain receives and processes all of the information that a child experiences in their environment. Early childhood is an important time as the brain is rapidly developing and needs stimulation in order to develop to its maximum potential. This early period is very important as the brain is growing and making connections in response to what it experiences. The brain is influenced by the social and psychological environment. This means that long-term development can be influenced by lack of stimulation or damage due to neglect or injury. At the same time the potential for growth and development in the early years means that if injury does occur there is potential for recovery over time. This is called plasticity.

The majority of the basic cognitive functions are developed from 2 to 6 years.

MEASURING COGNITION

There are many ways to formally measure the development of cognitive skills. Tests can measure difference between achievement (accomplished skills) and aptitude (measure of potential). All measures must be reliable (reproducible/consistent) and valid (measuring the right thing). For children under the age of 3 years parental reports can be used to assess successful completion of developmentally appropriate milestones. Paediatricians can use a range of checklists of developmental tasks that assess the number of tasks a child can perform (Table 7.1). These measures look at the extent to which a child passes or fails an item that the majority of children of a particular age can complete. The majority of these are relatively brief (for example Vineland Screening Scale), although there are longer and more comprehensive measures that require specialist training (Griffiths Developmental scales). These measures determine a specific level of achievement in one or more domain. Up to the age of 2 years, measures focus on motor skills and early pre-symbolic language skills.

From the age of 2–3 years more formal measures can be used to look at 'cognitive processes' and are geared to both achievement and predictors of potential. Vocabulary can be assessed using the British Picture Vocabulary Scale (BPVS) or phonetic skills (PAT) can indicate the potential for reading ability.

The Wechsler Intelligence Tests for children between 2:6 and 7 years (WPPSI-III[UK]), assess skills in verbal and non-verbal areas of intellectual functioning (including attention and memory) and requires no written English skills, so can be used in children with or without formal educational experience. However, standard IQ tests are inappropriate for very high- or low-functioning children, as they are unable to discriminate the children at the very bottom or top of the ability range (Table 7.1).

Clinical analysis involves observation of the child in a test situation. How they approach the tasks, how motivation changes and whether there are personality factors that might affect the achievement of correct answers, such as impulsiveness or a tendency to say the first thing that comes into the mind without careful consideration, are all relevant. A wide range of tests is available for assessment of specific populations using specific and appropriate reference groups. Cultural issues are also important as limited exposure to written and spoken English in the home will make interpretation of scores difficult as the tests are based on normative data from an English-speaking UK population. Therefore, test results for young people from different cultural backgrounds should be interpreted with caution.

Table 7.1   Some commonly used psychological tests to assess general development, cognitive function and specific aspects of cognition

Screening scales	Vineland Adaptive Behaviour Scales Griffiths Developmental Scales Schedule of Growing Skills
Language	British Picture Vocabulary Scale Phonological Abilities Test Clinical Evaluation of Language Fundamentals Wechsler Objective Language Dimensions The Renfrew Action Picture Test, 3rd edn The Bus Story (Renfrew)
Intellectual Ability	Wechsler Preschool and Primary Scale of Intelligence-III-UK Raven's Progressive Matrices
Attention	Test for Everyday Attention in Children Connors' Rating Scales
Literacy and Numeracy	Neale Analysis of British Reading Ability Wechsler Objective Reading Dimensions Wechsler Objective Numerical Dimensions

Assessing IQ can contribute to an understanding of why a child is struggling at school often because of emotional and behavioural difficulties. An IQ assessment will indicate possible global or specific learning difficulties and guide appropriate remedial strategies. IQ testing can also be helpful in monitoring treatment (for example treatment for attention deficit disorder can be shown to be increasing specific cognitive functions over time). In addition, where emotional or behavioural difficulties are framed as 'naughty, stupid or lazy' behaviour, IQ profiles can highlight specific cognitive difficulties associated with neurodevelopmental disorders like dyspraxia, dyslexia, or Asperger's or Tourette's syndrome, which are often exemplified by a complex IQ profile. As already mentioned, several abilities contribute to an overall measure of cognitive ability. These different areas are described in greater detail below.

Language

One of the most important functions is the development of speech and language. The human brain is organized to allow the acquisition of a symbolic communication system (speech). The part of the brain that is specialized for both the production and understanding of language is located in the left hemisphere of the brain. The right hemisphere is less capable of developing language skills; however, it can take over if the left is damaged during childhood. The correct development of the brain is essential for the development of language; however, social interaction with children and adults is also essential for the brain to be able to 'use' its ability. Lack of exposure to the spoken word in early childhood will result in impaired language development.

Language involves learning that objects and actions have labels, and that by using these labels young children are able to influence their environment. From 12 to 15 months children will use words in order to achieve a particular outcome. Saying a particular word will produce food, drink, desired objects or the appearance of certain people and the use of yes or no indicates a preference allowing increasing choice.

Over the next 12–24 months there is a rapid development of language with less reliance on gesture and the ability to put words together to form short phrases. The child can label actions and starts to begin to express abstract thought or future intent (for example 'me go'). As language develops, children can explain how words are similar in meaning to each other and give reasons for real (or hypothetical) actions or events ('girl cry' 'boy bad'). This higher order language is dependent upon understanding behaviour within a social context and being able to talk about issues that reflect ideas or the development of moral reasoning. The majority of children will have begun to use language to communicate fully by the age of 3 years. By the age of 5 or 6 children will have acquired a completely intelligible language system.

In the beginning, speech serves a basic communication function for children, helping to regulate their interactions with others in the world. Later, it also serves other functions and transforms the way in which children learn, think and understand. It becomes an instrument or tool of thought, not only providing a 'code' or system for representing the world, but also the means by which self-regulation comes about.

Memory

The ability of the infant to recognize another adult or parent is evidence of a basic memory system. The development of memory skills is essential for the normal development of other processes. Memory is a complex function with several interdependent components. The first part of memory is short-term memory. This is the ability to hold on to a certain amount of information for a short period of time. This is sometimes called working memory. A child might need to remember a brief instruction (go upstairs and bring down your hairbrush), a series of numbers (like a phone number) or non-verbal information (a clapping sequence in a song). Children gradually increase the number of chunks of information that they can hold in their heads from 2 or 3, and at the age of 3 years up, short-term memory increases its capacity to holding between five and nine bits of information by about the age of 12.

The next stage is the ability to store and recall information. Information (either verbal or non-verbal) is encoded then transferred to a short-term store and then to a long-term store. Memory can be disrupted at any of these stages. Memory problems can be due to a failure to efficiently code information as it is transferred between the short- and long-term stores. This failure might be due to the child not having the ability or capacity to code information efficiently; however, more often than not it is because they did not attend to the task and allowed the information to 'slip away'. A second problem may be in the ability to recall information that has been stored due to difficulty organizing information. This difficulty accessing information can be improved by learning efficient recall strategies.

During the pre-school years memory grows with language development. During the school-age years, more sophisticated strategies for processing information result in improved memory. School-age children remember more than pre-school children do

because they intuitively apply rules for recalling information. They have learned to sort information by time, place, category and other cues, all of which serve to organize memories and, thus, facilitate recall. As the ability to think in categories improves, so does memory, because categories allow for more effective storage of information. School tasks encourage children to intentionally remember information. The capacity for retrieval of information improves in middle childhood, but this ability is also reinforced by the emphasis on being able to retrieve information to answer questions in class. Motivated by school tasks, older school age children create strategies for remembering: repeating information to themselves or creating mental cues, categories, or images that help them remember.

Attention

Attention is the process of focussing on relevant information in the environment and the inhibition of responses to irrelevant intruding material. Attention can be sustained over time or selective for specific information and is a critical process for all other functions. Attention controls the amount and quality of information available for higher-order cognitive processes. The process of focussing our senses on what is happening in our environment allows us to make sense of information (and remember things) more efficiently. The development of attention requires the biological development of structures in the frontal lobes of the brain involved in this ability to focus as well as interaction with the environment where the child can learn to attend.

Like memory, attention is a complex process involving several components. Self-monitoring and regulation develops quickly in the infant; however, the child begins to develop the ability to focus on an external event (like reading a book or playing with a toy). By the age of 4 or 5 a child will be developing dual attention capabilities where there is a need to concentrate on two events and pick out the relevant information and appropriate response (for example in a busy classroom needing to listen to the teacher and not be distracted by other events or activities). Finally, around the age of 6 or 7 children start to develop the capacity to inhibit or prevent a response and produce an alternative response (wait to speak, not say an inappropriate comment). The developmental process involves children being able to bring attention under internal control, and to attend for longer periods.

As already mentioned, attention skills are closely dependent upon successful biological development. Difficulty with attention is a common impairment in many developmental conditions. However, it may also be that what is described as difficulty with attention is in fact due to excessive inquisitiveness! Children may be inattentive when they are bored while having the capacity to attend when they are engaged or inspired by a task.

Formal assessment of attention is difficult in children; however, there are a limited number of tests that measure different aspects of attention in order to determine the degree to which a child is capable of focussing on a specific task or attending to a task when there are distracters around (e.g. TEACH).

The ultimate mature expression of attention is sometimes called executive function. This process is involved in organizing information and directing attention. It is involved in complex memory and the inhibition of impulsive inappropriate (or antisocial) behaviour. Normal levels of executive function can usually be reliably measured in children by early adolescence.

Visuospatial skills

The right hemisphere of the infant's brain is preset to make sense of and manipulate visual and non-verbal information. The young child develops the ability to represent 3D objects initially as 2D figures, slowly developing perspective and depth. The child develops the ability to 'fill in' holes in partial images and make sense of complex patterns. We can see children developing these skills as they begin to complete jigsaw puzzles (by 30–33 months a child can recognize shapes and orient pieces in a nine-piece jigsaw) and make structures with blocks (from 15 to 24 months a child can increase the height of a tower of blocks from two to eight or more). From 33 months to 4 or 5 years the child can start to copy and construct matching models. Initially, these are from 3D models, but they quickly develop the ability to copy a 2D representation. In parallel with the

development of fine motor control, children develop the ability to copy straight lines in appropriate orientation (50% by 36 months) and draw basic figures like circles and squares (50% by 60 months).

Under 6 years of age a child tends to see only one dimension of a problem. Pre-school children asked to compare complex figures, such as two houses (alike except for the number of windows) will say the two are the same if they find only one similarity, without further exploration for possible discrepancies. In contrast, children of 7 or 8 will explore both houses systematically before deciding whether the two are alike or different. The ability to move back and forth between parts and wholes, between details and larger organizing ideas, is the basis of categorization and classification. As they move through middle childhood, children's ability to view reality in categories with multiple variables increases.

Awareness of time and space

By the age of 6 years a child will know right from left. By the age of 7 or 8 they will be able to accurately identify the right or left side of a person sitting opposite. Time orientation has also begun to develop by 7 and a clearer sense of how time is organized allows school-age children to think ahead and to plan their actions more efficiently than pre-schoolers. At this age, children become less bound by the organization or lack of organization of visual materials they look at, and can reorganize materials into patterns that are more interesting or satisfying. The school child can look beyond surface perceptions to imagine new patterns. An example of the child's visual organizational ability is demonstrated by a child's ability to clean up her room. A 5-year-old is likely to feel overwhelmed by toys strewn across the floor, because she is not yet able to construct an image of the room with everything in its place. While many children do not like to tidy their rooms, an 8-year-old is capable of doing it without assistance, because he/she can bring order out of chaos, mentally, thinking about where things go. As most parents know, this ability is strangely and tragically lost in adolescence then, hopefully, reappears in adulthood!

AUTONOMY AND INDEPENDENCE

In the early stages of life the infant is completely dependent upon parents for all aspects of care. As different skills develop and the infant becomes a toddler they develop the capacity to move away from their parents in order to explore their world. This is often a difficult time for parents, as very young children seem to have very little awareness of danger and may resist attempts to keep them safe (for example holding hands crossing roads or climbing on tables or chairs). The young child begins to physically and emotionally demand an increasing degree of autonomy and independence. This process is linked to the child's response to new stimuli and emotional development, which is a result of both biological predisposition and social learning.

PROBLEMS IN CHILDHOOD DEVELOPMENT

Enuresis

As motor systems develop in the young child they acquire the capacity to control their bladder and need to urinate during the day. The age at which this happens depends both on the child's biological capacity and environmental reinforcement for success from parents or peers at nursery or pre-school. Some children, particularly girls, rapidly become dry during the day and, with environmental manipulation (e.g. reducing fluid intake and lifting at night) reinforcing the development of bladder control, during the night. Eighty-five per cent of children are dry by the age of 5 years with 95% dry by 7. However, 3% of 10-year-olds and 1% of 14-year-olds continue to have primary enuresis either during the day (diurnal) or more commonly nocturnal (night time). This small group of affected children often comes from larger families; there may be a history of enuresis and an association with lower ability or social disadvantage.

Some children develop secondary enuresis, when they start bed-wetting after a period of dryness. In both cases, medical causes should be investigated in parallel with working with specialists who can advise on a range of psychological management techniques to help children develop the ability to stay dry. First-level approaches will involve simple environmental manipulations with a range of reinforcements for dryness. These approaches are simple and effective in up to 90% of children. Where children do not appear to respond to these approaches, a more thorough assessment of possible emotional factors must be addressed, both with regard to the possible causes as well as the effects of ongoing bedwetting in the older child.

Soiling

Nearly 50% of 2-year-olds will be able to ask for and use a potty or toilet, with the remainder capable of this before going to school as a rising 5. However, 1–2% of 7-year-olds (usually boys) have difficulty with soiling. This may be due to failure to ask for the toilet or overflow soiling due to excessive retention because of constipation, which in turn can be due to physical causes. Primary soiling may indicate developmental problems. These should be explored in parallel with bowel retraining methods. The first stage is to explore with the family and child the effect of soiling, and the impact it is having on family life and social relationships, with the objective of enhancing motivation to change and commitment to the management plan. A careful diet plan should be recorded with advice on increasing dietary fibre and fluid to prevent painful evacuation. It may be necessary to use laxatives or more radical medical interventions for children with long-term constipation or impacted bowels. A programme of small achievable steps will help the child move toward the goal. The family and child are then encouraged to practise and reward (a) sitting on the toilet, (b) bowel movements, (c) asking for the toilet and (d) using the toilet. Families should be encouraged to keep relaxed and positive in order to reduce anxiety and stress, which may exacerbate retention in the child.

Sleeping (see also Chapter 6)

It is common for infants and young children to wake during the night, however, the majority have established a regular sleeping pattern by the age of

3 years. The frequency of waking and degree to which children are able to settle easily after waking is a combination of biological, temperamental and environmental factors. Concerns about sleeping are usually about the child settling in their own room or settling down to sleep at a time that parents feel is reasonable. Other concerns may be around the time it takes for a child to settle, an inability to settle on their own or frequent waking, and an inability to then go back to sleep without reassurance and parental contact. The sleeping patterns are usually of greatest concern to the parents whose own sleep pattern is then disrupted. There are many effective self-help resources available for parents; however, the key to resolving these problems lies in developing an understanding of what has established the unacceptable pattern and what is maintaining it. Parents can then decide how best to change the pattern and establish an acceptable bedtime routine through reinforcement of preferred behaviours.

Feeding (see also Chapter 5)

The transition from milk to solids can be a difficult period. The majority of children successfully complete this transition; however, 10–20% of children are reported by mothers to be fussy, slow or faddy eaters.

Children who eat a limited range of food are considered to be selective eaters. The consequences are more often social problems than malnutrition: even those children who refuse to try more than about five or six carbohydrate-based foods rarely have difficulties with growth or physical development. However, between the ages of 7 and 11 selective eating can create social difficulties for a child if the limited range prevents eating with friends or going on school trips.

There are two kinds of restrictive eaters: those who just have limited appetite and those who have additional emotional difficulties (food avoidant emotional disorder). Young people that have experienced a traumatic experience related in some way to food (e.g. choking or sickness) may develop a phobic reaction and be unable to eat certain food textures or tastes.

While some children grow out of these eating difficulties, not all do. Psychological treatment for younger children and their parents can be successful, while for older children there will be a greater need to engage the child and ensure that they are motivated to make the changes. It is important to ensure that physical growth and development are not compromised by the refusal to eat a normal range/quantity of food.

Temper tantrums

The young child acquiring language and the ability to walk also begins to develop a curiosity about the environment and a demand for instant gratification. The 18–24-month-old wants to be able to explore or touch an object and does not yet have the cognitive capacity to understand the parental response that prevents the behaviour or offers a delay (for example sticking fingers in a plug socket, saying 'later' to sweets in the supermarket or preventing the child from running into a road). This period is culturally accepted as the 'terrible twos' and accepted as a part of a normal developmental trajectory. In addition to an inability to understand the concept of delayed gratification, there may also be an impact of frustration where the child feels they are struggling to communicate their desires and wishes. Volatile demands and emotional distress at refusal may also be part of a family pattern of behaviour that the child has learned. The usual course is for the child to improve their language skills and ability to communicate while at the same time understanding the concepts of danger or later reward as a consequence of acquiescence. This can be learned in different ways depending on families' approaches to discipline. For most families and teachers when the 'terrible twos' develop into the 'ferocious fours', there is a role for some kind of behavioural support in order to help parents work out whether too much, or too little, control is maintaining the behavioural demands. Encouraging parents to agree shared ground rules and develop consistent management approaches will enable them to gently reassert control and enable children to understand socially acceptable limits of behaviour. This becomes increasingly important as children get ready to enter school where they will need to have some self-control in a busy classroom and will no longer have the individual attention of a single adult.

Poor impulse control may also be an indicator of mild developmental difficulties, which should be discussed with a paediatrician, particularly if concerns still exist by the age of 5 years.

EMOTIONAL DEVELOPMENT

As cognitive skills develop in children there is a parallel development of the child's emotional repertoire. The development of language allows a greater precision in the development of words that could be used by a child to describe their internal emotional experiences. Early emotional responses in a newborn will be influenced (and made sense of) by an adult. Therefore, a baby may appear happy (because they are smiling) or distressed (because they are crying). As language develops, young children learn words to describe simple emotions like sad, angry, happy, bad and good that they can apply to both themselves and to others.

Anxiety and mood

Anxiety is a normal behavioural response to an event or object or person that is perceived as threatening or dangerous. A child may produce a panic reaction that is a consequence of a belief that they are unable to avoid or escape the real or imaginary danger. As the child develops the ability to recognize and differentiate familiar and non-familiar faces, the earliest expression of anxiety in an infant is distress when a parent leaves or when a new person approaches (fear of strangers). The child's temperament, as well as opportunities to learn that their mother always returns, will influence the capacity to be comforted and response to new situations. A similar expression of anxiety is separation anxiety, when children are separated from parents to whom they have developed an attachment. Crying or agitated distress in a new environment is so common that it is often thought unusual if children don't cry at the first day at nursery! However, the majority of children rapidly reduce the onset and frequency of distress as they develop new social relationships and become confident that

parents will reliably and predictably return. The abilities that underpin these emotional stages of development are linked with the development of underlying cognitive skills like memory, language and abstract concepts of present and future.

In very young children it can be difficult to differentiate between anxiety and depression. In older children and adolescents, however, it has been estimated that about 2% of children present with a range of behaviours that are consistent with the emotional distress that characterizes depression. While a persistent low mood is the key feature for children older than 12, younger children tend to look sad and report somatic symptoms like tummy pains or headaches. Boys in particular may demonstrate aggressive behaviour or high degrees of agitation. Social withdrawal is another symptom. The boundary between the levels of anxiety, frustration and low mood experienced by the normal child and the levels indicating a condition requiring intervention is often indistinct.

Other features of normal developmental anxiety are fears and phobias. These specific anxiety reactions are in response to normal everyday objects like animals, the dark or needles. The fear reaction is so common that, like separation anxiety, it is considered normal. There is a change in the events or objects that produce a fearful response that is linked to the bio-psycho-social development of the child. Fear of school or social situations may emerge as developmentally appropriate environmental challenges present themselves. For some young people anxiety associated with attending school can become extremely severe. This is often manifested in physical symptoms and peaks at the ages of 5 (starting school) and 11 (transition to secondary school). It is important to distinguish between school phobias and truancy as different psychological management approaches will be needed in order to support and help both groups of children. For the majority of children with anxiety, acknowledgement, reassurance and distraction can be sufficient to rapidly reduce the anxiety response. However, if the response persists or increases in severity and continues past the age it is normally seen, it may begin to interfere with social functioning and development and require specialist help and support.

Problems in emotional development

Obsessions

A repetitive focus on an idea, object or concept is a common feature of childhood, and almost all children have their comforting rituals, which are often evident around bedtime. About 1 in a 100 children, however, develop a condition called obsessive compulsive disorder (OCD), which involves the child having unwanted and intrusive thoughts, images and impulses or urges (obsessions) that are unpleasant and distressing. They appear in the child's head automatically and are distressing. The result of the obsession is that the child is compelled to carry out compulsive stereotyped behaviours in order to neutralize the anxiety caused by the obsessive thoughts. If this happens to the degree that it causes impairment in functioning due to time consumed with the symptoms, accompanied by distress and a subsequent interference in daily functioning, then professional help is needed.

Discussion of specific conditions like autistic spectrum disorders (ASD), Asperger's syndrome (AS), and attention deficit hyperactivity disorder (ADHD) is outwith the scope of this book, which focuses on the normal processes of development. Nonetheless, the features that distinguish these conditions illustrate the subtle balance of developmental skills that are required for normal social functioning. Impaired socialization, together with defective verbal/non-verbal communication and a restricted, repetitive pattern of behaviour, characterize ASD, whereas, unlike individuals with autism, sufferers of AS have good verbal skills and may be very bright academically. These children may show marked deficiencies in social skills, have difficulties with transitions or changes and prefer sameness, often having obsessive routines and preoccupations with a particular subject of interest. They have difficulty reading body language, impairing their ability to learn social rules. Children with ADHD lack the ability to focus on appropriate activity and inhibit the inappropriate. They are 'pushy', intrusive and impulsive, but around one-third (especially girls) are not hyperactive; this is when the term attention deficit disorder (ADD) may be used. There is an overlap with conduct disorder and the boundary between the end of the normal

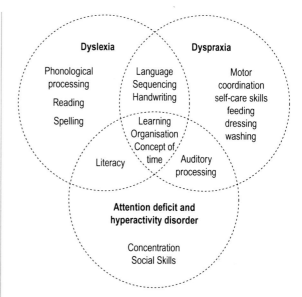

Figure 7.1 Overlap in psychological and communication components

range and the beginning of pathological disorder is unclear (Fig. 7.1).

Inattentiveness, impulsivity and over-activity can be noted at times in many children's lives. But when these features are excessive, long-term, pervasive and not present in children of the same developmental age, they may produce a significant hindrance to social and educational success, leading to a diagnosis of ADHD.

Inattention

Inattentive children may have a hard time keeping their mind on one thing and get bored with a task after only a few minutes (Table 7.2). Focusing deliberate conscious attention to organizing and completing a task or learning something new is often difficult. Paradoxically, they may give effortless, automatic attention to activities and things they enjoy.

Hyperactivity

Restlessness, fidgeting or inappropriate activity (running, wandering) when the child is expected to be quiet are characteristic of hyperactivity. Hyperactive children appear to always be in motion,

Table 7.2 Features of inattention
• Becoming easily distracted by irrelevant sights and sounds
• Failing to pay attention to details and making careless mistakes
• Difficulty in following instructions carefully and completely
• Losing or forgetting things like toys, or pencils, books and tools needed for a task
• Feeling restless, often fidgeting with hands or feet or squirming
• Running, climbing or leaving a seat in situations where sitting or quiet behaviour is expected
• Blurting out answers before hearing the whole question
• Having difficulty waiting in line or for a turn

dashing around or talking constantly. Sitting still through a whole lesson can be an impossible task as they might squirm in their seat or roam around the room. They may wiggle their feet, touch things or tap pencils.

Impulsivity

Impulsivity results in a child being unable to curb immediate reactions to events or take time to think before acting. Impulsive children may blurt out inappropriate comments and find it hard to wait for things or take turns in games.

Tics

Small involuntary movements (motor) or noises (vocal) are known as tics. These are usually simple movements located in the upper body or head region (eye blinks, head nod, sniffs and grunts). One feature of tics is their tendency to change over time. They may become more or less frequent or intense or may alter completely.

Tics are present in as much as 10–20% of the population, usually between the ages of 7 and 13 and mostly in boys. For most people these tics are not a matter for concern and they decline with time, although they can reappear under situations of severe stress or anxiety. In some children the increase in frequency and disruptive severity of tics may indicate a tic disorder, such as Tourette's syndrome, which can be very disabling and requires specialist management.

Further reading

Bellman M, Kennedy N (eds) 2000 Paediatrics and Child Health: a Textbook for the DCH. Churchill Livingstone, Edinburgh

Skuse D (ed) 2003 Child Psychology and Psychiatry: an Introduction. The Medicine Publishing Company, Oxford

Stirling J 2001 Introducing Neuropsychology. Psychology Press, Hove

8 Speech and communication

J. Jamieson

▼ OVERVIEW

This chapter will look at the way young children develop an elaborate system of communication in the first 5 years of their lives. During this time language progresses from random vocalizations to a vocabulary of approximately 2000 words that are clearly articulated and used in complex sentences. The linguistic terminology used for describing language and speech is discussed in the introduction.

A brief summary of the different approaches to child language acquisition is given before focusing on the development of communication from birth to 5 years. This section is divided into 10 stages where the development of receptive and expressive language and social interaction is outlined. The following section looks at the various environmental, medical and linguistic factors that affect language development.

The chapter concludes with guidelines on when it is appropriate to refer a child, with speech and language difficulties, for assessment by a speech and language therapist.

INTRODUCTION

There is often confusion about the use of the terms communication, language and speech, and the way these three areas overlap; the following will try to clarify their use in this chapter.

COMMUNICATION

Communication is interaction in its widest sense, including speech, gestures, signs and social behaviour. Much communication from young babies is without intent and is merely the result of reflexive responses; however, meaning can be inferred from these vocalizations and movements and, therefore, they may have a communicative function. We communicate with others non-verbally using eye contact, body posture, gesture, facial expression and verbally with speech. We interpret communication from others through hearing, listening, watching, understanding and our knowledge of social behaviour.

LANGUAGE

Language is the means by which humans communicate deliberately with others. Language can be verbal (speech) or non-verbal (sign language/writing). The usual vehicle for language is speech supported by gesture. Language is both symbolic and arbitrary, words are symbolic representations of an idea or concept and apart from words that represent the sound something makes, such as 'quack quack' for duck and 'brum brum' for car, there is usually no perceptual link between a word and the object it represents, for example the words 'table' and 'cat' are highly arbitrary symbols. Language can broadly be divided into two discrete components: receptive and expressive.

Receptive language (comprehension)

This refers to the ability to understand and interpret the communication of others. Expressive language is how we communicate with others (Fig. 8.1, Table 8.1).

Speech is only one aspect of expressive language; it involves the production of sounds (phonemes) that are combined to make meaningful words. In any language there are phonological rules that dictate how individual sounds can be combined to make words. Speech sounds are generated by coordinating an outward air stream, vibrating the vocal folds and changing the position of the soft palate, tongue and lips (speech articulators) (Fig. 8.2).

Consonant sounds are produced in a variety of ways (manner of articulation) and in different places in the mouth (place of articulation). Some consonants

Table 8.1   Essential components of receptive and expressive language and conversation

Components of receptive language	Components of expressive language	Components of conversation
Hearing	Crying (reflexive/ communicative)	Eye contact
Listening	Looking	Turn taking
Looking	Making eye contact	Timing
Understanding	Vocalizing	Shared attention
Interpreting	Pointing	Appropriate responses (e.g. answering sentences)
	Facial expression	Awareness of social context (e.g. casual, polite, formal)
	Gestures	Prosodic features e.g. the use of tone, volume and pitch of voice, rhythm, stress patterns, intonation
Reading	Writing	Eye contact
	Speech	Turn taking

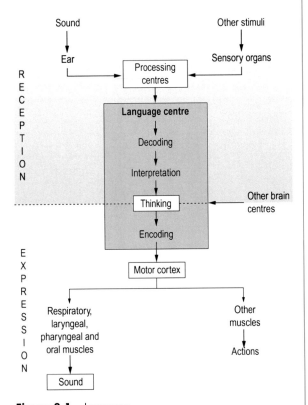

Figure 8.1   Language

use vibration of the vocal folds (voiced) while others do not (voiceless). When the articulators form a complete obstruction to the air stream, which is released suddenly, a **plosive** sound is produced (b d g = voiced and p t k = voiceless). A **fricative** sound is produced when there is a partial obstruction to the air stream, which causes friction when it is released (v z th [in that] = voiced and f s sh h and th [in thin] = voiceless).

Vowel sounds are also made by altering the position of the tongue and lips, but unlike consonants there is not an obstruction made to the air stream. The quality of the vowel depends on the part of the

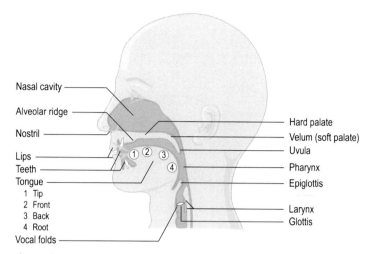

Figure 8.2 Anatomy of speech

tongue that is raised towards the palate (*front, central* or *back*), the proximity of the tongue towards the palate (*open*; away from the palate or *close*; near to the palate) and the presence or absence of lip rounding. All vowel sounds are *voiced*.

To make the '*ee*' sound in '*feet*' the *front* of the tongue is raised towards the palate and the tongue is *close* to the palate, but to make the '*ar*' sound in *car* the *back* of the tongue is arched towards the palate and the tongue is in an *open* position away from the palate.

Phonological development is the gradual process of acquiring adult speech patterns. Children follow predictable phonological processes or deviations in their attempts to acquire the accurate sound system of their own language. Certain generalizations can be made about the sequence of speech acquisition in children:

- consonants made at the front of the mouth appear before back sounds (p, b, m before k, g)
- plosives usually occur before fricatives (p/b, t/d and k/g before f/v, th, s/z and sh)
- consonant clusters appear at the end of a word before the beginning, e.g. la*st* before *st*op.

Components of language

There are rules that dictate how to combine words to make grammatical utterances – *syntax*, and rules that govern how to express meaning through vocabulary – *semantics*. These aspects of language are often referred to as form and content.

Syntax (form) refers to the set of rules that govern the grammatical arrangement of words in spoken or written sentences. In the sentence 'John chased Bill' the word order is essential for conveying a particular meaning, 'Bill chased John' has an entirely different meaning.

Morphology refers to the set of rules that governs word structure; how words are built out of meaningful units (morphemes.) For example; cat-s, walk-ed, un-explod-ed.

Semantics (content) refers to the meaning implicit in morphemes, words and sentences. Word recognition connects with a mental lexicon (an individual's intuitive knowledge of words and their meanings) to make the association between a given sound pattern and the meaning it conveys. For example: cat = animal, small, furry, purrs, meows; fish = animal, swims, slippery, scaly; table = furniture, legs, hard, flat surface. In sentences word order, grammatical inflections, information from the environment and the social context all combine to help the listener to interpret the speaker's meaning. For example, a parent might say, 'It's going to rain', but mean, 'Wear your coat!'

Pragmatics refers to the functional aspects of language, for example, its use in social contexts.

THEORIES OF CHILD LANGUAGE ACQUISITION

'In general, language acquisition is a stubbornly robust process; from what we can tell there is virtually no way to prevent it from happening short of raising a child in a barrel' (Pinker 1984).

Learning theory

Language is generally considered to be the most distinctive characteristic of human behaviour. Many psychologists and linguists have been concerned with trying to understand how children acquire the ability to speak and communicate meanings and thoughts to others.

Verbal behaviour theory

Learning theorists have attempted to explain language acquisition in terms of stimulus, response, rewards and reinforcements. Skinner (1957) maintained that language is learned through **operant conditioning**, where an infant's vocalizations and sounds are imitated and praised when they resemble recognizable words. This reinforcement continues to be given as the child's babble increases and the approximations to words are refined.

Skinner's theory was rejected by many psycholinguists at the time as being an inadequate explanation of language acquisition. This was primarily because it did not recognize any contribution from the child, who simply responded to external stimulation and reinforcement. Imitation undoubtedly plays a part in the child's learning of new vocabulary and grammatical structures. However, it does not take into account either the rate of language development or the fact that children's language is **creative**. Children understand and produce original novel sentences that they have not heard before.

Innate capacity theory

In the 1950s and '60s Noam Chomsky (1928–) rejected Skinner's theory that children acquire language purely as a result of imitation and reinforcement. He contended that humans are born with an innate capacity to develop language and that every child is born with a language acquisition device (LAD), which is programmed to recognize the universal rules common to all languages. He reasoned that children are inventive with their language and produce utterances that they have never heard before; therefore, their language could not simply be the result of learning or conditioning. Numerous experimental tests have shown that by the age of 3 years children have an implicit awareness of the grammatical rules of their language, which they apply to original utterances. The way children tackle irregular grammatical constructions also demonstrates that they do not learn language by imitating their parents; phrases such as 'I builded a tower' and 'Look at the sheeps' are derived from applying regular past tense and plural forms, not from imitating their parent's speech.

Cognitive theory

The model of cognitive development proposed by Jean Piaget (1896–1980) has also been used to explain language acquisition. This theory proposes that a child must have reached a particular stage in their concept formation before any meaningful language is possible. As language is a symbolic system, where one thing represents something else, a child needs to have an inner awareness that a word is a representation of an object. Piaget believed that this early stage of concept formation begins with the child's awareness of object permanence; the understanding that an object continues to exist even when it is out of sight. Piaget called this the *sensory motor stage*. Object permanence usually occurs at about 10 months of age and coincides with the emergence of naming objects. Many studies have looked at early language development and linked linguistic skills with Piaget's sensory motor stage. It is clear that there is a strong link between intellectual and language development. The child needs to have certain concepts to use language but similarly verbal labels facilitate concept formation. An early word may only have meaning for the child when it is applied to one particular object in a specific situation, for example, his/her own cup at mealtimes. Later the child will be able to generalize the 'cup' label to apply to any cup of any colour, shape or size. Conversely many children over-generalize the meanings of their first words, calling all men 'daddy' or all animals 'cat'.

LANGUAGE INPUT

It is now generally accepted that innateness is inherent in language development, in that, despite all manner of varying and sometimes adverse circumstances, the vast majority of humans acquire language. The way in which language is acquired and the level of linguistic competence achieved are determined by *genetic, neurological* and *cognitive* factors, each of these being influenced by *environment*.

Recent research has again focused on the importance of a child's *linguistic environment* and looked at the relevance of language input. Terms such as baby talk, motherese, parentese and child directed speech (CDS) have all been used to describe the distinctive nature of speech addressed to babies and young children. CDS is perhaps the least controversial and will be used in this chapter.

CDS refers to the particular style of speech that adults use when they talk to children and it is a matter of debate how much this type of interaction influences language development, in particular the fact that it is not used universally in all cultures. However, research has shown that babies attend to CDS for longer periods than they attend to speech intended for adults. Characteristics of CDS include:

- slow delivery of speech
- short sentences with key words stressed
- frequent repetition
- high voice pitch
- exaggerated intonation
- simple but accurate grammar
- frequent questions using rising intonation
- pauses to give the child an opportunity to 'reply'
- echoing the child's vocalizations
- running commentary to accompany activities
- exaggerated hand gesturing and facial expression
- phrases repeated during daily routines, e.g. mealtimes/bedtime
- being at the same level for face-to-face contact.

Interestingly, these speech patterns are not exclusive to adults; children from 3 years of age will address a baby (or a doll/pet) with their own version of CDS. Children with delayed speech and language benefit from this type of intense interaction, as it develops their attention and listening skills. There is well-documented evidence linking a child's language development with different styles of parenting behaviours. For example, the amount of speech directed at children has been related to children's vocabulary development. In addition there is evidence to suggest that children's language abilities influence parents' interaction. Mothers of language delayed children have been shown to use different speech styles than mothers of children following normal development. They may try to compensate for their child's reluctance to participate in conversations and they frequently try to teach language skills rather than interacting spontaneously.

THE DEVELOPMENT OF COMMUNICATION FROM BIRTH TO 5 YEARS

In addition to the innate element of language acquisition there are three prerequisites for normal language development that are inextricably linked:

1. The ability to understand the communication of others – *receptive language.*
2. The ability to convey meaning through non-verbal and verbal means – *expressive language.*
3. The instinctive drive and desire for *social interaction* that motivates the child to build relationships and characterizes human beings as social animals.

In this chapter the development of communication from birth to 5 years will be outlined, looking at these three areas separately. It is much easier to assess levels of expressive language than comprehension. It is possible to overestimate a child's understanding of language; for example, a child could be asked to 'Put the book on the table' and by using a natural gesture to accompany the command (pointing to the book and the table) the child could follow the instructions without understanding any of the six words in the sentence. Similarly, a child's *situational understanding* greatly assists their comprehension of language; when children hear, 'Bring me your coat and shoes' prior to leaving the house, the familiar situation will help them understand the words. This is analogous with an adult's experience of following instructions in a foreign language; slow delivery, gesture and familiar situations will enhance comprehension.

When discussing language it is important to remember that the rate of acquisition is unique to each child. Many factors will influence this, including genetic factors, cognitive profile and environment. However, language development is generally predictable and follows recognized stages; for example, generally children will babble before saying their first word and will need a vocabulary of

approximately 150 single words before they start joining two words together. Most children attain language milestones at roughly the same age, but there is a wide range that is still considered to be within normal parameters; for example, first words may appear at any time between 8 and 16 months.

Tables 8.2–8.11 show the development of communication skills from birth to 5 years.

FACTORS AFFECTING THE DEVELOPMENT OF COMMUNICATION

Numerous different factors, either on their own or combined, can influence language development (Fig. 8.3). About 10% of pre-school children have

Table 8.2   Communication: birth–2 months

Receptive language	Expressive communication	Social interaction
Distinguishes between mother's normal speaking voice and the voice of a stranger or the mother speaking in a monotone	Makes a variety of sounds and vocalizations; either *reflexive noises* indicating either hunger or pain, or *vegetative noises* such as sucking, swallowing or burping: these sounds are the beginnings of communication	Makes direct eye contact with people who speak to them (the distance from the mother's breast to her eyes is thought to be a new young baby's optimum focusing distance and during feeding babies make strong eye contact with their feeder)
Turns head towards sounds, particularly speech, and can be calmed by a friendly soothing voice	Reflexive cries show distinct patterns of length, pitch and quality depending on whether the cry indicates pain, hunger, discomfort or fear	Parents instinctively talk to their babies pausing to give time for the baby to respond. Mothers rarely speak when the baby is feeding, but resume the 'conversation' as soon as feeding stops and the baby is able to focus on the interaction
By 2 months, begins to locate people speaking nearby	Carers interpret cries and respond appropriately by feeding, changing or comforting; the baby has initiated a communication, and the parents have inferred meaning and responded. Early vocalizations require coordinating the air stream with the vibration of the vocal folds, both skills that are necessary for later speech development	Smiles at about 6 weeks; these early smiles are usually elicited by communication with parents or siblings and they encourage further interactions: this is the beginning of the virtuous circle of language development

Table 8.3   Communication: 2–5 months

Receptive language	Expressive communication	Social interaction
Responds to speech by looking directly into the speaker's face	Continues to make reflexive and vegetative noises, but in addition produces the first *cooing* sounds when content	Vocalizations occur when babies are *face to face* with a familiar adult
Attends to the movements of the speaker's mouth and lips rather than the face as a whole	Begins to move mouth and lips more deliberately and appears to experiment with sound making, for example, blowing raspberries	Usually smiles and vocalizes when spoken to
By 5 months begins to respond to the tone of voice being used (e.g. if a parent uses an angry voice to chastise an older sibling the baby may suddenly burst into tears)	Sounds become less random, the coordination between the vocal folds and speech articulators, becomes more controlled	Usually responds more readily to familiar people than strangers
	At about 4 months the cooing sounds increase in length and open vowels may be combined with a consonant made at the back of the mouth producing a 'gaa' or 'goo' sound	Varies facial expressions and will imitate mouth movements; sticking out tongue or opening and shutting mouth Simple interactive games such as peek-a-boo promote social exchanges

some problem with communication, language or speech and approximately 7% continue to have difficulties by school age.

It should be noted that speech and language may be either *delayed* or *disordered* and the distinction between these two conditions is very important. Generally, children with a language delay follow the predicted sequence of normal language development, but they are behind the level expected for their chronological age. These children may require speech and language therapy. Many (but not all) catch up with their peers by the age of 6–7 years. A proportion of children with delayed speech and language, encounter literacy difficulties at school. Children with a communication or language disorder present with features that are *not* seen in normal development. These children will require extensive speech and language therapy and, occasionally, specialist schooling. Many children with a language disorder will subsequently encounter literacy difficulties. Education places great emphasis on language competence and children with a language

disorder often lose out on educational opportunities and become socially isolated.

Language is a highly complex function and despite its robust nature there are many factors that contribute to and affect language development. These factors can be of a positive, adverse, inherent or developmental nature and all of them can greatly influence an individual's language competence. Many variables relate to the child's environment and these will be outlined before moving on to more specific disabilities and linguistic factors.

ENVIRONMENTAL FACTORS INFLUENCING SPEECH AND LANGUAGE DEVELOPMENT

Familial

A relatively high proportion of children with delayed language development or communication disorders have a family history of similar problems.

Table 8.4 Communication: 5–7 months

Receptive Language	Expressive communication	Social interaction
Begins to respond when called by name (but not consistently)	Begins *experimental vocal play* Often most vocal when alone, e.g. in the cot on waking	Looks for people when voices are heard in another room
Starts to respond to the word 'no'	Experiments with mouth and tongue movements, practises making sounds	Watches children playing and will vocalize and smile at them to gain their attention
Begins to be able to look and listen at the same time	Makes pre-babble vocalizations that have a wide range of sounds that occur in all languages including; gutturals, trills and clicks Early sounds not specific to baby's native language	Recoils and turns away when approached by a stranger
Starts to make the connection between speech, gestures and actions	Screams and moans when distressed or annoyed, in addition to crying	Rhymes and songs become an important part of social interaction Begins to learn familiar sequences and anticipate what is coming next, e.g. being tickled after 'This little piggy' Enjoys physical rough and tumble play and requests an activity to continue by vocalizing or moving

Gender

Boys are sometimes slower to develop language than girls. However, boys have a much higher incidence of speech and language problems that require therapy, generally outnumbering girls by 2 to 1. Some impairments such as, dysfluency (stammering) are four times more common in boys than in girls.

Family structure and size

Children in large families may be slightly slower to develop language than children with only one or two siblings. In large families there may be less interaction between parents and individual children and more interaction between siblings. For the same reason it follows that the first child in a family often speaks earlier and has a larger vocabulary than subsequent children. However, family size and structure on its own, does not have a significant or lasting effect on language development.

Multiple births

Twins and triplets generally speak slightly later than single children. Studies suggest that the majority of twins have delayed language development, particularly up to the age of 5 years. Caring for more than one baby influences the way parents interact, they tend to have fewer and shorter exchanges with one child on their own and are likely to be less responsive and more directive. Characteristically multiple birth children use more gesture than singletons and they often develop their own secret language that is incomprehensible to their parents or siblings. Most children of multiple births catch up

Table 8.5 Communication: 7–10 months

Receptive language	Expressive communication	Social interaction
Appears to listen to other's conversations, looking from one person to the other as they speak	Verbal and non-verbal attention seeking; greeting; refusing (pushing or turning away or shaking head for 'no'); requesting (opening and shutting hand/reaching/pointing); protesting	Adults will tune in to and repeat the babble sounds that most closely resemble real words, for example 'mama' and 'dada'
Begins to recognize names of family members or pets	Practises the specific sounds used in the environment that will form the basis of the first words	Shows *joint attention* by pointing or reaching for things that an adult can bring
Looks towards the source of a sound, for example, telephone or door bell	Produces repetitive consonant + vowel (C+V) sounds, e.g. 'dadada' 'mamama' (*reduplicated babble*)	Enjoys sharing an activity, such as, looking at a book or building a tower
Looks at pictures in a book	Most frequently uses the consonants; *t, d, p, b* and *m*, and vowels such as *a* (in *cat*) & *e* (in *bed*) (in most languages the word for mother and father usually begins with one of these early consonant sounds)	Requests a particular rhyme or activity by doing an associated action, for example, clapping hands for 'pat a cake' Imitates facial expressions, gestures and sounds
Understands 'no' and 'bye-bye'	Towards the end of this stage reduplicated babble changes to **variegated babble** where the consonants and vowel sounds are varied, e.g. 'dabooda' Shows interest in music (moving to its rhythm) and attempts to 'sing along' to familiar nursery rhymes	Seeks out an audience of people who will imitate their babble sounds and engage in 'conversations' with them Shows an interest in other babies and young children

with their peers by school age and do not require referral to speech therapy any more than singletons.

Bilingualism

In the UK, approximately 8% of children starting primary school have English as an additional language. Most children manage to learn two languages in a truly bilingual home, where they are exposed to both languages equally from birth. It seems important that children learn each language from a different source, for example, mother one language and father another. Comprehensive studies have shown that there is no correlation between bilingualism and language delay. Problems do occur, however, if the child has learning difficulties or if one language is favoured.

Neglect

Most children will develop language regardless of the amount of stimulation they are given. However, if the environment is severely socially and linguistically deprived, language development may suffer. Poor interaction, which may be a function of psychosocial deprivation, is unlikely to cause *severe* language problems, although it is likely to be associated with *milder* disturbances of language (Cantwell & Baker 1985). In any attempt to account for poor language development in abused or neglected children it is

Table 8.6   Communication: 10–13 months

Receptive language	Expressive communication	Social interaction
Develops an intense interest in speech	Expressive communication extends to become true language at this stage	Notices or even shows concern when another baby or child is heard crying
Shows understanding of several words that are used in a familiar context, by behaving appropriately, e.g. localizing common objects when they are named, such as spoon, cup and ball	Introduces the prosodic features of speech; rhythm, intonation and the tone and quality of voice are used in addition to speech sounds, these utterances are known as *jargon*	Develops a sense of humour; amused by an incongruous event, such as, an adult pretending to drink from a child's beaker
Understands at least 20 words by the age of 1 year	Uses first words, which often imitate the repetitive consonant + vowel syllables heard in babble, for example; 'mama', 'dada' or 'bye-bye' (sometimes the utterance sounds like a possible word, but the meaning is unclear; these are known as *proto words*)	Shows an interest in what other people are doing and has a desire to join them in a shared activity
Locates speaker when called by name	First words are usually labels for objects, people or acts, a single utterance may express many different meanings, which have to be inferred from the context, e.g. 'cup' may mean 'Where is my cup?' 'Give me my cup' or 'I've dropped my cup, pick it up for me!'	Initiates interaction with others, but ends an exchange by simply moving away
Begins to understand simple phrases and commands supported by context and gesture, e.g. 'Give it to Mummy' or 'Wave bye-bye to Daddy'	Uses gestures, in particularly pointing, in conjunction with vocalizations Attempts to say first words are often only approximations of the correct pronunciation, e.g. 'tup' for 'cup' Imitates animal sounds ('moo, woof and meow') and vehicle sounds ('brum-brum')	

vital to take into account the child's cognitive and developmental status.

Emotional

Emotional or behavioural problems and communication breakdown are frequently closely related. In *elective mutism* children talk selectively, for example, they may talk at home with their families, but refuse to speak outside their homes. The term selective mutism is sometimes used to indicate that the child chooses the environment where they are prepared to talk. Girls and boys are at equally at risk of developing selective mutism. It can be difficult to distinguish between this condition and extreme shyness.

Table 8.7   Communication: 13–18 months

Receptive language	Expressive communication	Social interaction
By 18 months most children have a receptive vocabulary of around 250 words	Between 13 and 18 months a child's expressive vocabulary increases from about five to 50 words	Between 13 and 18 months increased mobility gives a sense of independence and the ability to explore Learns to 'help' around the house; fetching things that are needed or copying actions, e.g. talking on telephone or tidying away toys
Shows *object recognition;* knows how to use objects such as a cup, spoon, brush or hat appropriately	Imbeds individual words in elaborate jargon, which sounds exactly like fluent adult speech; with melodic intonation, appropriate pauses, varied rhythm and stress patterns (*egocentric speech*)	Begins to want to do things independently, such as feeding self or getting dressed Looks for praise from an adult for achieving things on their own
Understands simple sentences, such as 'Bring me your shoes' or 'Give the book to Daddy', although comprehension is still assisted by the use of gesture and situational understanding	Uses intonation patterns to enhance the meanings of single word utterances, e.g. 'Mummy' could mean: 'Come here Mummy' (command) 'Where's Mummy' (question) or 'Look, there's Mummy' (observation)	Continues to develop a sense of humour, will do silly things to try and make others laugh
Understands vocabulary related to own experiences, e.g. the word 'dog' might only apply to the family pet, but not to other dogs they have seen in the park	Links two words to form one idea, e.g. 'All-gone', 'Whats-that?' or 'Go-now'	Continues to be interested in other children of a similar age and will occasionally offer them toys
Points to familiar pictures in a book when named	Sounds mastered by 18 months *m, p, b* and *w*	Enjoys sharing any activity with an adult and will start to take turns; turning the pages of a book or rolling a ball to and fro
Identifies named parts of the body on self and others	By 18 months speech is normally 25% intelligible	

COMMUNICATION DIFFICULTIES SECONDARY TO OTHER CONDITIONS (FIG. 8.3)

Hearing impairment

Many children have recurrent middle ear problems during their early years. This can cause fluctuating hearing loss making it difficult to discriminate between speech sounds which as a result limits comprehension. In addition, children's speech may be unclear, with the sounds they are not hearing being omitted from their speech. Children with a significant congenital or acquired hearing loss will have difficulty acquiring spoken language. Factors influencing the extent of communication difficulties resulting from hearing loss are as follows:

Table 8.8   Communication: 18 months–2 years

Receptive language	Expressive communication	Social interaction
Symbolic understanding extends to the appropriate or imaginative use of miniature toys such as small cars, farm animals or doll's house furniture	Often echoes words (*echolalia*) and may repeat the last word of a question rather than giving a considered reply, e.g. when asked 'Do you want a banana or an apple?' an echolalic child will say 'apple'. But if the question is rephrased to 'Do you want an apple or a banana?' the reply will be 'banana'	Uses communication to share experiences
Understands 2D representations – photographs or pictures Vocabulary increases, new words and phrases are understood every week	Vocabulary increases to between 100 and 200 words Begins to join two words together at around the age of 2 years Typical utterances are: 'Daddy garden', 'dog running', 'red brick', 'Mummy shoe'	Uses communication to share experiences Language is still egocentric with little awareness of another person's point of view
Selects a named object from a choice of five familiar items (e.g. cup, book, ball, keys and spoon)	Frequently imitates new words and occasionally repeat two- or three-word phrases	Recognizes familiar people by their voices alone, e.g. speaking on the telephone
Begins to understand and distinguish between personal pronouns, e.g. 'Give it to me/him/her'	Refers to self by using name rather than a pronoun, e.g. 'Tom do it'" not 'I do it'	Shows interest in being in the company of other children, and plays alongside them (*parallel play*) Will not necessarily attempt to talk to them
Understands some verbs used in context, e.g. 'Give teddy something to eat'	Sounds mastered by 2 years: *m, p, b, w + t* and *d* Frequently omits the final sound from words, e.g. 'be_' for bed and 'du_' for duck Changes a consonant to match another consonant in the word, e.g. 'Tat' for cat and 'Dod' for dog By 2 years speech is normally 50–75% intelligible	Engages in interactive, rough and tumble games with siblings

- the type of hearing loss (conductive [outer or middle ear], sensorineural, mixed conductive and sensorineural or central/cortical)
- management with hearing aids, for conductive loss, or cochlear implant for sensory neural loss
- the severity of the hearing loss and whether it is unilateral or bilateral
- whether it is congenital or acquired
- the child's age at the time of diagnosis
- whether parents also have a hearing loss

Table 8.9   Communication: 2–2½ years

Receptive language	Expressive communication	Social interaction
Relates two named objects, e.g. 'Put the car in the box'	Uses three- and four-word phrases often containing only key words – *telegraphic speech* (nouns, verbs and adjectives), e.g. the sentence 'I am going to the park with Daddy' becomes 'I park Daddy' In two- and three-word phrases the word order is nearly always preserved	Shows awareness of other people's feelings and will try to comfort them if they seem upset
Selects an object by use, e.g. 'Which one do we write/eat/ sweep/cook/cut with?'	Asks frequent questions These are often in the form of a statement but with a rising (questioning) intonation pattern, such as 'Daddy gone?' 'Shoes wet?'	Does not appreciate the need to be tactful and avoids commenting on people's appearance or behaviour
Identifies smaller body parts (finger, knee, chin, eyebrow, etc.)	Uses question words such as 'What? 'and 'Where?' e.g. 'What man doing?' and 'Where baby go?' (questions often very repetitive and more observational rather than true information seeking inquiries)	Learns some of the early rules of social behaviour
Understands concepts of size and quantity, e.g. 'Show me the little ball' and 'Give me one sweet'	Expresses negatives with 'no' and 'not'	Finds it difficult to share a game or a toy with peers
Understands some spatial concepts and prepositions, e.g. 'Put the books in the cupboard'	Uses personal pronouns correctly more often – I, you, me, he, she, they and it May still refer to self using own name Uses conjunctions (but, and, because) to join individual words or phrases together, e.g. 'Daddy and car and shops and Mummy come too' Uses plural 's' and possessive 's' – (sock**s**, cup**s**, Mummy'**s** coat) By 2½ begins to learn to count by rote (without a real concept of number) and name some colours Sounds mastered by 2½ : *m, n, p, b, t, d + w* and *h* Developing sounds: *k* and *g* Tends to omit the ends of words Has difficulty with consonant clusters, e.g. '<u>sp</u>oon, <u>st</u>op or <u>bl</u>ack' may become 'poon, top or back' **Common acceptable patterns:** k as t: 'tat' for 'cat' k as g: 'guddle' for 'cuddle' g as d: 'doat' for 'goat' p as b: 'big' for 'pig'	Becomes angry if does not get own way, but begins to learn the value of sharing and turn–taking as these experiences increase Social interactive play develops with other children in structured play situations, monitored by an adult

Table 8.10   Communication: 2½–3½ years

Receptive language	Expressive communication	Social interaction
Understands more complex instructions or requests	Uses language to describe what they have done in the recent past or to explain a picture they have drawn	Initiates and maintains a conversation by keeping the listener's attention
Follows language that includes the use of abstractions such as *colour, size, prepositions and negatives*, e.g. 'Show me the yellow flower', 'Give me the small ball', 'Put the book in front of the table' and 'Which teddy isn't on the floor?'	Language becomes much more complex and many grammatical constructions are used, although, they will not be accurate all the time	Understands the need to take conversational turns, saying something and then waiting for a response
Understands descriptive concepts such as opposites: heavy/light, wet/dry, hot/cold, same/different, empty/full	Prepositions (in, on, under), conjunctions (and, but), articles (a, the), auxiliary verbs (have, did), plural endings (dogs, boxes, children), tenses (talking, talked), pronouns (I, she, he, we, they), possessives (the cat's bowl)	Attempts to clarify speech if not understood by others
Understands that words can be categorized according to different groups, e.g. 'Tell me all the things you can; eat/ play with/wear'	Answers more complex questions such as, 'What do you do when you are cold/tired/hungry/wet/dirty?' Sounds mastered by 3½ : *m, n, p, b, t, d, k, g, w, h + y, l, f* and *s* Developing sounds: *r, ch, j, sh* and consonant clusters (e.g. **spl**ash) Common acceptable patterns: f as b or p; 'pat' or 'bat' for 'fat' s as t or d; 'tun' or 'dun' for 'sun' By 3½, 90% of speech can be understood by strangers	Converses with other children and plays cooperatively in a pretend play situation, such as the 'home corner' at play group or nursery

- the presence or absence of coexisting physical or cognitive problems.

Most children with hearing loss are excellent non-verbal communicators, using natural gesture, demonstrations, facial expression and sign language (for example. British Sign Language).

Learning difficulties

Learning difficulties are one of the commonest causes of speech and language difficulties in children. These children have a significant cognitive disability present from birth onwards. The learning disability may have an identified genetic basis such as; Down's syndrome or Fragile X. Learning disabilities vary in

Table 8.11   Communication: 3½–5 years

Receptive language	Expressive communication	Social interaction
Understands complex sentences including many different grammatical devices e.g.advanced, verbs (squeeze, pull, twist, fold), comparatives (smaller, heaviest), prepositions (under, beside)	Uses sentences containing more than one clause, frequently linked by 'and'	Knows how to mix and get along with other people without needing a family member present
More detailed vocabulary (eyelash, finger-nail)	90% of utterances are grammatically correct	Cooperates with others and asks permission before doing something
Questions ('Why?' and 'When?' questions understood)	Continues to make minor grammatical errors until about 7 years of age.	Makes firm friendships as school age approaches and often identifies with others of the same gender
Understands 'time' vocabulary (yesterday, today, later, after, while)	Approximately 4% of children under 5 years experience dysfluent speech while learning to talk; most of these will eventually speak fluently (normal non-fluency) The classic features of non-fluency at this stage are: tense and jerky speech often requiring extra effort, repeating parts of words (mu-mu-mu-mu-mummy) or whole words before continuing with an utterance or extending sounds within a word (s-s-s-s-school)	Becomes aware that social factors and contexts influence the success of conversations and uses the following devices: sensitivity to social context (cheeky, polite, quiet, formal), markers of politeness ('please, thank you, sorry'), conversational turns (not constantly interrupting or questioning), clarification ('What did you say?'), repetition, eye contact, ability to interpret meaning by matching words with tone of voice and facial expression, concluding a conversation (many younger children simply walk away when they have finished talking)
Follows more complex verbal instructions ('Show me the small brown dog that is sleeping')	Repeats a sentence of up to nine words	Uses language to tell jokes and relate stories
Conditional sentences ('If it is raining we won't go to the park'), inferences ('If you spill your drink what should you do'), predictions ('What would happen if you ran into the road'), analogies ('A mouse is small but an elephant is - - -')	Relates an experience that happened some time ago, tells a short story or says what will happen next in a simple sequence	Realizes that you can tell a lie and sometimes get away with it!

Table 8.11	Communication: 3½–5 years—Cont'd.	
Receptive language	**Expressive communication**	**Social interaction**
	Most speech sounds articulated correctly The last sounds to appear are *r* and *th*, which are often replaced by *w* or *l* and *f* respectively ('wabbit' or 'labbit' for 'rabbit' and 'fink' for 'think') Children often pronounce sounds in new words correctly before they update their pronunciation of old words, e.g. a child may continue to say 'wabbit' for rabbit, but they are able to say the initial 'r' sound correctly in new vocabulary they learn By 5 years children are usually completely intelligible to strangers	

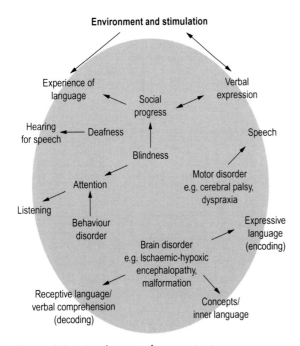

Figure 8.3   Development of communication

and 69) learning difficulties. Children with moderate learning difficulties usually achieve functional language sufficient to meet their individual needs, although language development is likely to be delayed. Children with severe learning difficulties may not ever develop functional speech and may rely on gestures or signing system (e.g. Makaton) for communication.

Neuromuscular disorders

Children with neuromuscular problems often present with a motor speech disorder, which impairs the ability to articulate speech sounds (*dysarthria*). Developmental dysarthria may occur with general motor disorders, such as cerebral palsy, or with a specific motor disorder, such as muscular dystrophy. Dysarthria is frequently associated with feeding and breathing problems.

Other causes of speech problems

Autism spectrum disorders (ASD), mentioned in Chapter 7, affect communication, social interaction and imagination. Acquired childhood aphasia (ACA) can follow conditions where there is severe cerebral dysfunction such as head injury, epilepsy

severity and characteristics as well as cause. Children will usually be categorized as having either *severe* (IQ of 50 or below) or *moderate* (IQ between 50 and more rarely Rett's and Landau–Kleffner syndrome.

PRIMARY COMMUNICATION DIFFICULTIES IN THE ABSENCE OF OTHER CONDITIONS

Specific language impairment

Some children fail to develop language normally; however, their difficulties cannot be attributed to hearing, cognitive ability, environmental or emotional difficulties. These children present with a language *disorder* that can affect receptive, expressive (impaired syntax and semantics) and phonological aspects of language. Typically their speech is slow and deliberate with significant word–finding difficulties, containing numerous grammatical errors, such as misuse of pronouns and the plural and past tense suffixes. Children with specific language impairment (SLI) often have a family history of similar problems and despite years of speech and language therapy, and possibly specialist education, subtle linguistic difficulties are likely to persist into adulthood.

Delayed and disordered speech production

Developmental speech disorders are considered to be either phonological or articulatory, but it can be difficult to differentiate between a pure phonological disorder and a more general speech disorder. There are various stages involved in speech production and problems can arise at various levels from *input* to *output*. Children normally acquire adult pronunciation patterns through hearing, listening, processing the received information, motor speech patterns and precise articulation.

There are various causes of delayed and disordered speech production:

1. Perceptual level – hearing and listening.
2. Cognitive level – difficulty with the processing of speech.
3. Neuromuscular level (see previous section).
4. Articulatory level – a malfunction of the speech production mechanism.
5. Oromotor, verbal or developmental *dyspraxia*.

Perceptual level – hearing and listening

Children need to hear and attend to the speech of others in order to acquire speech themselves. The first sounds that children produce are the sounds that occur most frequently in the language they hear; these sounds differ from one language to another. The '*v*' sound, which is a relatively uncommon sound in English, is late to be acquired by English-speaking children, but it is heard much earlier in the vocalizations of Swedish children, where '*v*' occurs more frequently in words. This indicates that sound frequency rather than difficulty of articulation influences the acquisition of sounds. Children with intermittent hearing loss due to otitis media score less well on speech and language tests than their peers, especially if it was during their first year of life, indicating that this time is a critical period for receiving, perceiving and assimilating auditory information.

Cognitive level

At this level children may have difficulty with the processing of speech. A faulty mental representation of speech sound can cause a *pure phonological disorder without* associated articulatory problems. In practical terms, it can be difficult to differentiate between a pure phonological disorder and a more general speech disorder, and, frequently, unclear speech will be caused by a combination of phonological and articulatory problems. A well specified mental representation of the sound (phonological) structure of words is necessary to process speech. Faulty representations will give rise to errors in pronunciation, for example, 'basketti', 'hopital' and 'hitapotamus' for spaghetti, hospital and hippopotamus respectively. These errors occur naturally in normal development and they are only considered to be a problem if they persist or if speech becomes unintelligible. Phonological representations are constantly updated with new representations being introduced for new words and old representations being updated. There may be a time lag between acquiring sounds in new words and updating existing phonological representations, for example, children may master the '**r**' sound in new vocabulary such as 'robot', but continue to pronounce 'rabbit' as '**w**abbit'. Children with a pure phonological disorder can often imitate a target sound in isolation, but they have difficulty producing the same sound in speech. This reduces the ability to signal meaning. For example, a child might be able to say the 's' sound in isolation but says 'tock' for sock and 'tea' for sea. Phonological disorders pose a particular risk for literacy difficulties.

Neuromuscular level (see above)

Articulatory level

A *pure articulation disorder* is characterized as a malfunction of the speech production mechanism. Children with articulation problems are not able to articulate a target sound and will substitute the desired sound with another. This reduces the ability to signal meaning differences and, therefore, can have phonological consequences. For example, a child who cannot articulate the sounds 's' and 'sh' and replaces both of them with the 't' sound will pronounce 'see/she/tea' as 'tea', and 'sin/shin/tin' as 'tin'.

Oromotor, verbal or developmental dyspraxia

This is an impairment of the ability to programme the position of the speech musculature and the sequence of muscle movements for the volitional production of phonemes (Stackhouse & Miller 1990). Children with verbal dyspraxia often present with extremely disordered articulation of speech sounds. Speech can be dysfluent and at times unintelligible, and there is often evidence of motor planning and coordination deficits. Comprehension of language is usually age appropriate. If children cannot be understood they may become socially withdrawn or develop other emotional or behaviour problems. These children often require intensive speech therapy possibly in a language unit and, in extreme cases, an alternative communication system, such as signing.

SEMANTIC AND PRAGMATIC LANGUAGE IMPAIRMENT

Children with semantic and pragmatic language impairments often present as fluent speakers, but their difficulties are with the meanings of words and sentences (semantics) and the use of language in context (pragmatics). It is often seen in children with ASD.

Children with these difficulties are likely to comprehend language literally and use stereotyped and empty language to communicate. They frequently have difficulty making friendships and fitting in with their peer group.

DYSFLUENCY (STAMMER/STUTTER)

Approximately 4% of children between the ages of 2 and 4 years go through a period of normal non-fluency. However, in about 1% of these children the problem does not resolve and the child will continue to have dysfluent speech. Dysfluency is a communication difficulty, not simply a speech problem. It can greatly undermine confidence and affects social, behavioural and educational performance. Boys are four times more likely to be dysfluent than girls. Early referral to a speech and language therapist is particularly important to ensure that assessment, advice and treatment can be given before the stammer becomes entrenched. There are several important features of dysfluency.

Guidelines for referral to speech and language therapy

Children with a clear medical condition or syndrome that is known to affect language development will usually be referred to speech and language therapy by their paediatrician. Other children with less obvious risk factors are usually referred by their health visitor or GP following the child's 21–month or 3$\frac{1}{2}$ year–developmental check. These two ages will be looked at separately and referral guidelines given for each respectively. When there are any concerns about a child's language development the first thing that needs to be tested is their hearing. It is vital to *exclude hearing loss* as a cause of delay before any other assessments are administered. Generally, if children's speech and language are at or below a level expected in children about two-thirds their age, there may be a problem that requires further investigation: e.g. a 21–month–old at a 14–month level or a 3$\frac{1}{2}$-year-old at a 28–month level. Babies may have a developmental check at 8 months

Table 8.12   Indications for speech and language therapy referral at 21 months

Receptive language	Expressive communication	Social interaction	Play
Not responding to own name			Persistent mouthing of objects
Unable to follow simple commands, such as, 'Give it to Mummy'	Not pointing or using gesture to communicate	Poor eye contact	Indiscriminate banging or casting of toys
Not able to identify common objects when named	Limited babble or jargon vocalizations	Socially withdrawn	No pretend or symbolic play such as, feeding a doll or pushing cars along an imaginary road
Unaware of the function of common objects (brush, spoon, cup)		Prolonged passive behaviour without attempting to interact or play with others	

Table 8.13   Indications for speech and language therapy referral at 3½ years

Receptive language	Expressive communication	Social interaction
Not understanding a command such as 'Give me the *little* ball' or 'Put it *under* the table'	Only using single words or two-word phrases	Limited eye contact and facial expressions
Unable to identify body parts such as eyes, hair and toes	Not using any grammatical markers such as verb endings or plurals	Lack of awareness of other people's presence or feelings
Unable to identify objects by colour such as 'red ball' or 'blue cup'	Not asking questions	Shows no interest in playing with other children
Parents comment that child does not appear to understand what people say	Frustrated by inability to communicate, may use gesture such as pulling people by the hand to something they want	Does not want to share an activity and would prefer to be alone
Not interested in stories	Echolalia – repeating words or phrases they hear Speech is very unclear and cannot be understood by people outside the family Sounds omitted from words, e.g. not saying the beginning or ends of words When dysfluency persists after 4 years of age and there is a family history plus raised anxiety in the child or parent	Poor symbolic or imaginative play skills

and, although some babies might be babbling at this stage, it is not unusual for babies to still be making open vowels sounds. However, if babies are not vocalizing at all and seem reluctant to interact, they should be referred for a hearing or general developmental assessment. Referral to speech and language therapy at any age is indicated if there is a *family history* of speech and language problems, *combined with specific concerns about the child.*

21-month developmental check

Although many children have a large vocabulary and may have started to join two words together by 21 months, some may only be beginning to develop communicative speech and yet still be developing within normal limits. It is, therefore, much more important to look at the child's social, interactive and play skills as a whole rather than simply counting words. Often children who are slow to speak are skilled communicators, showing a desire for interaction, using eye contact, gesture (particularly pointing) and vocalizations to get their message across. It would be inappropriate to refer these children as this would cause unnecessary anxiety for the parents and child. Referrals should **not** be made for inaccurate or poorly articulated speech sounds at 21 months (Table 8.12).

3½–year developmental check

By 3½ most children will be speaking in sentences that are 90% grammatically correct and 90% intelligible to others. They are able to understand increasingly complex instructions including prepositions and comparatives. It is important to remember that this is a common age for normal non-fluency and, where possible, this should be excluded before a referral for dysfluency is made (Table 8.13).

Children are likely to have a number of immature speech patterns at 3½. Referrals are not appropriate at this age for lisping, consonant cluster reduction (e.g. 'tamp' for 'stamp') or for difficulty articulating – *r, l, h, th, sh, ch* and *j*.

References

Cantwell DP, Baker L 1985 Psychiatric and learning disorders in children with speech and language disorders. Advances in Learning and Behavior Disabilities, 4:29–47

Pinker S 1994 The Language Instinct: The New Science of Language and Mind. Penguin Books, London

Skinner BF 1957 Verbal Learning. Appleton-Century-Crofts, New York

Stackhouse J, Miller C 1990 The nature of speech and language problems in children: module 2, course text 2. HMSO London,

Further reading

Crystal D 1987 The Cambridge Encyclopedia of Language. Cambridge University Press, New York

Lynch C, Kidd J 1999 Early Communication Skills. Bicester: Winslow Press/Speechmark

Websites

www.ican.org.uk (I CAN is a charity which helps children to communicate)

9 Play

S. Scott-Roberts, L. Westcott

▼ OVERVIEW

The study of play is said to be crucial to the understanding of the developing child. This chapter will discuss and examine a range of themes that contribute to this important area of activity in human development. Influenced by Western European understanding, the meaning of play will first be explored and then discussed in terms of skills used and impact of environmental influences on play, looking at how play occurs and asking the question 'Why play?'

In order to achieve this, some influential theorists will be introduced that have specialized in this interesting area. So that the fullest implications of play and its potential within child development are recognized, the chapter considers relevant biological, psychological and social concepts. This holistic perspective is influenced by the professional philosophy of the authors as occupational therapists. A brief overview of the enduring nature of play beyond childhood will also be included.

Blunden (1991) states that there is no such thing as a normal child, but each is a different and unique individual. This chapter will explore what play is, the skills needed and developed within play and the environmental influences that impact on the child.

WHAT IS PLAY?

This seemingly straightforward question is in fact a complex and difficult area that has triggered much work and debate amongst theorists and researchers.

Difficulties in defining play

Since the late nineteenth century, play has been recognized as a meaningful rather than a trivial behaviour. Over the years there have been numerous attempts to define what play is, but attempts have struggled due to various degrees of duplication and contradiction. This may be because play cannot be narrowed simply to a single set of behaviours, undertaken in specific conditions or situations (play need not be confined to 'play times'). It is true to say that everyone reading this chapter will have their own ideas of what play includes and be able to recognize many examples in action. However, vast amounts of ambiguity remain as to what may be considered play and what may not.

In an attempt to define play, we may in fact be adding unhelpful boundaries that serve to restrict the shaping and understanding of childhood activities. With that in mind, this section does not attempt to define play, but instead will explore some of these ambiguities in order to identify key elements of what play is about.

CATEGORIZATION PLAY THEORIES

Categorizing play activities appears to be a useful way to break down the topic area into clearly delineated groups. One influential worker in this area was Jean Piaget (1896–1980), a Swiss psychologist who is best known for his stage theory of cognitive development in childhood. Piaget saw play as a functional set of activities in which children could assimilate skills. He worked to categorize and organize play activities, naming each one. Some critics see this theory as struggling to capture the real essence of play in an attempt to impose an academic framework onto a non-academic pursuit.

Playfulness theories

This group of theories is devised by outlining criteria of what may be considered as playful and non-playful actions. This suggests that a level of playfulness can be derived simply by outlining the behaviours used to engage in activities of all sorts. It would seem that examining some key characteristics of playful behaviour, rather than the activities that may be seen as types of play, allows a better opportunity to try and define the broadness of what can be called play. Criteria for playfulness can even be determined to decide if a particular activity could be considered play or not. This is useful in allowing for the huge diversity of human activity that could be seen as play or playful in kind.

Developmental theories of play

A common view of play is that it forms a means to further development. Vygotsky regarded play as the leading source of development in the pre-school years. He was able to link play with ideas of learning and motivation. Through play, children are motivated to learn, so learning that occurs in meaningful contexts becomes a spur to further motivation and, hence, to further learning. Within the educational system this developmental view has been embraced and utilized in the design of school curricula. Play has been categorized into domains of development.

Psychological theories of play: behaviourism

From a behaviourist viewpoint, human learning is regarded purely in terms of stimuli from the environment evoking learned behaviour. Play can be seen as a learned phenomenon that results from positive interaction with the child's surroundings. A positive sense of fun or excitement gained from involvement in play can be seen as a form of operant conditioning. Enjoyment and excitement act as positive reinforcers or rewards for engaging in play situations, which means that the child will be likely to respond to potential stimuli for enjoyable types of play with playful behaviours.

The play becomes the reward for itself, explaining why having the chance to be 'just playing' is in fact enough to engage children into doing it, rather than seeking opportunities for play in order to achieve a finite end result. On the other hand, low levels of enjoyment discourage further pursuit as the positive reinforcer to continue is absent. In behavioural terms the desire to continue with the behaviour or activity can be said to have been extinguished: the child gets bored and the activity stops or changes to something more rewarding. As well as being a self-reinforcing activity, play can also be used as a reinforcer for other behaviours desired by adults, such as a reward for finishing homework or tidying a bedroom. Play only works as an effective reinforcer in this respect because it is something desired by the child.

Psychological theories of play: psychodynamic ideas

Psychodynamic theorists influenced by the ideas of Sigmund Freud (1856–1939) and his successors (notably his daughter Anna Freud [1895–1982]) have proved influential in the study and explanation of children's behaviour in play. Influenced by ideas of the power of the unconscious and unresolved internal conflicts, theorists of this tradition examine and analyse how these themes are translated into action. For children the action is play. Psychodynamic theorists believe that children play out situations and think through their meaning (Winnicott 1971). Play is an activity where the unconscious internal world of the child is put on show and the child can work through solutions to problems or difficulties that disturb the internal world. In therapy this approach is used as a tool to explore and resolve difficulties.

Psychological theories of play: humanism

The most influential thinker about play within this tradition of psychology was Virginia Axline (1947–1989) who viewed the child as an innate force for change engaged in perpetual self-development. Within a context of unconditional positive regard, Axline recognized that play is the natural medium for children to express themselves. She developed eight key principles of play therapy that are still upheld as an influential practical guide for play therapists. The use of these can be seen in the readable account of play therapy with a young boy, 'Dibs' (Axline 1964).

CHARACTERISTICS OF PLAY

Blunden (1991) noted that there is no right or wrong way to play. For the child the play process is more important than the outcome achieved. This observation also points to the importance of playful behaviour rather than the activity itself. It stands true irrespective of whether a product emerges from the play. Thus children could engage in a self–care activity such as bathing in a playful way, holding their breath under water or blowing bubbles and enjoying the experience. On the other hand they could participate in a structured 'play' activity like a board game without demonstrating any playfulness behaviours at all.

It is important to stress that playfulness has a useful purpose and play is a most meaningful activity for children (and many adults). For children, play can be seen as serious activity, not just a diversion from the rest of their life or something to fill idle time. The vital point to note from this is that the key purpose of play in childhood is to enhance a child's development and this constitutes the serious activity. Part of the serious purpose of play occurs as the child acquires the skills necessary to move successfully in adulthood through the development gained from deriving fun, enjoyment and excitement from play activities.

Despite the serious purpose of play, Garvey (1977) delineates some key factors that are critical to defining what play is. Play is characterized by being positively valued by the player, giving pleasure and a sense of enjoyment. Play is spontaneous, children cannot be forced to play and in this sense it is an optional not obligatory activity.

This sense of spontaneity and the ad hoc way in which people engage in and out of play can be at odds to the declared 'official' purpose of a task. This has the potential to lead to confusion that can sometimes enhance the sense of fun for those engaged in the play, even if conflict is the result. Consider children winking and waving to members of a wedding gathering during the peak of the ceremony or flicking paper around a classroom when the teacher is writing on the blackboard. In these kinds of situation a blurred understanding seems to operate of what is acceptable and what is not. The protagonists consider the pleasure of engaging in play to outweigh the risk of consequences. Adults who participate in work-environment pranks also illustrate this point well. Often in these circumstances players can appeal to a generalized understanding of the nature of play. The well used excuse 'I was only playing around', infers that play should be condoned or forgiven even if a particular behaviour may be regarded as unacceptable in that situation. The implication is that the concept called 'play' forms part of an understandable and acceptable side of human behaviour without harmful intent.

Acting to seek a sense of satisfaction from participating in play activities can be viewed as an intrinsic motivator for playing. Even in the absence of external extrinsic goals there still exists a strong internal drive or need to play (Garvey 1977). The child, therefore, can be viewed as active in seeking engagement in further episodes of playfulness. This is different, however, if children perpetually derive no enjoyment from activities than might be seen by some people as play, such as learning a musical instrument or a sporting activity. What is important to note here, is that any activity in itself needs to be considered enjoyable by the individual for them to consider it as play. The range and type of activities will vary from individual to individual. This is why parents or adults can provide children with numerous toys only to find them neglected and untouched. It is the adult who sees the toy as affording potential fun not the child. Consider for example the caricature of a father buying his son a train set or electric car track only to play with it himself!

Excitement and stimulation also reinforce the desire to engage in play activities even if the level of excitement experienced is mixed with other emotions such as fear. Children like to experiment and risk–take with fear-inducing play or leisure activities, especially when the risk is also acknowledged as being within some kind of safe limit. A child may, therefore, repeatedly use thrill-seeking fairground rides, combining experiences of excitement, enjoyment and fear. Scary movies are seen as enjoyable and games that make participants jump are joined in with a sense of endless fun. Some children seem to be more likely to engage in such thrill-seeking play, especially those with more extroverted characteristics. As children pass into adolescence, thrill-seeking play may also be linked with a wish to demonstrate braveness and spirit to other people.

The child's level of playfulness is dependent upon the balance of three elements:

1. The amount of control a child perceives to have over what and with whom they play.
2. The intrinsic drive and motivation to participate.
3. The freedom to suspend reality.

Bundy (1996) believes that a child's level of playfulness is dependent on all of these behaviours, seeing each on a continuum. Their position on this scale may alter playfulness. Alterations may occur if the child perceives the play opportunity as being controlled by an adult or if the only reason to participate is to gain an external award, for example stars or sweets.

In conclusion, despite the ambiguities that exist, play has key characteristics. These are playfulness, fun, excitement, enjoyment and stimulation. Participation in play can be at odds sometimes with the overt purpose of an activity. Engagement in play has the important consequence of enhancing a child's development.

SKILLS USED IN PLAY (WHY PLAY?)

Although difficulties can be encountered in defining what the characteristics of play actually are, a useful way of advancing our understanding it is to examine key component skills that are developed through this childhood activity. This provides an insight into why children play from a developmental perspective. Play provides opportunities for children to practise and develop a wide range of skills that will ultimately prepare them for adult life. This process means that play is now commonly used as a core treatment modality for children with a wide range of problems.

This section considers groups of key component skills and, although these have been considered under distinct headings, this has been done for the benefit of the reader. Human learning and development is so very complex that no single area of study can account for all the processes involved. In reality, individual skill components do not develop alone and a child instinctively utilizes an appropriate mixture of skills when engaging in any activity. It is fair to say that the stage of development will govern a child's level of competence at any particular activity. It is, therefore, important when working with children to consider how the developmental level can affect play or be improved by offering appropriate play opportunities.

Component skills developed through play

Sensorimotor

There is a rapid acquisition of motor skills in the first few years of life after which development of new skills slows down and a period of refining appears to go on until adulthood. During the first years of their life the infant gains voluntary control of movements by firstly integrating some of the primitive reflexes present since before birth. For example, prior to the integration of the asymmetric tonic reflex, during the first few months of life, when a baby turns the head to the side the arm on the same side straightens or extends while the other arm bends or flexes. This makes it difficult for the infant to explore a toy fixed on the side of the cot with both hands, as arm movements are controlled by the position of the head.

The voluntary control of the movements of the limbs is gained as the central nervous system matures. Control develops in a cephalocaudal direction (meaning motor skills develop in a head to toe direction) and from proximal to distal (nearest to the body to furthest away). This is reflected in the play activities a child engages in. The baby that has not yet gained head control will need their head and trunk supported if they are going to attempt to reach for the mobile hanging above them. This pattern of development means that head control and trunk control needs to be gained before the child can walk or use hands purposefully.

Control of the joints nearest the body (proximal), needs to be gained before control can be achieved of the joints furthest away (distal). At about 18 months the child has sufficient shoulder stability to begin to gain control of the elbow, wrist and joints of the hand. A child of this age will have sufficient control to be able to hold a large crayon in a gross grasp, in the palm of the hand, and can make large arm movements to form random/scribble marks on paper. The child's older sister of 4 years, however, has continued to gain increasing control of her upper limb joints. She now has more control over the movements she makes with her pencil. She now holds her pencil between her thumb, index and middle finger and carefully selects movements that will allow her to draw straight lines and stop and change the direction of the pencil, so giving her sufficient control to draw shapes or form letters to write her name. She enjoys the praise she receives for colouring between the lines and she has begun to seek more complex tasks that utilize tools, for example cutting with scissors.

The control and quality of a child's movement is dependent on the interpretation and integration of the sensory information received from the environment. In early childhood the child makes sense of their world directly from sensations. The child of 7 years and below can be described as a sensory processing machine that does not have many thoughts and ideas about things, but is mainly concerned with sensing them and moving its body in response to the sensation. The child responds to a sensory experience by performing a purposeful goal–directed movement, known as an adaptive response. The formation of an adaptive response allows the brain to develop and organize itself. The toddler who first sits on a rocking horse is often initially nervous about being rocked backwards and forwards on the toy. However, the game quickly becomes enjoyable and repetition of the action is sought again and again until they can initiate the movement themselves. The child has gained sufficient adaptation to the sensory input received while on the toy and has mastered the necessary motor skills not only to cope with the movement, but begin to gain control of it.

Children have an innate desire to make sense of their world, and play ensures that sensorimotor processing opportunities are in abundance. Through play the foundations are laid so that more complex tasks, which demand a higher level of sensory processing, such as writing and driving a car, can be achieved in later life.

As children begin to move about in their environment they begin to build up an idea of how their body is spatially related to objects in the environment. The development of motor skills is accompanied by the development of the perception of space. The small child who crawls or cruises around the room begins to develop a sense of where its body finishes and objects in the environment start. Toddlers quickly learn to negotiate doorways and gaps between furniture and pleasure is gained from play activities that involve positioning their body in, under or through objects in the room (Fig. 9.1).

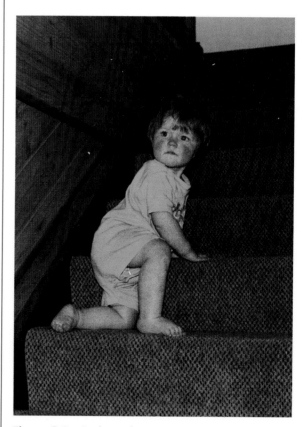

Figure 9.1 Exploring the environment

The ability to make accurate spatial judgements and relate ourselves to that space is dependent upon the integration of sensory information. Tactile, visual, auditory, proprioceptive and vestibular information need to be integrated to give the child an accurate perception of position and orientation within their environment. In the early years these skills are reflected in the play choices children make. Commercially purchased play tunnels and tents offer opportunities to develop and refine spatial judgements; however, just as much fun can be had with a large cardboard box that can be climbed in and out of or a den made from a blanket draped over two chairs. During the later years of childhood the ability to make more accurate spatial judgements is reflected in neatly sized and spaced handwriting, play choices that include complex construction and model building and the ability to play sports with friends in confined places, for example indoor football.

Cognitive

Piaget (1951) considered play to be the way children practise cognitive skills. He attempted to discuss the development of play through the classification of games. He described three types of games linking them to key stages in cognitive development. The first stage, 'practice play', occurs during the first 2 years of infancy but also throughout life when new skills are acquired and practised. It does not involve following shared rules or demand any form of make-believe. Bouncing on a bed or playing in a water trough is engaged in purely for the sensorimotor experience and the child repeats the game just for the pleasure of practising it. From approximately 12 months onwards children have identified and remembered how objects are used. They will pick up everyday objects and imitate their use, for example pick up a spoon and take it to their mouth. The play may also include someone else, for example feeding mummy or the doll with the empty spoon. By 24 months of age the child uses unrealistic or invisible objects in their play, for example dolly is now fed with a stick that is meant to represent the spoon. This form of pretend play is described by Piaget as 'symbolic play'. If you visit any nursery or infant school you will observe complex pretend play scenarios, often involving a number of children.

Their play is not dependent on props and they will quickly utilize all manner of things to act out the pretend scene.

According to Piaget, between the age of 7 and 11 years both practice and symbolic play in the main are replaced by 'games with rules'. These games have socially constructed rules and are played by more than one person; they are considered to be important in the development of socialization. These rules can be previously determined such as those that are followed to complete board games or play team sports such as football or the rules can be devised by a group of children involved in the development of their own game. Skills such as turn taking, sequencing and the ability to negotiate are certainly practised during this stage of play. Piaget felt that it was this mode of play that we continue to be involved in throughout our lives. Certainly most adults' leisure time is spent involved in some form of gaming, whether it be in organized sports or playing the latest game on the computer.

Gardner (1983) agreed with Piaget that during late childhood there was a desire to conform and comply with convention, but feels that symbolic play is just submerged and is not replaced by rule-based play. Gardner believes that this stage is essential for the development of creativity as children begin to take on and master the rules and techniques of an art form. This is typified by the child spending time trying to replicate drawings or models rather than designing their own. Prior to this age, the younger child utilizes their newly gained knowledge of their environment and communicates this through the imaginative unique use of play resources. Paintings are colourful and singing and dancing are enthusiastically embraced. This creativity, although submerged during primary school years, is believed to reappear during adolescence and carry on into adulthood. A number of other theorists believe that the continued involvement of the individual in some form of symbolic play, whether that is through an artistic medium or by fantasizing, helps to ensure a flexible, creative and innovative approach to problem solving throughout the life-span.

What Piaget and his counterparts agreed upon, however, was that the learning process is dependent upon active participation in playful activity. Children should be afforded the opportunity to learn through discovery.

Social development and communication

Play has long been highlighted as providing an experiential springboard for social development. Through the medium of play children have opportunities to develop and practise their interactive skills. These interactive skills will ensure that the child can successfully participate with others in their environment. Essentially play is social in origin, is mediated by language and is learned with other people.

It has been suggested that play offers the child opportunity to rehearse and integrate a wide range of skills necessary for communicating with others. Communicating is a complex task that requires the people involved to be able to delineate both the verbal and non-verbal components as well as the interface between them. In order to master this task

children have to learn that communication is about using and understanding words said to them, how they are said and also about the non-verbal cues that may or may not accompany the spoken word (see also Chapter 8).

In play younger children may struggle to understand the language complexities presented by older children or adults, especially if they have used subtleties such as irony, sarcasm or specific body language. The child who fails to understand the joke or to follow the complex verbal and non-verbal instructions of a game may demonstrate their frustration by becoming indifferent, aggressive or withdrawn. As with any other developing skill, the child requires a safe environment to practise within and they will tend to select opportunities when their own communication levels are matched or accommodated. Observation of nursery-aged children playing in the home corner will show that a wide range of communication is taking place. The conversation often mimics the language they have heard spoken at home and is accompanied by

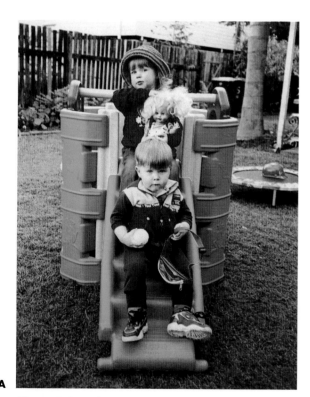

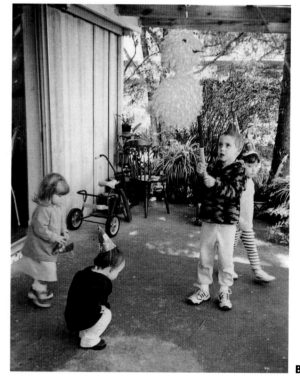

A   B

Figure 9.2 Taking turns

gestures that are used by the significant adults in their life, for example finger wagging to accompany words of warning. Also more subtle skills such as turn taking and listening that are also essential for successful communication, are practised between children or even on toys such as dolls and teddy bears (Fig. 9.2).

The children playing in the home corner will also make decisions about what is and is not acceptable behaviour in this setting. This experience allows them to develop and test out ideas and begin to internalize rules or codes of interactive behaviour. They are forced to acknowledge their playmate's point of view and to consider their own perspective. This broadens their concepts of the real world as well as enriching their social skills. Play experience can thus be seen to be important in the development of cooperative behaviour, performance in team problem-solving tasks and leads to more sensitive role taking in social groups. Children who have difficulties accommodating their play within the social demands of other children, perhaps because they find it difficult to understand these subtle social rules or norms (often seen in Asperger's syndrome) are more likely to become isolated from their peers or to withdraw from opportunities where social skills can be practised, and may continue to experience social interaction difficulties into later life.

At a young age the primary mode of communication between parents and their children is play. The mother, who bounces her baby on her knee while singing a nursery rhyme, will note that she has engaged the baby in two-way communication. The baby will provide the mother with eye contact and listen to the song being sung, intermittently vocalizing in response. The mother monitors the baby's reaction and continues to respond to the child's interactions in a meaningful way by smiling and continuing the song. The need to accommodate and respond appropriately to children's communications becomes increasingly harder as they become older and a unique opportunity for adults to understand how the child views and interprets the world around them can be lost. The older child who constantly asks 'why?' and receives an understandable answer will continue to be interested and inquisitive and make continued efforts to communicate. The child who is consistently told to be quiet will eventually cease in their efforts to make conversation.

Social development theory considers the child's increasing ability to interact within a variety of demanding social environments. Throughout their childhood, children form and develop a number of different friendships. The nature of these friendships has been noted to change as the child develops. Young children have transient playmates anywhere they find themselves at play, while older children form lasting bonds based on trust and recognition of need. During play children can observe, assimilate and try out their emerging social skills and link with others, thus play affords a medium for forming and sharing relationships.

Children sometimes include imaginary characters such as an animal or person in their play. This is often a transient occurrence, although some may become a more established phenomenon in the form of an imaginary friend. It is well known that some young children develop the persona of their imaginary friend, including and consulting the opinion of the 'friend' in many activities involving family members or peers. This is thought to provide companionship for some children, especially those with no similarly aged siblings. Friendship plays a vital role in developing a child's social skills and sense of self. Another interpretation of such imaginary companions is that they allow the child a creative outlet. A 'friend' can even provide an opportunity for the child to disassociate from aspects of the self as naughty or disapproved of behaviour may be blamed on the imaginary friend. The 'friend' offers a safe context to play with socialization issues or lay blame. Children do tend to lose their imaginary friends as they develop and form a wider range of meaningful relationship with peers, for example. when they start attending school. For most children pretend play is particularly important for development up to and around 6 years of age.

It is important to note that children can be highly adaptable in the roles they choose to use and demonstrate in play. They may for instance choose to use only the skill levels of a younger child within play activities. This might be seen when an older child plays alongside a younger sibling, adopting the behavioural and even the speech patterns of the younger child. This ability to choose to regress to the expected behaviour of someone younger is widely recognized in play therapy.

Self-development

Children need to develop a positive view of themselves to enable them to make successful social relationships and manage the social environment around them. Play allows a child to develop an awareness of self-identity. Through the praise derived from being engaged in play given by other children and significant adults, children begin to build a picture of how others perceive them. Their success and failure to access and gain pleasure from the play activity itself will also impact upon their confidence and feelings of self-worth.

Developments during the first decade of life, particularly in the areas of cognition and language, allow children to begin to understand, evaluate and express how they feel about themselves. Through play children can develop and practise the skills needed to shape an emerging sense of the self. It allows them to interact with a range of objects, experience an array of locations and come in contact with a variety of people. A young child at play may tell you that his teacher has said he is good at colouring and he may also claim to be good at an array of other tasks, often not associated with the initial activity, for example running or football. He has taken on board the positive feedback given by his teacher and has generalized it to other activities as he is still too young to make differentiated judgements of ability. This global judgment of the self is reflected in the approach most children take to trying out new play equipment or taking part in play activities, for example 'I can run and kick a ball so I can play football with the older boys on the play ground'. Positive feedback helps the children build up a picture of how others view them; however, negative feedback will also have an impact and this may result in the child not trying new activities.

A significant developmental transition occurring approximately between the ages of 7 and 11 years, labelled by Piaget as the concrete operational period, coincides with the child's increased ability to make differentiated judgements about their own competence in an everyday activity. The emergence of logical thinking, that enables the child to classify and logically organize the concrete experiences in their life, potentially allows the child to begin to define what their attributes are, for example. 'I have a lot of friends who want to play with me in the playground because I am good at football'.

It is also at this stage that the child becomes conscious of being judged by others: 'self-consciousness'. As a consequence of this process a new skill emerges, the ability for self-evaluation. As children become more able and accurate at comparing selves with peers, they begin to recognize that they are good at some skills, but not others, and play choices reflect these evaluations of abilities and difficulties. Play activities chosen will often utilize skills that a child feels capable of carrying out successfully. Children who do not consider themselves to be artistic and/or musical will avoid such play activities. They are less likely to enjoy those activities perceived as offering potential for failure. In this way play allows children to come to a realization of who they are by giving them opportunities to experience emotion and consider their position in the world.

By the onset of adolescence the individual is able to think abstractly about his or her attributes, behaviours, emotions and motives. Being prepared to pursue activities that require practice, they can be more persistent in attempts to master skills as initial failure is recognized as transient and part of the learning process.

Role development

Play can be viewed as a medium in which children and young people imitate and experiment with potential roles for adult life. Some of this can be seen as a selection process in which a range of roles can be tried out within the safety of the play environment and some of these will inevitably become a rehearsal for adulthood.

This area of development is important to discuss as a discrete entity. It has been placed at the end of this section, however, because it also demonstrates how the component skills explored above can be integrated effectively to facilitate the emergence of more complex skill areas.

Children often mirror what they see in the world around them within their play. For young children this may be explicitly encouraged, such as the home corner of most nursery or school reception classes. Here children are encouraged to play adopting various adult and children's roles within a familiar domestic setting. Observation of young children can show both imitative play, reflecting say a family mealtime or 'adults' dealing with a 'naughty child'. Sometimes the boundaries of normality may be altered or push into fantasy. A child with younger siblings may become the baby in playing at families; young children may take cross-gender roles or experiment with exaggerated patterns of behaviour such as being the naughtiest child, a child with magic powers, a parent who is secretly magic or Superman! This tendency to imitate and reflect the world at home may be used in play therapy to show and work through difficult experiences with the child.

The lasting impact of such imitative play on a child's psychological development has been widely debated. Imitation, particularly of violent behaviour seen on television and other visual media like consul games have been cited as a cause for concern. Some links have been made between crime and deviance in the young and exposure to violent role models from television and film. Evidence such as Bandura's classic experiments (1986), where children were seen to imitate adult violence towards a large doll, have been used to support this argument. There is not a simple relationship, however, between levels of exposure to violent role models, the amount of imitative play seen in childhood and engaging in violence in adult life. It is true to say that many children will be exposed to violent television programmes and imitate or reflect some of this in their play, but not go onto adult violence or crime; for others, however, this may be different.

For older children and adolescents, role imitation and rehearsal can reflect the stage of development marked by the need to establish an autonomous more adult self. This need was highlighted by Erikson (1968), who described adolescents as feeling a need to attain autonomy versus experiences of guilt. This idea of conflicting psychological experiences can be reflected in the wide range of play or experimental leisure activities that young people engage in during this stage of the life-cycle. Play may reflect behaviours seen in the world around the young person, and can include experimentation with activities perceived as more risky as boundaries are explored and the consequences evaluated by the individual.

The innate need to develop autonomy and an adult identity may lead to idolization of older peers or celebrities and their behaviour (a phenomenon well recognized by the advertising industry).

Activities that can be seen to demonstrate achievement may be valued, with competitive occupations becoming important as a process to maintain levels of self esteem. This may be through leisure activities approved of by adults such as competitive sports activities or engaging in established award-based organizations like Scouts or Guides. Conversely such activities may evoke adult concern including sexual behaviours, experimenting with substances, gang involvement, graffiti art and other activities that might be considered risky, antisocial or delinquent.

Despite the drive to develop an adult self identity, activity can often lapse from role playing 'adult'-type behaviours to playfulness. Sometimes this can be considered excessive, for example washing the car becomes a lengthy water fight. The range of play activities and behaviours are particularly influenced during adolescence by the strength of friendship bonds to peers. Young people value highly the company and bonds with their friends; however, it can lead to conflict or anxiety within their families who may find their own plans or values being considered less desirable than those of the peer group! This can be seen with adolescents who want to stay at home with their friends rather than travel on the annual family holiday.

In conclusion, most play activities incorporate a wealth of different skills, hence the use of play as an assessment medium by health and education professionals. Children do not discriminate between these domains, integrating their actions to the demands of the situation. Many children will, however, adapt their environment to ensure that the play activity will be a positive experience for them, for example a child who struggles to concentrate in a busy home by retreating behind the sofa to read a book.

ENVIRONMENTAL INFLUENCES ON PLAY (HOW AND WHERE PLAY CAN OCCUR)

The ability to gain pleasure from play opportunities is dependent upon the interplay of the individual's growth and development and the physical and social environment that they find themselves in. Through play the child is able to act upon and learn to control aspects of their environment. It is also possible, however, for the environment to impact upon the child's play experiences.

Physical environment

Children do not need an elaborate playroom full of commercially produced toys to become engaged in playful activity. Most children offered time, space and objects to explore will turn any everyday activity into an opportunity to be playful, for example bath time becomes fun if the child is offered a range of empty containers and time to play. The innate desire to explore their surrounding environment ensures that the most unusual objects become toys. The child who sits happily in the garden making pretend cakes and pies out of mud is gaining a wealth of sensory experiences that will contribute to the refinement of skills and future learning, but is also having fun. A lack of sensory stimulation affording play opportunities and access to objects that could be used as toys is believed to be responsible for much of the retardation found in institutionalized and deprived children like those found in Eastern European orphanages after the removal of the Iron Curtain.

To classify what makes an object a toy is difficult. It appears that any object that can be explored and offers the child a sense of excitement and pleasure can be considered a toy. Commercially purchased toys on the whole come with guidelines, for example a board game comes with rules. However, even with a set of guidelines for use the playful child will change the rules and design their own game. This is most obvious when everyday objects become toys. No regard is paid to the original use of the object and saucepans are explored for their musical properties, cardboard boxes quickly become cars, dens, spaceships or boats. Children appear to be able to separate thoughts of sole purpose from an object, so a box can become a car. They develop actions from ideas rather than from things, so can accurately role play being a policeman without the necessary uniform or equipment and without ever having had contact with one.

The novelty or newness of an object can be the lure for the younger child to play with it. Almost all new objects that lend themselves to investigation will offer a challenge to the child. This in turn maintains their motivation to utilize it in a playful way. If the object offers the right challenge for the child's developmental level it will be utilized, but if the toy fails to offer the child sufficient challenge or is beyond their developmental level, it will be abandoned for something more suitable. A Jack-in-the-box offers an appropriate level of novelty and complexity to keep a toddler occupied for some time; however, this toy is quickly discarded by an older child once they have completed the necessary procedure once. This is because it no longer offers the right level of challenge.

The opportunity to play is not just dependent upon the provision of suitable objects, but also upon the child's ability to access and master the physical environment. We have already discussed how the need to explore the wider environment is necessary for the development of skills. This is illustrated by negative effect on play development that may be imposed by simple environmental restrictions such as not allowing a young child to play on the floor. It is often the case that in an attempt to ensure that their child is safe, a parent will place them in a play-pen, disregarding that this confinement may restrict the exploration that is needed for learning through play. The balance between ensuring safety and allowing the exploration opportunities each child needs is, at times, difficult for all parents to maintain and is not restricted to just early childhood.

When children become ambulant the stairs become an area of concern for carers and also have the effect of luring the child towards them. Left unattended the child could be in danger, but the supervised exploration of this unusual 'toy' offers opportunities to introduce and refine skills needed for independent living. The older child who wishes to play outside on their bicycle with friends does so often at risk from passing traffic or rough terrain that challenges both cognitive and motor skills. Parents can place boundaries to try and increase their child's safety without restricting an opportunity for play thus allowing their child the scope for interaction and competition with their peers and mastery of their new environment, for example. the child stays within a certain radius of their home, comes home at an agreed time and wears safety gear.

Social and cultural environment

Play often reflects the social encounters that children experience. The younger child will model the adult behaviours they observe daily during their play. A group of 5–year–olds playing school will repeat the instructions they hear from their class teacher daily. This social modelling also allows them to develop a perception of what is and isn't acceptable behaviour. The anthropologist Margaret Mead believed that the social rules and norms that regulate the conduct of society are learnt through play.

By middle childhood the variety of settings in which the child plays has increased and so have the social encounters. Children are involved with more adults other than their family members. These adults are often in a position of authority, for example teachers, and they will make more complex demands of the child. Play at this stage reflects the increasing expectation to conform and is often dominated by games with rules and play activities, such as craft and construction play, which have clear sequences of instructions to follow. By 7 years of age, children begin to compare themselves with their peers. The impact of success and failure to measure up to the expectations of others or to their peers is now important for the developing self-concept.

The child's perception of social support is an important part of self-evaluation. A consistent approach by adults to things such as discipline, active listening, and encouragement to be involved in decision making, is important for the development of high self worth.

Young children initially move from playing in isolation, to playing alongside other children and eventually working cooperatively with their peers. By 6 years of age children are considered to spend over 40% of their waking time with their peers; it is hardly surprising, then, that most play occurs within groups. There is a desire to be with other children and look like one another, with the role of the leader fluctuating during play. As the child moves towards adolescence the groups become more selective and a clear peer culture begins to emerge. Play activities also may become more selective and mastery of hobbies and interests is now starting to be experienced. Play occurs mainly outside the supervision of adults, this autonomy taking place alongside the adolescent's ever increasing awareness of self compared with others, and can mean that some children are excluded from peer groups and are vulnerable to bullying.

What a child might choose to play at or what they ask Santa for at Christmas is not just the result of an independent individual judgement of desire at that time. It is a complicated decision that is influenced and shaped by the values of those surrounding the child. These influences may come from peers, family members, media advertising and culture. A boy at 2–or 3–years–old, for example, may ask for a pink–clad doll of a teenage girl, which may or may not be approved of by their carers. The child will only be given the doll if the carers view it to be a harmless part of the child's development. By the age of 7–8 years the demand by boys for these dolls will have greatly decreased. Their choices will now have been shaped by cultural expectations. Action figures that emphasize traditional masculine qualities such as fitness, strength and skilful fighting will be chosen.

Media and topical elements of the times affect trends in play. Different generations will be influenced by the play fashions of the day, reinforced by advertising especially now on the numerous television channels aimed at children. Many parents will queue for the fashionable toy at Christmas to ensure their child has the latest trend only to find that the trend is short–lived and the toy abandoned within weeks. In contrast, more traditional play activities seem to pass from generation to generation, for example tag and skipping rope games. A number of traditional toys have earned themselves a seemingly perpetual place in the toys shop, with children enjoying play with toys their parents and grandparents valued, for example balls, teddy bears, construction kits and dolls' houses.

Cultural pressures on activity choices can vary according to locality, the social grouping of the family and religious practices. Most children choose to engage in those activities that meet the approval of those around them. This accords positive reinforcement and helps encourage social networks based on shared values and beliefs. This strong pattern of influence on the events in play may be challenged from time to time, although the cost of this for the child can be to meet with conflict. The movie 'Billy Elliot' for example told the story of a young boy in Northern England who joined ballet classes while his family thought he was attending boxing lessons. In the film his father was clear in his disapproval of this choice of activity, despite his son's talent for dance. This may have been different had 'Billy' been brought up in a home that valued achievement in the arts and/or disapproved of fighting as a sport. Most conflicts of this type are avoided, especially by younger children so that they maintain adult and peer approval.

Desire for adult approval may be subsumed during adolescence when the positive opinion of peers is highly valued and young people participate in leisure activities within groups. Adolescents are more likely to choose leisure activities that their peers would value or even make choices that will challenge those of their family or culture. These choices can change again and become more conformist when young people enter adulthood. Over the years many young people's preferences have been described by adults as 'a passing phase'. This was demonstrated during the 1970s and 1980s by the large number of teenagers who chose to become 'punk rockers', adopting a strict dress code and listening to a single genre of music. There are, however, far fewer middle–aged punk rockers in British society!

ADULTS AND PLAY

Although the focus of this book is children, it seems unfair not to include a brief section on adults and play. Play is an important lifelong occupation, the ability to play does not cease with the end of childhood! The skills used by adults to engage in playful behaviour and have fun, begin in childhood. Although adults do not need the full range of developmental potential from play, like children, their involvement in fun activities still serves many important functions for the self in the context of a social environment and creativity. Play not only includes activities with extrinsic motivators like playing squash with the boss, but also includes intrinsically driven activities like spontaneous practical jokes.

Play gives adults an opportunity to form and maintain friendships away from the agendas of other activities such as work. This enhances self-esteem and happiness and consolidates an adult's place within a social group. Engagement in playful or fun activities marks a level of acceptance by others that can be more meaningful than that gained in paid activity. The beneficial effects of play on staff morale, productivity, creativity, and team problem solving are acknowledged increasingly by employers. It is now common to find that employees are offered perks like social or health club membership, or even outdoor pursuit courses to allow people to form social bonds away from the normal workplace. Some enjoy flexible working patterns to make the best of leisure opportunities.

As well as being an important balance to work, play allows adults to relax, facilitating the balance of activity that is essential for wellbeing. The positive use of leisure time in adulthood is increasingly recognized as important for health with an ageing population. Pre-retirement courses focus on positive use of leisure time, as those who are able to learn balanced patterns of activity throughout their adult lives are more likely to enjoy a long and active retirement.

References

Axline V 1964 Dibs; in search of self. Penguin, London
Bandura A 1986 Social Foundations of Thought and Action: a Social Cognitive Theory. Prentice-Hall, New Jersey
Blunden P 2001 The therapeutic use of play. In: Lougher L (ed.) Occupational Therapy for Child and Adolescent Mental Health. Churchill Livingstone, Edinburgh
Erikson E 1968 Identity: Youth and Crisis. Norton, New York
Gardner H 1983 Frames of Mind. Basic Books, New York
Garvey C 1977 Play. Fontana, London
Piaget J 1951 Play, Dreams and Imitation in Childhood. Routledge and Kegan Paul, London
Winnicott DW 1971 Playing and Reality. Pelican, Harmondsworth, Middlesex

Further reading

Axline V 1947 Play Therapy. Ballantyne, New York
Frost JL 2001 Play and Child Development. Prentice Hall, Upper Saddle River
Garvey C 1990 Play. Harvard University Press, Cambridge, Mass
Jeffrey LIJ 2002 Therapeutic play. In: Creek J (ed.) Occupational Therapy and Mental Health, 3rd edn. Churchill Livingstone, London
Lougher L (ed.) 2001 Occupational Therapy for Child and Adolescent Mental Health. Churchill Livingstone, Edinburgh
Mellou E 1994 Play theories: a contemporary review. Early Child Development and Care 102: 91–100
Parham LD 1997 Play in Occupational Therapy for Children. Mosby, St Louis
Pelligini AD 1991 Applied Child Study: a Developmental Approach. Erlbaum Associates, New Jersey
Reilly M (ed.) 1974 Play as Exploratory Learning. Sage, Beverley Hills
Sheridan MD 1999 Play in Early Childhood: from Birth to Six Years. Routledge, London
Wood E, Attfield J 1996 Play, Learning and the Early Childhood Curriculum. Paul Chapman, London

10 Motor skills, gait and coordination

J. Brownson

▼ OVERVIEW

A 'broad but orderly sequence' of development entails that 'all aspects of child development are interdependent' (Bellman & Kennedy 2000). This chapter will focus on motor skills, gait and coordination as key milestones in the development of the normal child.

The key stages of motor development lead to the development of a gait pattern and, ultimately, the attainment of sophisticated coordinated skills. 'Normal' can span across a wide range, from the child who is a reluctant participant in formal sporting activities, to the talented gymnast, athlete or team player, and somewhere between these poles there may be the enthusiastic but unskilled players who set themselves unrealistic goals. The examination of motor skills, gait and coordination within this chapter will enable us to understand the significance of their interdependence in the development of the normal child (Table 10.1).

INTRODUCTION

The hierarchy of learning (Haring et al 1978) can be applied to children's development of motor skills, gait and coordination (Tables 10.2–4). Practice, concentration, and effective performance will lead to consolidation of a skill through the following stages:

- acquisition
- fluency
- maintenance
- generalization
- adaptation.

DEVELOPMENTAL THEORIES

The two dominant developmental theories are the neuromaturational theory and the systems theory.

Table 10.1 Domains of development
Gross motor abilities – posture and large movement
Fine motor abilities – motor-adaptive skills
Hearing
Language comprehension
Expressive language
Vision
Social skills
Play skills
Behaviour and emotional development
Cognitive abilities

Table 10.2   Key points in early motor development

Lying on the floor in supine is an ideal position for a baby to 'learn' the movement, truncal stability and control that will be needed for sitting/crawling/walking
Sitting or being placed in a seat is not the best preparation for independent sitting
Babies need the opportunities to lie on firm surfaces
Sleeping in a cot is an ideal place for babies to move and meet resistance, as they can use that resistance in the same way that they use the resistance of the floor to move into or away from positions, and pull themselves onto their knees or up into standing
The age bands reflected in surveillance charts give the opportunity to relate normal ranges of development and should be considered within the sub-scale units of prone, supine, sitting and standing development
Motor skills evolve in a fluid, changing way, but are often noted and recorded as a static evaluation
It is essential to be able to draw a line between what is normal development and what requires further investigation
Age-related clusters of skills provide a useful point of reference; it is the absence of a cluster of skills that is cause for concern

Table 10.3   Key points about gait

Mature gait parameters occur at about 7 years of age
A 4-year–old should be able to hop three steps
Balance on one leg for at least 10 s is achieved by the age of 5 years
Hopping is achieved by 6 years
During the 2nd year of life, genu varum (bow legs) is a common, but normal presentation as is genu valgum (knock knees) during the 3rd year. At 3 years of age 80% of children are said to have knock knees; both features gradually decrease throughout childhood
Knock knees (genu valgum), bow legs (genu varum), flexible flat feet, in-toeing and out-toeing in children often cause parental concern and require strong reassurance
Joint laxity generally diminishes with age, although ethnic differences in joint laxity have been recorded
Orthotic management of flat feet by the provision of in-soles is rarely appropriate; pain or deformity are the indicators for intervention

The neuromaturational theory

This describes changes in gross motor abilities that result from neurological maturation of the central nervous system. It assumes that a 'blue-print' exists in the brain and that the environment plays a secondary role in the emergence of motor skills.

The systems theory

This theory, on the other hand, encompasses all areas of development and is derived from developmental psychology. It recognizes the requirement for maturation of the central nervous system, but includes motivation, cognitive awareness

Table 10.4   Key points in locomotor screening markers

At 2 years of age the young child walks well, but with steps that are rather short and constrained; can be observed to enjoy the pleasure of movement through running, climbing up and down stairs and beginning to jump off the bottom step; and can kick a ball and steer a push-toy

At 2 $\frac{1}{2}$ years the child can walk on tip toes, jump with both feet, stand on one foot, throw and catch a ball using the hands and body together, and practise galloping

At 3 years a child can go up stairs reciprocally (but comes down with two feet to a step), rides a tricycle and hopping may emerge

At 3 $\frac{1}{2}$ years the child is less stable, less secure and less physically coordinated, and may show more fear of falling

4-year-olds can generally go up and down stairs reciprocally, run well and often display great exuberance

A simple screening test for 4-year-olds could look at abilities in:
stair climbing
balancing on one leg
hopping, skipping and running
independent dressing and undressing

and emotional state, which are acknowledged to provide feed-back into the 'blue–print'.

MOTOR DEVELOPMENT

Motor development is one of the best indicators of developmental wellbeing in the first year of life. The rapid changes in motor development occurring in the first few years of life are often compared with stepping stones, building blocks or a series of jigsaws or layers that fit together. One analogy describes the result as being 'a repertoire of jigsaws on different layers from which a child can select to perform different tasks and activities throughout life.'

In order to assess infants and children it is imperative to have a clear understanding and knowledge of development. The expected age-related abilities need to be viewed with recognition of individual characteristics of performance.

When combined with cognitive and communication competence, it becomes clear that motor development is an assemblage of skills that transform a totally dependent infant, whose movements are reflex controlled, to a (comparatively)

independent 5–year–old ready for school, who just requires sophisticated modifications to the repertoire of skills and abilities.

The reflex activity of normal infants becomes modified as they respond to the impact of gravity, handling, movement and the demands placed upon them, and in this way, primitive reflexes become integrated as normal movement takes over under cortical control. However, the premature infant is not neurologically prepared for any of these external pressures. Having been deprived of the opportunity to 'practise' flexion activity in utero, the sudden impact of gravity will significantly alter motor development. Hence the patterns of abnormal movement are emphasized and prolonged when 'normal' influences are not, or cannot, be accommodated.

INTEGRATION OF MOTOR AND SENSORY DEVELOPMENT

Sensory and motor developments are entirely interdependent: a baby will experience sensations both from the environment and from his/her own movement in relation to the environment.

Movement against a firm surface, a soft surface, being held in the mother's arms or being held by an unfamiliar adult all contribute to the continuous sensory/motor loop and, therefore, to the development of the baby's own movement. For example: 5-month-old babies who do not lie on their back and play with their feet are not building up a sensory and motor database of memories of themselves, and this lack of body image could influence and distort their ability to move and learn.

The development of selected movements, for example index finger isolation and segmental rotation, is the key to learning sophisticated movements. For example, an 8–month–old will attempt to explore an object by using all extended fingers. By 10 months, this movement will have been refined by the ability to select just the index finger to successfully poke and prod the object of attention. By 10 months the skill of using the index finger jointly with the thumb to pick up tiny crumbs and morsels will also have been mastered. However, it is not till the age of $4^1/_2$–6 years that this will develop into a mature pencil grip when complex control of the interphalangeal joints has been learnt.

REQUIREMENTS FOR NORMAL MOVEMENT

The movement abilities of the very young baby are generally considered as having reflexes as their foundation. Maturation of the nervous system has been considered to allow motor development, and reflexes have formed the basis of assessment of maturational levels. Early normal movement abilities have been described as being the result of neurological development from a primitive reflex controlled state to a state of posture control against gravity. Righting reactions become modified and develop into equilibrium reactions. A more in-depth look at the way groups of muscles become stronger and work together to use or influence reflex activity alongside sensory and proprioceptive feedback and behavioural aspects has led developmental specialists to see a much more comprehensive picture of motor development.

Rotation

Developmental therapists generally agree that, aside from motivation, rotation is the most important requirement for normal movement and the development of motor skills. The ability to fix one segment of the body while rotating another, not only provides us with balance and control, but also facilitates cognition.

We know that the ability to fix segments of the body is learnt from a supine position in babyhood from where the baby masters head control.

Head turning

At 3 months, when supine, a baby can briefly maintain the head in midline and rotate it from side to side. The control of the neck flexors is improving, but the relatively reduced cervical spine mobility means that head rotation easily elicits the neck righting reaction. This may lead to the baby 'accidently' rolling onto one side, but because, characteristically, a 3–month baby lies with arms abducted the risk of this inadvertent rolling is reduced.

When pulled to sit a head lag will be seen during the early stage of the movement, but becomes controlled midway through the movement. This head lag and the absence of chin tucking demonstrates that the neck flexors are still not strong enough to provide complete head control. Neither is there synergist control from other larger groups of trunk muscles, which, when more developed, will stabilize the shoulders. Increased control of the neck flexor muscles will lead to shoulder girdle stability so that the asymmetrical tonic neck reflex is stimulated less often and may only be seen at rest.

Bringing hands to midline

A 3–month–old will bring hands to the side and feel the body, and will fleetingly regard the hands in midline and may bring them together. At 4 months midline orientation is much stronger; with more active control of the shoulder girdle the hands are more readily brought together to reach for toys. Accuracy is increasing, but controlled release of a toy and the ability to transfer from hand to hand have not yet developed. This developing voluntary control of the hands enables exploration of the face, body and the upper parts of the legs. A mind map of the body is being created. Alongside this is the steady build up of a sensory memory of different textures when other objects are touched.

Moving out of the midline

Rolling to the side from supine occurs from 4 months (although more voluntarily from $5^{1}/_{2}$ months). In the early stages rolling often occurs to visually follow a stimulus; extension of the head and neck initiates the movement, extension appears exaggerated, and the different side–lying position that ensues is generally considered not to help the development of antigravity side flexion of the trunk. This is, therefore, described as a more primitive rolling movement. Rolling through flexion (that is initiated by hip flexion and neck flexion) is considered a much more sophisticated contribution to the development of segmental antigravity rotation.

Flexing hips to reach and touch feet

The controlled symmetrical flexion of the legs that is achieved at about 5 months brings the feet and toes into the visual field. More of that mind map of the body can be created; not only can the feet and toes be touched, but they can be seen (provided that chin tucking can occur) and brought to the mouth with the hands in order for real exploration to occur. A progression is the selective choice to hold only one leg: dissociation of the upper limbs from the lower limbs has begun a real progression towards flexing the upper limbs while maintaining active extension of the hips. The muscle control demanded for this controlled activity is synergic activity of the large trunk muscles. Sitting independently will soon be the natural progression from this newly acquired ability.

Accidental rolling to the side

Until the synergic control is fully active, the result will often be accidental rolling to the side. Initially, a flexed side-lying position results, but the repeated practice in supine of disassociating limb movements (that is flexing and holding one leg while keeping the other straight) leads to using this posture and rolling onto the side so that the bottom leg can be extended while keeping the upper leg flexed. The result is a more stable position from which the lower arm becomes the supporting arm and the upper arm can reach forward for toys,

The action of rolling the upper trunk to reach or to look, soon becomes integrated with controlled flexion of the hips and knees, and by the age of approximately $5^{1}/_{2}$ to 6 months, develops into a purposeful roll.

Observe the 'corkscrewing' of a $5^{1}/_{2}$–month-old, supine on the floor, anxious to reach or look for the mother. The head is arched turning to the contralateral side, but with hips firmly rooted to the supine position.

Sitting to crawling

Many babies will sit unsupported briefly at 6 months, but the time frame for this skill is broad and independent sitting at 9 months is well within normal limits. Initially the base of support is wide, with the legs abducted and externally rotated. The natural development of this ability utilizes rotation as the young child uses the hands as props for the sitting position, then turns to reach up high outside a stable base and centre of gravity. Side sitting becomes

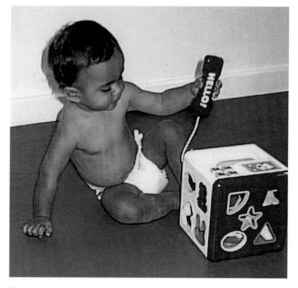

Figure 10.1 Side sitting

another option as the base of support diminishes; one leg remains externally rotated while the other comes to a neutral position, usually to enable the baby to rotate the trunk to reach for a toy (Fig. 10.1).

As children grow, their development is characterized by an increasing ability to consciously control their own movement. Compare the active learning potential of a normally developing 9-month-old child, sat in a pushchair, who eagerly pulls forward from a semi-reclined position and rotates the upper trunk in order to watch and follow a stimulus (e.g. dog or bus), versus the passive learning of the developmentally delayed peer, who is only able to learn passively from stimuli which cross the field of vision.

Standing and walking

The route to walking, for most children, is through crawling on all fours. The adoption of 'all fours' follows naturally from the counterbalance required to reach across the body and move out of the midline. Side sitting, necessary for this movement, is a transitional movement (Fig. 10.1).

The movement in and out of this position is practised again and again, and coupled with the simultaneous inhibition of the symmetrical tonic neck reflex (which is influenced by the baby rocking on all fours and moving backwards), four point

crawling is soon established (Fig. 10.2).

Variations such as commando crawling and bottom shuffling (which is often a family trait) are usually normal, unless associated with variances in other areas of development. Modified crawling and bottom shuffling include the use of a foot to aid propulsion. Bottom shufflers invariably achieve walking later than babies who crawl. This is principally because, not having used the transitional movements to get into four-point kneeling, they have not 'learnt' to feel and experience this shift of their centre of gravity. They have become accustomed to their centre of gravity being behind their legs (as in sitting) rather than forward of their legs (as in four-point kneeling). Some babies miss out this stage altogether, although it is reasonable to assume that they achieve some sort of weight shift and movement from a sitting position in order to get to a standing position.

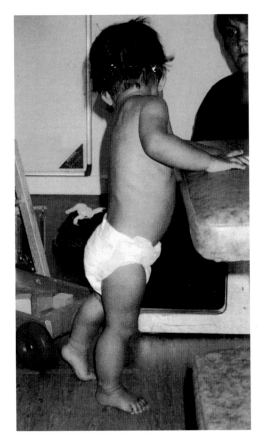

Figure 10.3   Standing

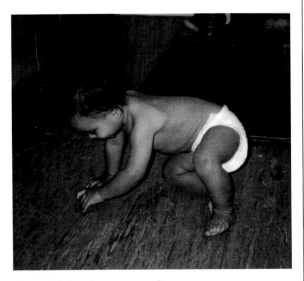

Figure 10.2   Four-point crawling

In standing, segmental rotation of the trunk is necessary for the development of balance and coordination (Fig. 10.3). An essential prerequisite of walking is the ability to take the weight off one leg without collapsing or losing balance in order to progress sideways (cruising) or forwards (walking).

A 10-month-old child who may enjoy bouncing and weight-bearing on the feet will allow the parents to 'walk' them with both hands held high above the head, but will not allow one hand to be held. When the parents attempt this, the child's whole body turns towards the held hand in an attempt to feel safe. A couple of months later the child will readily allow one hand to be held, but by then will have been prepared by the repeated practice of getting up and down from the floor from the crawling position to the standing position, practising the ability to weight shift, 'bear' walking or playing on the floor in a half-kneeling position (Fig. 10.4).

Independent walking (Fig. 10.5) is variously described as being achieved by or during the 12th month (Sutherland et al. 1988), between 11–18 months (Bellman et al 1996), 15 months (Illingworth 1991).

Baby–walkers do not encourage or promote walking. A baby–walker may occupy a child, by allowing access to forward and backward movement, but encourages leaning rather than the crucial development of lateral weight shift or rotation of one segment upon another.

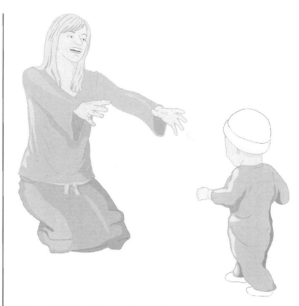

Figure 10.5 Independent walking

In cultures where babies are swaddled (cocooned) and carried with their mothers, development may be different, although not delayed, as the babies might be held, carried, bounced or rocked on a family member's knees, but not necessarily put on the floor. These babies make adaptive postural changes while held in their mother's arms or carried on her back.

Traditionally, in Western cultures, babies were put to sleep in cots, prams or carrycots, and on the floor or in playpens to play. Feeding took place on the lap and progressed to a high chair or at the table. In moving away from these traditions we should be cautious about social and commercial trends that replace these customs with baby seats and baby-walkers, as research suggests that attention deficit and coordination difficulties in children may be the result of babies not having the same experiences of movement as in previous generations.

ATTENTION

It is the baby who leads the mother from her protective holding towards robust handling and boisterous games, but it is the mother who can direct her child towards attention and concentration by

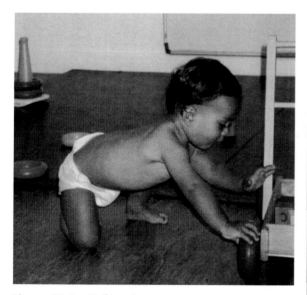

Figure 10.4 Half kneeling position

interacting with the child: talking, playing, smiling and 'demanding' eye contact. This interactive 'reward' system has considerable impact on the bonding process, and the attitude of the parent can significantly affect the developing child. Babies who are not given this attention are likely to find it harder as children to maintain attention.

Psychologists have stressed the importance of reinforcement from trusted adults to encourage exploration and activity. Purpose, motivation and curiosity are considered to be inextricably linked with movement and learning, thus the absence of any one of these is cause for concern. This concept can be contrasted with the use of developmental charts that are task–or skill–orientated: a deficit or delay in any one area within a developmental chart will not necessarily be a cause for concern, rather it is the picture of an array of delays or deficits across a wide range of factors (motor, fine motor, communication, cognitive, feeding, social interaction) that becomes a cause for concern.

The absence of so-called 'transitional movements' and the sequence of acquisition of motor skills may be a clearer marker for identifying concern. The child who is able to lie, sit unattended and be placed in a standing position and 'walked' with hands held, but who is not able to move between any of these positions himself, should alert concern, not for his physical abilities, for he undoubtedly will walk, but for his learning ability.

GAIT

Gait is as unique to an individual as is handwriting. It is not just walking (which can be defined as ' the progress made by advancing each foot alternately, never having both feet off the ground at once'), but rather, walking influenced by the way gravity acts upon the variety of shapes and forms of the human body and the subjective influences of mood or conscious control (Table 10.3).

Development of gait

At certain stages in the development of a mature gait pattern particular characteristics are distinguishable.

As with other aspects of motor development, the development of walking requires mechanical, neurological, cognitive and perceptual factors. The average child crawls at approximately 9 months, walks with support at 12 months, walks without support at 15 months and begins to attempt to run at 18 months.

The physiological changes in the structures of the hip, knees and feet, coupled with growth and developing coordination, present a changing picture of gait. Knowledge of this is required in order to be able to accurately assess normal development.

Early stages: 12–18 months

Early gait is represented by a jerky, wide-based, unsteady movement. The arms are abducted and extended at the elbows (described as 'high guard'); the manner of initial ground contact can be observed to be variable. It is not reproducible as a gait cycle and often resembles the kicking and stepping action that will first have been seen in early infancy. It is useful to note that new walkers often have a transient tip-toe walking phase, while maintaining the ability to stand still with both feet flat; early weight bearing will be with physiological bow legs (genu varum) often exaggerated by the coexistence of a degree of tibial torsion.

Established walkers: 18–24 months

The typical gait of a toddler is wide-based, flat-footed, stiff-legged, and often bow legged. The efficiency of locomotion improves from around 18 to 24 months as the child's centre of mass descends to being close to the chief motor power in the legs. Studies have shown that heel strike and reciprocal swing are consistently in place 22 weeks after starting to walk. Genu varum generally resolves towards the end of the second year, and because there is a general lessening in the range of hip abduction the base of support in standing tends to narrow.

All the basics of mature gait are said to be in place at approximately 40 weeks of independent walking. Thus, by 2 years of age the young child will generally have achieved heel strike, midstance knee flexion and an efficient ankle knee mechanism. Together, these produce a heel–toe gait, but it will be abrupt and look unskilful.

Maturation of gait

Any observation of a group of children within an age range of 2–5 years will show that younger children tend to expend much more energy with extraneous movements and variations in speed, stride and rhythm.

2–3 years

Maturation of gait at 2-3 years of age allows for the base to diminish and movement to become smoother. Knock-knees (genu valgum) may become a transient feature due to a valgus tibiofemoral alignment and the foot will seem pronated with apparent out-toeing.

Between 2 and 3 years, the young child learns to gallop, usually leading with a preferred foot; and they may walk up stairs reciprocally. Their balance reactions improve, the relevant medial connective tissue of the foot strengthens and the compensatory pronation of the foot gradually decreases.

A reciprocal arm swing develops, and the step length and walking velocity increase; in practice, the reciprocal arm swing comes well before mature cadence, step length and walking velocity.

3–4 years

By 3 years of age muscle control and balance will have improved so that there is more uniformity of step length, width and weight transfer. They may now be able to come down stairs reciprocally, but their relative joint laxity and hyperextension of the knee present as genu varum.

At 4 years they will have a more fluid looking gait; smooth, easy and rhythmical, it will be more energy cost-effective and the child will be able to run fast on flat surfaces. Adult patterns are described variously as being established by 3 or 4 years.

4–7 years

It is the skilful achievement of hopping, jumping and skipping and changes in velocity and cadence that lead to the mature gait pattern of a 7–year–old, which can be modified and adapted to changing need. The changes accommodating for and relating specifically to height and the changing centre of mass probably account for the disequilibrium, which is often seen between the ages of 4 and 6 years.

7–9 years

The progress from immature to adult gait, achieved at 7–9 years, will reflect age, environmental experience, skeletal structure, body proportion, energy levels and muscle power. The immense range from 2 to 7 years of age allows for a huge variance in achievement of this maturity.

'Patterns of early walking can be compared to that of an experienced walker on a slippery surface, i.e. very small steps, a widened base of support and maintenance of the body and limbs very upright and in an extended stiff position' (Jean Stout 1995).

Postural alignment

It is very difficult to successfully observe children's gait (particularly when looking for an anomaly) within a consulting room. Children will 'perform', but rarely with the gait pattern that has given their family or teacher the initial cause for concern. Children whom you suspect of doing their 'best ' (or worst) should, if they are able, be asked to run, jump or hop before being asked to ' walk'. By then they may have settled into their habitual pattern and assessment can then effectively evaluate static and active postures as well as walking and running.

Parental concerns

Foot deformities such as curly toes, in-toeing, out-toeing and flat feet are the common causes of parental concern. Physiological bow legs and knock knees need to be differentiated from pathological presentations (see Chapter 13 for further discussion).

When to refer

Most of these anomalies will correct themselves without treatment. A consultation with a physiotherapy orthopaedic practitioner or paediatric physiotherapist will allay fears and if normal ranges of variability are not met, and/or if there is pain, then the therapist can refer to an orthopaedic surgeon.

Mechanical forces affect musculoskeletal development throughout childhood, and so-called 'muscle and joint problems' may just be a variation from the normal presentation and considered to be due to muscle imbalance associated with bone growth. Because of the interdependence between the musculoskeletal system and the nervous system, a physiotherapist is generally in a much better position to identify the actual nature of the child's problem.

A paediatric physiotherapist will be familiar with the various presentations of gait, ranging from flat footed, in-toeing, tibial torsion, and femoral anteversion, to those influenced by low tone or high tone. Assessment of any presentation of tip-toe walking must identify whether a normal walking pattern had been present before its onset in order to eliminate pathological causes.

Paediatric physiotherapists are very skilled at assessing gait. They view it in combination with assessment of maturity of motor skills and a functional assessment.

Their assessment looks at the components of gait: the subtleties of posture, range of limb joint movement, muscle tone and muscle power. If necessary, the gait is analyzed using computer video analysis, and any recommendation that it may be necessary to investigate the child with an in-depth, formal 3D gait analysis should lead to appropriate and timely referral.

Full gait analysis, which comprises 3D analysis with kinematics and dynamic electromyography, is becoming a vital part of the early management of children with cerebral palsy and other significant motor problems.

COORDINATION

Coordination can be defined as the result of movement performed in an optimal way. This may mean that it will be organized, have rhythm, be performed smoothly, or be an adequate and efficient use of the sensorimotor systems to produce a quality movement. It is sometimes easier to describe *lack* of coordination; except that the variations are so great that this can result in confusion.

A poorly coordinated movement is usually described as 'clumsy'; this led to the term 'clumsy children' being applied to those with difficulties in coordination. A variety of terms ensued, all with slightly different meanings and interpretations: minimal brain damage, minor coordination dysfunction, motor dyspraxia and developmental coordination disorder. DSM IV and ICD10 both classify developmental coordination disorder.

Inclusion criteria have been and will continue to be debated. Identification, management and treatment are complex areas for discussion; however, the fact remains that there are children (and adults) who have difficulties both with their organizational skills, as well as with performance of smooth coordinated movements. The wide range of 'normal' should be taken into account, but more importantly, whether or not the difficulties interfere with learning or, indeed, are part of a learning disability, needs to be considered.

For some children their difficulties are further complicated by language and comprehension difficulties but for others it is because they have a sensory system that appears to differ from the norm so that they are either hyper–or hyposensitive. For example a child may seemingly not be aware of his shirt being untucked or his socks being on back to front. It seems that for some children not only do they not feel that it is wrong, but they are also unable to sort it out. Sometimes the difficulties are with specific types of tasks, at other times they are clearly linked with listening and information processing skills. They may find it hard to stand still, constantly seeking more sensory and proprioceptive input to 'top up' their feedback system. Other children will be seen to always join the back of the queue, not being able to tolerate being jostled.

Identification

Identification is rarely valid before 4 years of age, when the ability to imitate postures and true hand dominance is established. Figure 10.6 shows an example of cross laterality. Knowledge of the functional skills of pre-school children helps in

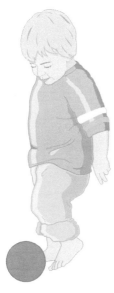
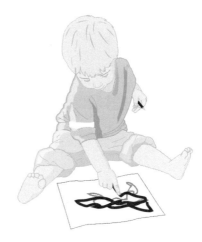

Figure 10.6 Cross-laterality

the preliminary assessment of difficulties with coordination. It is particularly useful to be aware of the peaks and dips in the development of mature balance and coordination. An example of typical presentation of a significant difficulty identified at school is the inability to cross the midline with a dominant hand. Writing commences with the left hand to the middle of the page where the pencil is changed to the right hand to complete the line. Alternatively the right hand commences the writing in the correct place on the paper, but gradually 'forgets' to cross the mid-line.

Parents may identify a whole range of difficulties; history taking will often reveal that the child has always been a messy feeder, was slow to establish speech, cannot dress himself and 'falls over nothing'. Specific questioning might reveal an inability to pedal a tricycle, difficulty in hopping or jumping, poor manipulative fine motor skills. Anecdotal theories abound and many theories and ideas for management approaches have been formulated, some falling well outside the parameters of conventional therapy.

Occupational therapists and physiotherapists use a number of tests to establish the extent of the difficulties, and offer appropriate intervention programmes. Some work closely within the education system to allow for a more integrated approach.

They often record great success with children whose overall abilities are below their expected ability, particularly if the programme can be implemented in association with teachers. Some children with a learning difficulty present as uncoordinated, and if this is commensurate with their cognitive ability then any intervention will need to take that into account.

The greatest difficulty is in the identification of the most appropriate treatment approach for any child whose difficulties seem to be outside the norm. Some children seem able to work out their own strategies and presumably become the adults we are all familiar with who function within their own limits, never, perhaps, participating in sports etc., but otherwise following a perfectly normal way of life. Others are described as never achieving their educational potential because of their very specific difficulties. There are theories that it is this group of children who become very troubled (and trouble-making) adolescents. Other theories suggest that new style physical education (PE) lessons or classroom layouts or changes in social patterns have affected the adaptive learning patterns of children. There is some debate about whether this should be regarded as a health or an educational issue.

Difficulty with coordinated movement is often identified in children who display autistic spectrum disorders; this may be a behavioural manifestation of the disorder and intervention should be planned and evaluated as part of the whole management, rather than an isolated intervention.

References

Bellman M, Kennedy N 2000 Paediatrics and Child Health. Churchill Livingstone, Edinburgh

Bellman M, Lingham S, Aukett A 1996 Schedule of Growing Skills, 2nd edn. NFER-Nelson, Windsor

Haring NG, Lovitt TC, Eaton MD, Hansel CL 1978 The Fourth R: Research in the Classroom. Charles E Merril Publishing Co, Columbus, Ohio

Illingworth RS 1991 The Normal child, 10th edn. Churchill Livingstone, Edinburgh

Sutherland DH, Olshen R, Biden E, Wyatt M 1988 The Development of Mature Walking. Mackeith Press, Oxford, Blackwell Scientific Publications Ltd

Further reading

Bly L 1994 Motor Skills acquisition in the First Year. The Psychological Corporation, San Antonio, Texas

Campbell SK, van der Linden DW, Palisano RJ (eds) 1994 Physical Therapy for children. WB Saunders, Philadelphia

Gordon N, McKinlay I (eds) 1980 The Clumsy Child. Churchill Livingstone, Edinburgh

Hall DMB, Elliman D 2003. Health for All Children, 4th edn. Oxford University Press, Oxford

Hall DMB, Hill P Elliman D 1991 The Child Surveillance Handbook, 2nd edn. Radcliffe Medical Press, Oxford

Knobloch H, Stevens F, Malone A 1980 Manual of Developmental Diagnosis. Gesell Revised developmental Schedules. Harper & Row, Hagerston, MA

Meisels SJ 1989 Can developmental screening tests identify children who are developmentally at risk? Paediatrics 83: 572

Staheli LT 1977 Torsional deformity. Paediatric Clinics of North America 24: 799–811

11

Special senses: vision, hearing and skills integration

M. Bellman

▼ OVERVIEW

Traditionally it is considered that there are five special senses, namely: sight, hearing, taste, smell and touch. It can be argued that balance should be included but as it is part of inner ear function, it is described together with hearing. However, there is a further sensory mechanism that is very important in child care and satisfies the above criteria for a special sense. It is the maternal ability to detect threats to her children and protect them from danger, described here as a 'mother's sixth sense'.

This chapter describes important aspects of normal sensory systems including basic anatomy and physiology together with their clinical applications. References are made to some abnormal situations to illustrate deviations from normal.

INTRODUCTION

The special senses evolved as defence systems in animals to alert them to dangers from external sources. They consist of highly specialized mechanisms for detecting various stimuli and transferring them through the peripheral nervous system to the brain, for analysis and interpretation. The brain builds up a memory bank of sensory images and through a combination of this experience and instinct, each input receives an appropriate output response.

VISION

The eyes are said to be the 'gateway to the soul' and whether or not that is true, they are, indeed, the organs through which much environmental experience is sensed and are thus vital for normal childhood development. In addition, the eyes provide 'windows' that show many patterns associated with various health indicators and are, therefore, included in routine medical examinations.

Structure of the eye (Fig. 11.1)

The globe of the eye is roughly a sphere 2.5 cm in diameter suspended in a cushion of fat within the bony orbit, which protects it from indirect trauma. The unprotected anterior surface of the eye ball (the cornea) has partial protection by the upper and, to a lesser extent, the lower eyelid. The cornea is lubricated and cleansed by tears secreted by the lacrimal glands. Tears contain antibacterial enzymes to prevent infection and they drain via the lacrimal canals into the nose.

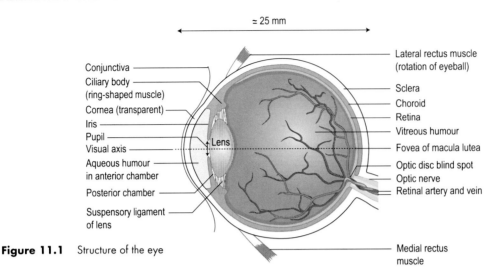

Figure 11.1 Structure of the eye

The globe is contained within a tough membrane called the sclera, which is pierced posteriorly by the optic nerve. The sclera is opaque, but anteriorly it is continuous with the cornea, which is more convex than the rest of the globe and is transparent to allow transmission of light. The inner surface of the sclera (the uveal tract) is highly vascular and in the posterior two-thirds of the eye forms the choroid, which is deeply pigmented (except in albinos) to absorb light. Anteriorly, the choroid is continuous with the ciliary body, from which the lens is suspended, and the iris, which is a circular muscular sheet that contracts or relaxes to dilate or constrict the pupil in order to control the amount of light rays that enter the eye (acting like a camera shutter). The lens is composed of a transparent matrix enclosed within an elastic capsule. It is suspended by a ligament to the ciliary body and muscle, which can contract and pull the outside edge of the circular lens so that it becomes less convex. This is the method by which the eye accommodates and changes its focal length so that objects at varying distances can be imaged accurately.

Lining the inner surface of the posterior two-thirds of the choroid is the retina, which contains the photoreceptor nerve cells, which convert light energy into neural energy for transmission to the visual cortex in the occipital lobes of the brain. The photoreceptor cells contain photosensitive discs of pigment, which absorb light and generate a change in electrical potential within the nerve cell. The photoreceptor cells are of two types:

1. Rods, which are rich in photo-pigment and hence function in low light situations.
2. Cones, which contain less pigment and so are more adapted for bright light.

A major component of photo-pigment in rods is rhodopsin (visual purple), which has a different spectrum of light wave length absorption to other pigments and which helps to distinguish colours. Formation of rhodopsin depends upon retinol, which is not synthesized in the body, but is derived from carotene in food. Severe retinol (vitamin A) deficiency is associated with night blindness. There are three types of cone each of which contains isodopsin sensitive to light wavelengths in a specific range. If all three are stimulated equally white is perceived.

The axons of the retinal photoreceptor cells are transparent so that light rays pass through them. They run across the inner surface of the retina towards a central point posteriorly where they collect at the optic disc before running into the optic nerve. The optic disc contains no photoreceptors and is a blind spot in the retina. It is usually not noticed

Figure 11.2 Demonstration of blind spot
Close one eye and look at the figure from a distance of 30 cm. With the right eye look at the dot and with the left eye look at the cross. When the page is moved nearer and further away, the other symbol disappears when its image is focused on the macula (blind spot)

because of binocular vision, but can be demonstrated (Fig. 11.2).

The fovea is a spot slightly lateral to the optic disc, which has a very high concentration of cones and no overlying fibres or blood vessels. The fovea is within the macula, which is the fixation point during normal vision in order to maximize visual acuity and reduce distortion. Hence the visual axis of the eye is approximately 5° eccentric to the optic axis.

The globe of the eye behind the lens is filled with vitreous humour. This is a viscous jellylike material and must be totally transparent so that light rays can pass through the lens to the retina unimpeded. In front of the lens in the anterior and posterior chambers is the aqueous humour, which is less viscous. It is secreted by the ciliary body and circulates in the anterior chamber and through the pupil to the posterior chamber from where it is drained through the canal of Schlemm into the blood circulation. If this canal becomes blocked the intraocular pressure increases, causing glaucoma and, if not treated, blindness.

Eye movements

The eyes must be able to move quickly and accurately in order to track a moving object and the movements of both eyes must be in precise synchrony to maintain binocular vision. The globe of the eye functions as a ball joint within the socket of the orbit. The movements are controlled by six muscles, which combine to move the globe in any plane. The internal (medial) and external (lateral) rectus muscles move the globe horizontally, the superior and inferior rectus muscles move it vertically and the superior and inferior oblique muscles move it diagonally.

The superior oblique muscle is innervated by the 4th cranial nerve, the lateral rectus by the 6th cranial nerve (abducens) and the others by the 3rd (oculomotor) nerve. A paralytic (non-concomitant) squint can occur if one of the muscles does not function correctly.

Eye movements must be very rapid and are controlled by a brainstem reflex mechanism with relays to the motor cortex in the frontal lobes for voluntary fixation and relays to the visual cortex in the occipital lobe for smooth pursuit (tracking) movements. Saccades are rapid movements from one point of fixation to another and can be observed when watching a series of moving objects, for example looking out of the window of a train. They also occur during rapid eye movement (REM) sleep.

Nystagmus

Sometimes jerky movements of both eyes occur due to an abnormality of the visual pathway. It can be caused by defective vision or a neurological abnormality in the brain stem pathways. The movements are usually identical in both eyes and are rapid and small in amplitude.

Squint (strabismus)

Paralysis of a muscle causes deficiency of movement in that particular direction. The most frequent is paralysis of the lateral rectus muscle due to a lesion of the abducens nerve so that the affected eye is unable to move laterally (abduct). A concomitant squint is when a squint in one eye remains constant in relation to the other eye in all directions of gaze. This is the commonest type of squint seen in young children due to an abnormality of visual acuity (e.g. astigmatism or refraction error) in the affected eye.

Stereoscopic vision

The benefit of two eyes is that each receives an image that is slightly different to the other due to parallax. These two retinal images are transmitted to the visual cortex where they are interpreted to give a 3D picture of the scene. This allows judgement of depth as well as the two linear dimensions of height and width. Binocular vision is established in the first few years of life and if one eye is not functioning perfectly and the image received by the visual cortex is not identical with that from the other eye, than the image is suppressed. This results in monocular vision, which is only in 2D.

Infants with a squint learn quickly to suppress the image from the squinting eye to avoid the diplopia (double vision) that would otherwise result and if this suppression continues for more than 2 or 3 years, the visual cortex does not develop properly and the acuity cannot be regained. Hence, children who have a suspected squint need urgent expert assessment (usually by an orthoptist) so that timely treatment can be started at least before the age of 7 years. The aim of the treatment is to restore the quality of the visual image in the squinting eye to normal so that it can take up equal fixation on a target in order to maintain binocular vision. Loss of vision in one eye, resulting in monocular vision causes amblyopia. Although amblyopia means that only one eye is functioning normally and there is therefore a remote risk of severe visual loss if the normal eye is damaged, most people with amblyopia have remarkably little visual dysfunction. They quickly learn to use other clues to the depth of visual field such as the contrast between light and shade, colour differentials, perspective and parallax when the head is moved from side to side.

Optics

Normally, light rays from the visual target are focused accurately onto the retina by the cornea and lens. The cornea has a greater refractive power than the lens; however, the latter can change shape and thus vary its refractivity in order to accommodate to targets at varying distances. The image of the target is upside down and horizontally reversed (Fig. 11.3).

Figures 11.3a and b show how light rays from distant or near objects are refracted by a lens of different convexities in order to focus the image on the retina.

Figures 11.3c and d show how an eyeball that is too long causes short–sightedness (myopia) and an eyeball that is too short causes short-sightedness (hypermetropia). In the former case an extra convex lens is needed and in the latter, a concave lens.

Visible light includes a spectrum from approximately 400 to 800 nm (Fig. 11.4). It includes all colours of the rainbow (red, orange, yellow, green, blue, indigo, violet), which together are seen as white light. Individual colours are best detected in bright light by cones, which are of three separate types with different photo-spectral sensitivities. When all three are stimulated equally the light is interpreted as

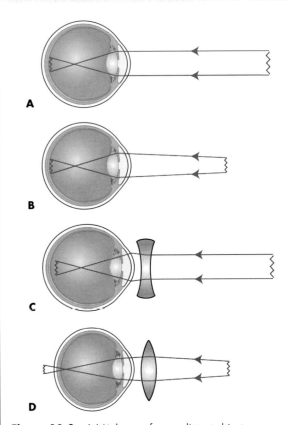

A

B

C

D

Figure 11.3 (a) Light rays from a distant object are parallel and are refracted by a stretched lens with low refractive power (contracted ciliary muscle) to focus the image on the retina. (b) Light rays from a near object diverge and need a more convex lens with high refractive power (relaxed ciliary muscle) to focus on the retina. (c) In myopia the globe is too long and the image from a distant object is focused in front of the retina. Only near objects can be seen clearly. An additional concave lens is required for distant vision. (d) In hypermetropia the globe is too short and despite accommodation to a maximally convex lens the image from a near object is focused behind the retina. Only distant objects can be seen clearly. An additional convex lens is required for near vision, e.g. reading.

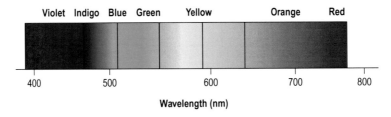

| Violet | Indigo | Blue | Green | | Yellow | | Orange | | Red |

400   500   600   700   800

Wavelength (nm)

Figure 11.4 Visible spectrum

white. As seen above, rods contain a single pigment (rhodopsin), which gives monochromatic vision, but is active in dim light.

Visual sensation

The dependence of the sensation of vision upon photosensitive chemicals has three important effects:

1. Light/dark adaptation – when rhodopsin is bleached by light, it must be regenerated again before it can re-function and during that time light sensitivity is reduced. This is experienced as dazzle after looking at a bright light.
2. Visual persistence – the photosensitivity effects in the chemoreceptors last for a significant amount of time during which the image persists. This is the reason why films, which are composed of multiple rapidly sequenced frames are seen as 'movies'. It can also be experienced by looking at a bright object and shutting the eyes when the image will persist transiently.
3. Complementary colours – certain pairs of colours stimulate different combinations of photosensitive pigments. There are three types of cone pigments that absorb light best in the blue, green or red sections of visible light spectrums. The pairs of colours that stimulate complementary neuroprocesses are green/red, yellow/blue, black/white. This can be experienced by looking at a well illuminated green or yellow object and than shutting the eyes when the image will be seen as red or blue respectively. Black is also a positive sensation in contrast to white and is not simply the absence of light stimulation. In colour blindness, which is relatively common (approximately 8% of males), one of the three cone pigments has been lost and the light wavelength of that particular sensitivity is poorly sensed. The most common disorder is red/green colour blindness.

Neuro-ophthalmology

Light (pupillary) reflex

The iris adjusts the amount of light entering the eye and is controlled by a reflex action, via the 3rd (oculo-motor) nerve, without having to go through the visual cortex. Light strikes the retina and nerve impulses pass down the optic nerve to relays in the brainstem and back via autonomic nerves to the iris, which causes the pupils to constrict. The direct light reflex refers to pupillary constriction on the same side, but the reflex also passes to the iris of the other eye by a consensual light reflex. This is a protective mechanism to prevent excessive amounts of light entering the eye and potentially damaging the retina. It also increases the depth of focus and, therefore, the sharpness of the image on the retina (similar to a camera shutter).

The retinal nerve fibres collect at the optic disc to form the optic nerve which passes through the sphenoid bone into the cranial cavity. The left and right optic nerves join at the optic chiasma where approximately 50% of the nerve fibres (mainly from the medial side of the retina) cross to the opposite optic tract running to the visual cortex in the occipital lobes of the brain (Fig. 11.5).

Vision tests

During child health surveillance normal children will have several different visual tests and procedures performed on them.

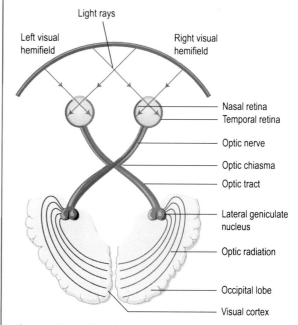

Figure 11.5   Visual pathway

Red reflex

When a bright light is shone into the eye the light rays travel through the globe and are reflected from the retina, which appears red (as in a flash photograph). If the red reflex is not seen, or has a black area in it, there may be opacity in the eye. The test should be performed in the neonatal examination and at the 6–week check so that opacity, like a cataract, is quickly identified and surgically removed as soon as possible so that the visual cortex is exposed to images and develops normally.

Tests for strabismus (squint)

The visual axes of very young infants may not consistently be parallel, but by 3–4 months they should be well aligned. Squint beyond that age needs diagnosis and treatment. A constant squint at any age should be investigated. The best test is family observation and if a parent is worried, the baby's eyes should be carefully examined. The simplest test is the *corneal light reflection*, which can be done easily in a clinic. The spot of light reflected from the corneas from a pen-torch shone at a distance of 50 cm should be symmetrical in both eyes. If not, it indicates that the axes are not parallel. A more detailed test that detects both manifest and latent squint is the *cover test*, which involves covering and uncovering each eye in turn while the child fixates on an object held 33 cm away. If there is a squint the axis will change and the eye will move as fixation occurs. This test is difficult and should only be performed by specially trained staff such as orthoptists.

Acuity tests

Accurate testing of visual acuity in an infant is very difficult and can only be done in a specialized clinic. Blind children smile and may appear to look towards their mother during feeding, but will not follow a moving object with their eyes, which, therefore, can be used as a simple test with a face or bright light (for example pen torch) in the first few weeks or a dangling toy at 2–3 months. At approximately 3 months children start to reach out towards objects and these can be offered, using a 2 cm cube at 6

months, a raisin at 12 months and a '100 & 1000' (small sugar strand cake decoration 1–2 mm in length) at 18 months. All these techniques are crude and will only detect severe visual impairment. If there is concern a referral should be made to an eye clinic where specialist tests such as preferential looking are available.

Around 2$^1/_2$–3 years of age many children will be able to match shapes on a keycard, which they hold, to those on a test card that the examiner holds at a distance of 3 or 6 m. By 3 years of age, children can usually match letters on STYCAR or Sheridan–Gardener cards (single letter optotypes). These techniques underestimate visual difficulties because of the absence of competing visual stimuli and a more sensitive method is to use a linear letter chart, for example Sonksen Silver system or the Cambridge crowded letter test, in which the target letter is confounded by other surrounding letters. When children are able to recognize and name letters visual acuity can be measured accurately with a standard 6 m letter (for example Snellen) chart.

HEARING AND BALANCE

Hearing

The ability to hear is one of the marvels of the animal kingdom and, in humans, this sense has become so sophisticated that it has enabled the human species to develop the ability to communicate interactively through spoken language, which has allowed them to dominate all other animal species. The fetus can hear, as shown by ultrasound imaging of movements in response to sounds, which is a phenomenon well known to pregnant women and has been confirmed by ultrasound scan studies. It has been shown that fetuses can be affected by exposing them to different sounds during intrauterine life, for example music, and that babies can remember some such sounds, for example their mother's voice and heart beat. Infants are avid auditory learners and it is highly unlikely that it is a skill that emerges only after birth.

The ear is fully formed at birth and consists of three main parts: outer, middle, and inner ear (Fig. 11.6).

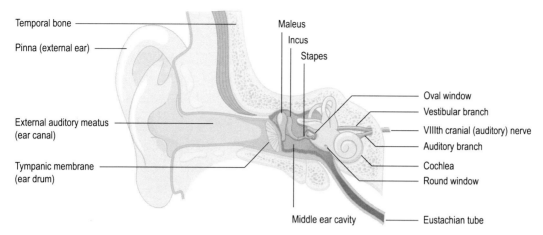

Figure 11.6 Structure of the ear

Outer ear

The most obvious part of the outer (external) ear is the pinna (auricle), which is conical in order to funnel sound into the ear canal, although this function is marginal in humans. The external auditory canal is a tube approximately 5 cm by 1 cm (unfortunately large enough to admit small objects such as beads, which children may insert) and extends into the temporal bone to the tympanic membrane. Some protection against admission of foreign objects, for example insects, is offered by hairs at the entrance to the canal. The canal lining contains cerumen glands that produce wax, which has bactericidal qualities as well as being a further sticky barrier. Wax is produced from infancy in variable quantities and mothers should be advised that it is absolutely normal and essential and should not be cleaned out of the ear by inserting objects such as cotton buds. The growth of the skin of the external auditory canal is from inside to outside, so that there should be a constant extrusion of material from the external auditory meatus, which again mothers need reassurance about.

Middle ear

The tympanic membrane is the interface between the external auditory canal and the middle ear. It is 0.01 mm thick and hence very fragile. It is the transformer mechanism for conducting sound waves from air to the fluid of the inner ear. It is concave in order to enhance its acoustic qualities. Internal to the tympanic membrane are the three ossicles (malleus, incus and stapes), which are a lever system to transmit vibrations from the tympanic membrane to the oval window and thus to the inner ear fluid of the cochlea. The mechanics of the transmission chain through the middle ear amplifies the sound vibrations approximately 18 times.

The middle ear is air-filled and the pressure is maintained at atmospheric level via the Eustachian tube, which connects to the back of the nose. This enlarges with age and during childhood is narrow and easily blocked at the nasal end. Obstruction to the Eustachian tube reduces ventilation of the middle ear and is thought to be the main reason for the high incidence of secretory otitis media (otitis media with effusion/glue ear) in young children. During relaxation, the Eustachian tube is closed, but opens briefly during swallowing, yawning and chewing, hence the beneficial effect of eating to equalize middle ear and ambient air pressure. Obstruction to the Eustachian tube ('blocked ear') can be cleared by forcibly increasing intranasal air pressure (Valsalva manoeuvre).

Inner ear

This comprises the cochlea (organ of hearing) and the labyrinth (the organ of balance). It is very fragile and is deeply imbedded in the temporal bone, which is the hardest bone of the body.

The cochlea is a tube curled 2.5 times and is said to look like a snail. It is divided into three inner tubes, which contain endolymph, which is the medium for conducting sound vibrations to the organ of Corti in the middle of the inner tube (cochlear duct). The organ of Corti is the sensory end organ of hearing and contains approximately 23 000 hair cells, which vibrate in resonance to the sound frequency and intensity and transduce the mechanical energy into electrical stimuli that travels up the cochlear nerve to the brain. The hair cells have different frequency responses, so that low frequencies are received at the apex of the cochlea and high frequencies at the base. This differential frequency (tonotopic) spectrum is maintained into the auditory nerve and the ascending afferent tracts.

The labyrinth is also filled with endolymph and consists of three semicircular canals at right angles to each other in order to detect the 3D movements of the head. The motion of the endolymph stimulates the sensory organ (crista) at the base of each semicircular canal, which also connects to the cochlear nerve. The labyrinth has rich connections to the cerebellum and other areas of the brain and is essential for identification of orientation of the body and movement in space. Labyrinthine dysfunction causes dizziness and impairment of balance, which is extremely disabling.

Acoustics

Sound waves Sound is transmitted by sinusoidal pressure waves of vibrating molecules in a transmitting medium: usually air. These acoustic waves emanate in 3D from the sound source as an expanding sphere.

Figure 11.7 shows the physical characteristics of a sound wave such as that produced by a loudspeaker in which the diaphragm vibrates successively increasing and decreasing the adjacent air pressure. The rapidity of the vibration (measured as cycles per second or Hertz) determines the frequency of the sound and the amplitude of the vibration determines the volume (measured in decibels [dB]). At any one point sound waves have a longitudinal velocity of approximately 340 m/s in air (1500 m/s in seawater because of its higher density). As the acoustic energy is dispersed spherically the volume diminishes in proportion to the square of the distance from the sound source (inverse square law). Thus, the decibel scale on an audiogram is logarithmic.

Ambient noise Figure 11.8 shows the volume of some common sounds. Workers in occupations involving noise levels of 100 dB and above will inevitably become deaf if precautions are not taken. The cochlea becomes more vulnerable with increasing age, but teenagers who regularly attend discos or pop concerts should be advised to wear ear plugs or keep as far away as possible from the loudspeakers.

When a sound wave hits a surface some of the energy is absorbed and some is reflected.

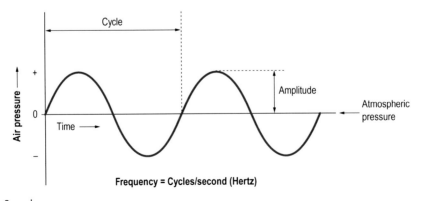

Figure 11.7 Sound waves

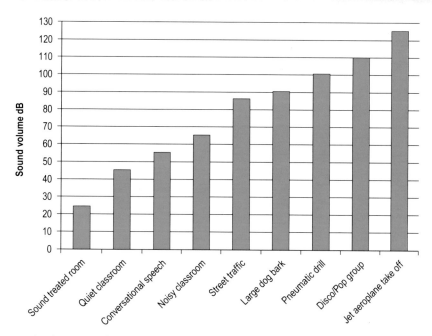

Figure 11.8 Noise levels compared

The proportions depend upon the characteristics of the material. Absorption is greater in lightweight materials as well as human bodies. In concert halls, the walls are made of wood and the seats are well padded so that acoustically there is little difference whether or not someone is in the seat. Reflected sound waves enhance the volume of sound, but their quality is different due to their longer pathway and frequency diffraction. Thus reflection of sound waves may significantly pollute the original sound and make it more difficult to interpret. This is often the situation in classrooms if there are bare walls and may be made even worse by reverberation from other surfaces such as cupboards and desks.

Auditory processing

The outer, middle and inner ear are basically a mechanism for detecting sound waves in air and converting acoustic energy to neural energy in the auditory nerve.

This mechanism can be duplicated by an artificial microphone and amplifier and is relatively simple (Fig. 11.9). It is a means of hearing, which is a passive process. However, the auditory processing system, which transmits neural energy to the language centre of the brain, is much more complicated and has not been duplicated by a man-made system. It is the means of listening that is an active process and has evolved to a very high level in the human species, as noted above.

The central auditory nervous system (CANS) is a distinct pathway through the brainstem that starts at the cochlear nucleus on the auditory nerve and ends in the auditory cortex in the temporal lobe. Most of the afferent auditory nerve fibres cross over at the level of the cochlear nucleus and so connect to the auditory cortex of the hemisphere opposite

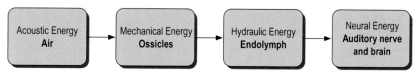

Figure 11.9 Converting sounds into nerve impulses

to the side of the ear where the sound is received. In most people, including left handers, the main language centre is in the left hemisphere and so information from the left ear, which is received in the right auditory cortex, has to be transferred back to the left side of the brain through the corpus callosum before it is interpreted as language. The integrity of the brainstem pathway can be measured by electrophysiological tests (brainstem evoked response), which show a steady maturation with age due to progressive myelination of the nerves that is not completed until the age of around 12 years.

The CANS is very complex and relatively fragile and can be damaged by various brain insults including developmental, inflammatory and traumatic events. Fortunately, the young brain is very plastic and particularly before myelination has been completed, the auditory pathways appear to be able to compensate for deficits. The structure of the CANS is highly tonotopic, that is arrayed systematically according to the sound frequencies relayed from the cochlear. Thus, at the end of the auditory pathway in Heschl's gyrus, cortical neurones receive specific frequencies, which is the basis for cognitive analysis of the sound spectrum.

Speech sound patterns are learned during the first year of life and the cortical neurones become 'tuned' to their specific frequency. If the sound spectrum subsequently changes, it may be difficult for the brain to adapt and auditory difficulties may result.

It has been shown that from around 3 months of age infants can distinguish and eventually reproduce sounds specific to their language environment. If there is a hearing impairment at a young age and the learned sounds are distorted, the child may subsequently have auditory and language difficulties if the hearing loss later resolves.

Auditory processing abilities are highly complex, but the sophistication of the human brain is such that they rapidly become automatic during early childhood.

Figure 11.10 represents the whole process diagrammatically between sound reception in the ear, central processing and sound production, that is speech.

Central auditory processing (CAP) enables humans to function in complex auditory situations, such as

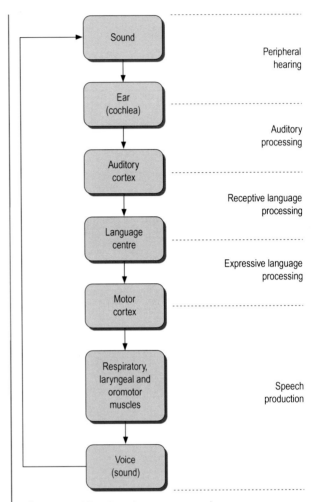

Figure 11.10 From hearing to speech

listening to a conversation in a crowded classroom. The listener is able to attend to a selected conversation even though other similar speakers may be talking nearby, which may also be monitored so that attention can be diverted if something relevant is heard. This process requires the simultaneous monitoring and selection of many streams of incoming information and analyzing them according to changing spatial and temporal dynamics (Table 11.1). Auditory processing overlaps with language processing (see Fig. 8.1).

Given the complexity of CAP, it is not surprising that occasionally it does not work perfectly. Auditory processing disorder (APD) is being increasingly recognized as a cause of poor attention, difficulty

Table 11.1 Central auditory processing (CAP) abilities	
Localization	Ability to identify a sound source
Auditory attention	Ability to attend to a sound signal
Auditory discrimination	Ability to discriminate frequencies and harmonics
Auditory closure	Ability to complete an auditory message if part of the signal is missing
Auditory integration	Ability to synthesize complex signals, e.g. words, from separate signals
Auditory figure–ground	Ability to isolate and focus on one signal in the presence of others
Auditory association	Ability to correlate a sound signal with another cognitive symbol (the basis of language), including written letters
Auditory memory	Ability to store and recall sounds and their associations

following oral instructions, problems with listening (especially in background noise), poor educational progress and behavioural problems.

If APD is suspected for any of these reasons, a child should be evaluated by a specialist audiology team, which can analyze the problem using a battery of auditory behavioural and electrophysiological tests. Many of the children can be helped by interventions such as enhancing the sound signal-to-noise ratio by improving the auditory environment (for example eliminating background noise and sitting the child near the teacher), provision of a personal or soundfield amplification system or oral or computer-based auditory training.

Hearing tests

A child's hearing is tested in different ways at different ages during the normal UK Child Health Surveillance Schedule.

Otoacoustic emissions When a sound is received by the cochlear it generates a sound in response that is called an otoacoustic emission (OAE); this is an automatic response if the conduction pathway from the outer ear to the cochlear hair cells is intact and so is very useful in patients who cannot actively cooperate. It is very effective in infants and has been adapted as a neonatal hearing screening test that is offered within a few weeks of birth to all babies born in the UK.

Distraction test By the age of 8 or 9 months, children can respond behaviourally to sounds by turning the head in order to localize the sound source. This response is the basis of the distraction test that is no longer used for screening purposes since the introduction of a universal OAE neonatal screen, but is useful for selected children during early childhood if there is concern about their hearing. The distraction test can be used to obtain an auditory threshold as the sound intensity can be progressively lowered to minimal levels.

Visual reinforcement audiometry Some children who cannot cooperate for distraction testing, for example because of learning difficulties, are able to show responses when the target sound is reinforced by a visual stimulus such as a moving toy.

Play audiometry From the age of about 3 years, children are able to respond to freefield audiometry when puretones are generated by an audiometer at varying frequencies and intensities by carrying out a specific task such as inserting wooden men into a boat or balls into a bucket, even though they cannot give a verbal response. The sounds are produced by a freefield audiometer and thus an accurate pure tone audiogram can be produced.

Pure tone audiometry The 'gold standard' audiological test is a pure tone audiogram delivered to individual ears through headphones. Each sound is first made at a fairly loud level and quickly reduced progressively to a point at which the child cannot hear it. The quietest level that is heard at each frequency is the hearing threshold. This is the only method that can generate an accurate pure tone audiogram for both ears separately and so identify a unilateral deafness.

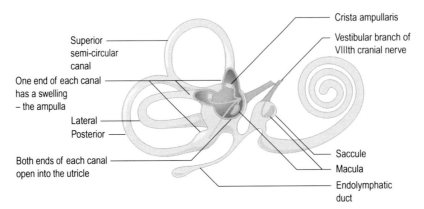

Superior semi-circular canal

One end of each canal has a swelling – the ampulla

Lateral

Posterior

Both ends of each canal open into the utricle

Crista ampullaris

Vestibular branch of VIIIth cranial nerve

Saccule

Macula

Endolymphatic duct

Figure 11.11 Balance mechanisms

Balance

The sense of balance (equilibrium) is detected in the labyrinths of the inner ears within the temporal bones (Fig. 11.11). There are two different mechanisms for identifying balance.

Static equilibrium

This determines the position of the head in relation to the rest of the body when both are still. The receptor organ is the macula located inside the utricle and saccule, which are expansions of the membranous labyrinths within the bony vestibule. The macula is a collection of hair cells in contact with a collection of gelatinous material holding otoliths. These move under the influence of gravity bending the hair cells, which generates a change in electrical potential and initiates a nervous impulse that travels centrally up the vestibular branch of the eighth cranial nerve.

Dynamic equilibrium

This is the mechanism for maintaining balance when the head and body are moving. Movement is detected by motion of endolymph in three semicircular canals at right angles to each other within the bony labyrinth. The receptor organ that detects fluid motion is the crista ampullaris located in the ampulla of each semicircular canal. The crista consists of a number of hair cells ending in a dome-shaped gelatinous cupula, which is displaced by the movement of the endolymph. This generates a nervous impulse as above. Dynamic

equilibrium is rapid and is very effective at detecting sudden movements of the head. Additionally, body movement is sensed by mechanoreceptors in joints and this information is integrated, together with visual input, in the cerebellum and others centres of the brain.

SOMATOSENSORY SYSTEM

The somatosensory system is the first-line mechanism in animals for detecting pressure internally and externally. It consists of sensory receptor organs in skin, muscles, joints and viscera, which transmit stimuli centrally to the brain. The receptors connect by first-order afferent neurones to the spinal cord or brain stem. Second-order neurones cross over and transmit information to the thalamus and synapse with third-order neurones, which project to the sensory cerebral cortex in the parietal lobe. In some areas, fourth- and higher-order neurones connect to other parts of the brain.

In the spinal cord, the ascending (afferent) fibres are grouped into distinct pathways, which carry specific types of information such as touch, vibration, proprioception (position sense and joint movement), temperature, pain and visceral sensation.

Receptor organs

Several different types of cutaneous receptors are located in skin covering the whole body in varying concentrations.

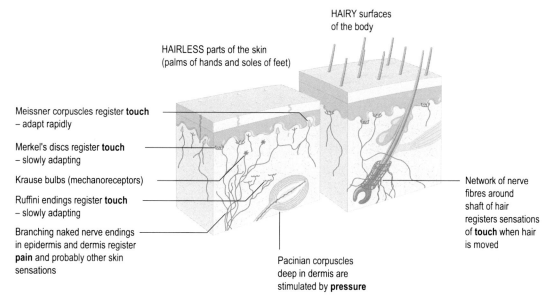

HAIRY surfaces
of the body

HAIRLESS parts of the skin
(palms of hands and soles of feet)

Meissner corpuscles register **touch**
– adapt rapidly

Merkel's discs register **touch**
– slowly adapting

Krause bulbs (mechanoreceptors)

Ruffini endings register **touch**
– slowly adapting

Branching naked nerve endings
in epidermis and dermis register
pain and probably other skin
sensations

Network of nerve
fibres around
shaft of hair
registers sensations
of **touch** when hair
is moved

Pacinian corpuscles
deep in dermis are
stimulated by **pressure**

Figure 11.12 Cutaneous receptors

Cutaneous receptors (Fig. 11.12, Table 11.2)

Muscle, joint and visceral receptors As well as mechanoreceptors and nociceptors, skeletal muscle contains stretch receptors, which are important for motor control. Nociceptors in muscle respond to chemical stimulation, for example during ischaemia. Joint capsules contain articular receptors, which respond to movement and vibration and nociceptors activated by excessive movement, which could damage the joint. Viscera have a low density of sensory receptors, which can detect stretching and distension and, in some organs, for example pancreas and mesentery, pain due to inflammation or chemical stimulation.

Spinal pathways The peripheral nervous system sensory axons join the spinal cord via the dorsal root before synapsing to the second order neurones. The cutaneous sensation of the body is conventionally divided into serial dermatomes, or sensory areas, which correspond to the position on the spinal cord where the dorsal root enters. There are six cervical dermatomes, twelve thoracic dermatomes, five lumbar dermatomes and five sacral dermatomes. (There is a similar arrangement of motor dermatomes which pass through the ventral spinal route.)

Table 11.2	Functions of cutaneous receptors
Mechanoreceptors	These respond to light pressure, which indents the skin They may function rapidly, e.g. those attached to hairs or particularly sensitive areas such as fingertips or slowly in less sensitive areas of skin
Thermoreceptors	These are receptive to temperature and basically detect cold and warmth In contrast to other receptors, thermal receptors are constantly functioning Cold receptors become inactive above normal skin temperature (approximately 37°C) and warm receptors stop discharging above 45°C
Nociceptors	These respond to potentially damaging stimuli such as laceration or crushing and thermal or chemical burn Occasionally, nociceptors overreact to stimuli resulting in persisting high-intensity pain (hyperalgesia), which may not necessarily be related directly to the degree of stimulation

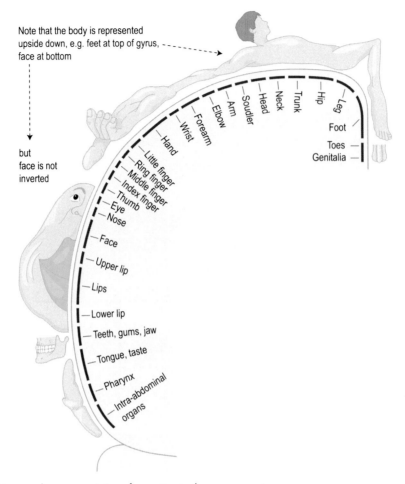

Note that the body is represented upside down, e.g. feet at top of gyrus, face at bottom

but face is not inverted

Little finger
Ring finger
Middle finger
Index finger
Thumb
Eye
Nose
Face
Upper lip
Lips
Lower lip
Teeth, gums, jaw
Tongue, taste
Pharynx
Intra-abdominal organs

Hand
Wrist
Forearm
Elbow
Arm
Soudler
Head
Neck
Trunk
Hip
Leg

Foot
Toes
Genitalia

Figure 11.13   Homunculus representation of sensation in the sensory cortex

Dorsal column One of the main sensory pathways lies in the dorsal column of the spinal cord which accumulates sensory fibres from successive dermatomes as it ascends to the sensory cerebral cortex which is arranged in a specific way, proportional to the relative importance of sensation from various parts of the body. This is represented schematically by the homunculus which shows that large sections of the cortex are devoted to sensation from the face, especially lips, and the hand, especially the thumb and fingers (Fig. 11.13 & Table 11.3).

Interruption to the dorsal columns in the spinal cord, for example by trauma, causes deficits in tactile discrimination, vibration and position sense and visceral sensation, in the dermatomes below the level of the lesion.

Spinothalamic tract The spinothalamic tract is a very important sensory pathway for pain and temperature from nociceptors, thermoreceptors and mechanoreceptors. They are strongly stimulated by potentially dangerous events and provide the main protective alerting mechanism of the body to immediate danger.

Interruption of the spinothalamic tract occurs due to ventral lesions of the spinal cord and results in loss of pain and temperature sensation on the opposite side of the body below the level of the

Table 11.3   Sensory modalities passing via the dorsal column

Flutter (low-frequency mechanical stimulation)	Detected by receptors in hair follicles and Meissner corpuscles in skin. Flutter is tested by gently tapping the skin with a finger or cotton wool
Vibration (high-frequency stimulation)	Mainly detected by Pacinian corpuscles in subcutaneous tissue. It is tested by holding a vibrating tuning fork against a bony prominence
Light touch	Skin indentation is recognized as touch detected mainly by slowly adapting Merkel cells and Ruffini endings in the skin
Proprioception	Receptors in muscles, joints and skin relay sensory information, which is interpreted in the cerebrum and cerebellum to analyze the position of each part of the body in relation to others
Visceral sensation	Receptors in the walls of internal organs relay information about stretch, which is interpreted as indicating relaxation or distention of the organ, e.g. the urinary bladder

lesion. This can be performed surgically in order to relieve intractable pain from conditions such as cancer.

Trigeminothalamic tract The trigeminal nerve supplies the sensation from the face, teeth, nasopharynx, oropharynx and dura mater (outer meningeal membrane surrounding the brain). The trigeminal tract is very important in identifying oral pain (including toothache) and tension/stretch in facial and head muscles and meninges, which may be interpreted as headache and possibly migraine.

Pain

Pain is an extremely important defensive mechanism and loss of pain sensation prevents the body from protecting itself against major injury. The different receptors allow analysis of pain sensation so that the brain can interpret likely causes such as penetration or burning of skin, which cause sudden severe pain, or ischaemia and overstretching of muscles and ligaments, which cause persistent ache. The pain pathways are associated with many other centres of the brain and cause various somatic, autonomic, hormonal and emotional reactions. The nature of the pain influences the way that it is analyzed in the brain and interpreted as an unpleasant stimulus. It is well known that the threshold of pain varies widely and some people seem to be able to withstand degrees of pain that would be intolerable to others.

Hyperalgesia

This occurs when receptors (particularly nociceptors) become extra–sensitized after injury. Subsequent pain at the same site may then be interpreted as even more painful. Injury can sometimes cause sensitization to surrounding receptors even though they have not been directly damaged, causing secondary tenderness.

Referred pain

Sometimes pain is localized to a part of the body even though the source of injury is somewhere else. It may occur because the injury is in deep parts of the body that cannot be imaged directly by the cerebral cortex so the site is projected to the corresponding dermatome on the body surface. This occurs in abdominal pain when the site is often felt to be periumbilical even though it may arise from other parts of the abdominal cavity such as in appendicitis.

Neuropathic pain

This occurs when the nerves themselves are damaged and the stimulus does not arise from the nerve endings in the receptors. It may occur from an abnormality in a dorsal root ganglion when it is localized to that particular dermatome. Central neuropathic pain is sometimes caused by lesions of the thalamus or higher spinothalamic-cortical pathway. Another example is phantom limb pain when the source is projected to a part of the body such as an arm or leg that has been amputated. Neuropathic pain can be very severe, but difficult to treat.

Pain inhibition

Occasionally, pain sensation is inhibited when large areas of nociceptors are stimulated. This can be triggered by relatively weak mechanical stimuli and may work by inhibiting the discharge of selective receptors and synapses. A commonly used mechanism to relieve pain is rubbing around the site of an injury and is well appreciated by children, particularly when accompanied by a cuddle. Transcutaneous electrical nerve stimulation (TENS) systems use the same principle to relieve pain from joints and muscles or in childbirth. They work by applying weak electrical shocks to the skin near the site of pain.

Pain control

Pain can be treated by a variety of analgesic drugs that block the transmission of neuro-information at various levels. There is an important higher centre control reflex mechanism that can inhibit pain under certain circumstances. This may happen in highly emotional or stressful situations such as intense sporting competition, or traumatic accidents. Older children who have been injured characteristically say that even after severe injury, such as bone fracture, they felt no immediate pain, but that the pain came on after the acute event had passed. This endogenous analgesia system is mediated by production of opioid peptides, which include endorphins and encephalin. These activate opiate receptors that inhibit the normal pain pathways. This effect can be mimicked artificially by administration of opiate drugs such as morphine. Other mechanisms in the endogenous analgesia system probably include secretion of various neurotransmitters under stress, such as serotonin, adrenaline and noradrenaline.

MOTHER'S SIXTH SENSE

In general, newborn infants of mammalian species are immature and need care for survival. Their main requirements are for nutrition, warmth and protection and these are usually provided instinctively by the mother. Human infants are particularly helpless and require adult care for longer than most other species. In addition to these physical essentials, human babies need emotional care, which is also programmed into human mothers' instincts.

Bonding

In 1976 Klaus and Kennell in San Francisco, USA proposed that there is a 'sensitive' period immediately after birth when a mother becomes emotionally *bonded* to her baby. This process is facilitated by skin-to-skin contact and is compromised by separation. It is significantly enhanced by breast feeding. It is now accepted practice in many maternity units that infants are handed straight to their mother after birth, preferably before washing so that she can hold and cuddle her baby and start the post-natal bonding process. It is reinforced by 'rooming-in' of the baby rather than sleeping in a cot in a separate nursery. Bonding is greatest in the mother but is not exclusive to her and also develops in fathers who have close contact with a newborn infant. Bonding is a very powerful force and induces parents to make sacrifices (metaphorically nowadays) for their baby. In modern times these include financial hardship, loss of sleep and curtailment of career and recreational ambition. In ancient times, when newborns would invariably have been kept close to their mother (as long as she survived), bonding was the force that ensured that the infant's protection was her top priority. Bonding probably occurs in most mammalian species and makes a major contribution to the persistence of the species.

Attachment

The first descriptions of child behaviour following separation from their mothers followed observations done in the Hampstead War Nurseries (later the Anna Freud Clinic) on infants and children during World War II. Subsequently, detailed analysis was made from classic filmed records of looked after toddlers by James and Joyce Roberton. They found that the behaviour followed a consistent pattern:

1. *Protest* and acute distress with verbal and physical expression of anger. This phase seems to be an attempt to forcefully communicate the need to regain the mother's presence with the expectation that she will immediately reappear.
2. *Despair* when the child becomes progressively less active, quiet and withdrawn. This is a phase of mourning, but may be misinterpreted as a diminution of distress because of the lack of demands and silence.
3. *Detachment* is the phase when the child becomes more interested in surroundings, which is often erroneously interpreted as indicative of recovery. There is no longer rejection of advances from substitute carers with some social responses, such as smiles and physical interaction. However, when mother returns she does not receive the enthusiastic welcome that is expected and the child remains remote and apathetic and may appear to reject her. If the separation from mother is prolonged and the child has a succession of temporary carers, transient attachments are likely to be formed with progressively less commitment. Eventually the child may be unable to form a meaningful attachment and become self-centred. This harmful process can be mitigated by placement with a consistent carer, such as a grandparent, other relative or long-term foster parent.

Attachment was well described by John Bowlby (1907–1990). It is seen in many animals, for example ewes and lambs, ducks and ducklings, when the term *imprinting* (which can occur with any moving object) has been used. This happens very quickly, often within hours, and the mother and infant learn to recognize each other and behave in a mutually special and specific way. In humans it develops much more slowly: most human infants show attachment behaviour (specific smiling and vocalizing, which induces close proximity) to a mother figure around 6 months and have a strong attachment by the age of 12 months. The speed at which this develops depends mainly on the proximity of the mother and the duration of intimate contact with her. At first mother and child remain close to each other in dynamic equilibrium, but their distance apart increases as long as they are they are in visual contact.

As in other animals, attachment in humans diminishes in intensity as the child becomes more mobile. Dependence remains strong until the age of approximately 3 years and subsequently wanes gradually and disappears in adolescence, although emotional attachment continues. This sequence is one of the reasons that the normal age for entering nursery in the UK is 3 years. Prior to that children are very upset by the departure of their mother and greatly demanding for attention from the nursery staff (the 'protest' phase of separation – see above), whereas after the age of 3, most children accept a temporary mother substitute once they have become familiar with them, preferably in the presence of their mother. Deviation from this normal pattern is suggestive of abnormal emotional development and demands further investigation. Excessive separation anxiety and 'clinging' to mother in a 4–or more year–old may occur during illness or emotional trauma, such as the birth of a sibling. Attachment behaviour between two individuals is arguably the most powerful human emotion and endures despite interference by conflict, physical trauma (for example child abuse) and temporary separation.

Mother as caretaker

The newborn infant of all mammals requires physical care at first, which is usually provided by the mother. *Retrieval* is the action of keeping the infant close, which in many animals is done with the mouth, but primates use hands and arms. In humans this may mean cuddling, which, if not just for feeding, demonstrates an emotional interaction, or it may be physically protective if a mobile infant strays beyond a certain distance or signals distress. If the infant is threatened the mother's action is urgent and strenuous and only ceases when the infant is safely retrieved.

Mothers are very busy people and care of the infant has to compete with many other activities, for example housework. This, and most other maternal tasks, can be dropped at short notice and so are not incompatible with mothering. There are a few activities that are not so easily deferred, such as care of other children and relatives. A small number of mothers may have insuperable difficulties that interfere with their caretaker role, such as physical or mental illness, and they need special support and treatment.

One of the first proponents of the special relationship between a mother and her infant was Donald Winnicott (1896–1971). He said 'without maternal care there would be no infant'. Infancy is a crucial period for development of self and personality and the mother is normally the facilitator. At first, mother and infant are intimately adapted to each other, but as time goes by and the infant develops his or her own personality and independence, the mother's adaptation becomes progressively less complete. Winnicott proposed the term 'good-enough-mother' for the mother who is able to care appropriately for her child, recognize and respond to needs and allow the child to develop a healthy 'self'. *Holding* is the way the good-enough-mother shows her love; initially physically as well as emotionally, but over time she progressively lets go and the emotional component becomes more important, until, eventually, that too is released. Holding has three phases:

1. Absolute dependence – when the infant is unaware of the mother as a separate being and has no control.
2. Relative dependence – when the infant becomes aware of mother and maternal care.
3. Towards independence – when the infant does not need maternal care for everything and develops some self-determination through a combination of memory, cognition and increasing self-confidence.

During the first phase of absolute dependence the infant and mother are, in effect, *merged* and, by empathy, mother knows exactly what her infant needs. Gradually the infant separates and gives signals, which the mother interprets through sympathy, allowing the infant to progress to the next phase of holding. An experienced mother may be so good at understanding and anticipating her child's needs that she prolongs the merged state and the infant is unable to gain any control and separate from her. However, more recent research suggests that the child plays a much more active role and exerts a powerful influence on the mother–child relationship even from very early infancy.

Mother as child

When a professional is asked for advice about an infant or young child it is invariably the mother who makes the initial approach, relates the history of the concern, gives the background information, and implements recommendations and treatment. In effect, the mother is a proxy for the child and, in many ways, from a medical perspective, is the patient. In the management of some common problems of early childhood, for example feeding and sleeping disorders or oppositional behaviour, the treatment strategies are aimed mainly at the parents rather than the child.

It is a fairly common experience of child-care professionals that a mother may appear to identify too much with her child and her level of anxiety can interfere with best management from the professional's point of view. Winnicott used the term 'too-good-mother' to describe the mother who finds care of her baby too gratifying and is really meeting her own needs rather than those of the baby (Hopkins 1996). If it goes too far she can become a 'smothering' mother who completely swamps her child with her own needs for gratification and disregards the child's interests. The only way of dealing with this situation is to understand the mother's level of emotional identification and to work with it. Adopting an adversarial position is almost always counter-productive and does not help the child. This often requires patience, but the time is usually well spent. A major part of the art of the good children's advisor is to distinguish the mother who is appropriately anxious about her child for good reason from the mother who is inappropriately overanxious.

Mother as witness

A good witness is someone who has first hand experience of the situation under investigation and can give a accurate account of the events and circumstances leading up to them. A child's mother is uniquely placed to do that for several reasons:

- During pregnancy the fetus was physically part of the mother.
- Many substances including hormones and neurotransmitters cross the placenta and are shared in the body fluids of mother and fetus.
- As the fetus grows it becomes an increasingly strong component of mother's self-image.
- Half the child's genetic endowment is derived from mother so they will share many physical and psychological characteristics.
- The mother has known her child for approximately 9 months longer than anyone else during the antenatal period.
- Feeding, especially by breast, is the most intimate contact and reinforces the special relationship.
- After birth the mother usually spends more time with her baby than anyone else.
- A child's progress depends upon nature and nurture and mother is a major contributor to both.

Mothers quickly learn their child's normal pattern of behaviour and they are usually the first to recognize any deviation from it. If they have older children they know what to expect and they similarly will be suspicious if there is a change compared with their previous experience. Sometimes 'significant others' who know the child well, such as a grandmother, child-minder or nanny are the first to raise a concern. If a mother has a worry that she feels is important enough to bring to the attention of a childcare professional, she must be taken very seriously indeed. She must be listened to very carefully so that her anxieties are understood. It is wise for an assumption to be made that *mother is right* and her concerns should be dismissed only after great consideration. The reasons for reaching a different conclusion must be explained to her so that she understands and accepts them. Experienced professionals know that a mother's anxieties are ignored at great peril, and that a course of action with which she does not agree is most unlikely to work and is probably wrong.

References

Hopkins J 1996 The dangers and deprivations of too-good mothering. Journal of Psychotherapy 22: 407–422

Further reading

Baloh RW 1998 Dizziness, Hearing Loss and Tinnitus. FA Davis, Philadelphia
Grierson I 2000 The Eye Book. Liverpool University Press, Liverpool
Katz J (ed) 2002 Handbook of Clinical Audiology, 5th edn. Lippincott, Williams and Wilkins, Philadelphia

Social environment

R. Crowther

▼ OVERVIEW

This chapter summarizes the impact of different features of the social environment on the normal child and explores the impact of socioeconomic and environmental inequalities on children. This is a vast subject that cannot be covered in any detail in a chapter of this length: the aim is to encourage all those working with children to look beyond the child and appreciate the social circumstances that have helped to shape the child, and to consider the ways in which they – as adults, parents and professionals – can positively influence the social environment of all our children.

INTRODUCTION

No child is born or grows up in isolation, but is part of a complex social web that has a profound influence on life, health and development. This web of relationships and organizations includes the family and local community, home and school, and the wider world of the media, social policy and even international relations. How children perceive and experience the world, and how they perceive themselves as part of it, are vital parts of growing up and establishing an individual identity. The values and social conventions of the child's world and their impact, both direct and indirect, have a powerful effect on the child's experience and beliefs. But the child is also a *part* of the social environment: how people behave towards the child is important, but so too is how the child behaves towards others. As any parent knows, even the newest of newborn babies has a dramatic impact, influencing the lives, and the health and wellbeing, of others in the family. As children grow, so too does their influence on the social world.

The range of circumstances within which 'normal' children live is vast, even within the UK and other developed countries; indeed, the definition of normality may vary substantially from one community, faith group or family to another, and it is often through studying the effects of children's differing situations that we can explore and analyze the impact of social and environmental factors on their health and wellbeing. Most normal children grow up happily and healthily in a wide variety of different families and communities, and this social and cultural diversity adds richness to our collective experience. However, certain types of variation in children's social circumstances are clearly deleterious and are quite properly the concern of government and of all professionals working with children.

One example is poverty and socio-economic inequality, which lead to stark differences between the expectation of life and health of children from different ends of the social scale. Another is the difficulties experienced by a diverse range of children who are, for various reasons, vulnerable or in need: these include children at risk of abuse, children who take on a caring role for parents with health problems, children who are asylum seekers or refugees and others from socially excluded families; all of them 'normal', but experiencing more than normally difficult lives.

It is of course important to promote the health and happiness of children, who, as a vulnerable and dependent section of the population, deserve the help and protection of adults. We increasingly understand, however, that it is not just children's health that is at stake, but the health and happiness of the adults they will become. The dividends are potentially immense.

DETERMINANTS OF HEALTH IN CHILDREN

It is perhaps helpful at this stage to take a step backwards, considering briefly the state of children's health at the start of the twenty-first century and then setting in context the role and significance of the social environment by examining the different factors that affect the health and wellbeing of children and young people.

The health of Britain's children today

British children are in many ways healthier now than they have ever been. There has been a significant drop in infant and child mortality over the last century, and rates of illness (especially acute illness) have also fallen. Children are living longer, growing taller, and playing a more significant role in society. Improvements in medical science account for part of the difference, especially preventive measures such as immunization, the introduction of antibiotics to treat infectious diseases, and specialized medical and surgical treatments such as those for childhood cancer or congenital heart disease; however, social and environmental factors have been even more significant. These include increased prosperity and improved nutrition; the availability of birth control,

resulting in smaller families; public health measures such as improved housing, water supplies and sewage treatment; and action to tackle accidents.

But at the same time new child health problems have begun to emerge, the morbidities of a modern, prosperous, sedentary and 'high tech' society. Like the largely vanquished diseases of the nineteenth century, these new problems reflect the social, economic and environmental circumstances in which children now live. Many of the social advances of the last century have brought with them unwelcome side effects. As food (especially processed food with high levels of fat, sugar and salt) has become more and more readily available, obesity among children has risen to reach epidemic proportions. Because children's views are now seen to be important, they are increasingly targeted by advertisers wanting to take advantage of their vulnerability and spending power and to promote unhealthy products, from fast food to sexualized images. Changes in social attitudes and advances in equality of opportunity have led to changes in family composition and childcare patterns that may have an effect on children's wellbeing. Ironically, increased prosperity has brought with it greater inequalities in both income and health. Social and environmental change will be just as important in tackling the 'new morbidities' of child health such as obesity, substance misuse and the rise in emotional and behavioural difficulties as they were in addressing the child health problems of the last century.

The UK is at the top of the European league table for child poverty, injury rates for child pedestrians, and teenage pregnancy and sexually transmitted infection. Emotional and behavioural problems are increasingly common. Teachers in many inner city areas find it hard to teach, even in primary schools, and may be physically threatened by pupils. Among older children, smoking and binge–drinking continue to rise and suicide is more common, now accounting for one-third of deaths in 15–24 year olds. Meanwhile, fewer children walk to school, and their dependence on television, electronic games, mobile phones and the Internet increases. There are important health risks, as well as some benefits, associated with these changes in patterns of behaviour and interaction. Even if children are healthier, on balance, their adult selves may not be, as the time-bomb of risk factors set ticking in childhood reaches the end of its fuse: the gains in life expectancy of the last century could be lost if the rise in childhood obesity is not halted, and a generation of children risk dying before their parents.

FACTORS INFLUENCING CHILD HEALTH
(Fig. 12.1)

The social environment is only one of a wide range of factors affecting the health of children, but many of the others either influence the child's environment or are influenced by it. For example, the availability of public services, the quality of the physical environment and a family's economic circumstances are all substantially influenced by social policy, which

in turn reflects the values, beliefs and priorities of society. Individual choices about lifestyle and behaviour are heavily affected by social norms and pressures, environmental constraints and, indeed, policy decisions, which shape the costs and incentives associated with varying activities, e.g. smoking cigarettes or buying fresh fruit. This chapter takes a broad view, arguing that there are significant interconnections between different determinants of health and that most of the factors in the diagram below can legitimately be included in a discussion of social and environmental influences on health. This argument is even more pertinent when it is not just the child's health, but also growth, development and whole experience of life that is under consideration. Figure 12.2 illustrates this broadly defined social world as a series of layers surrounding the child.

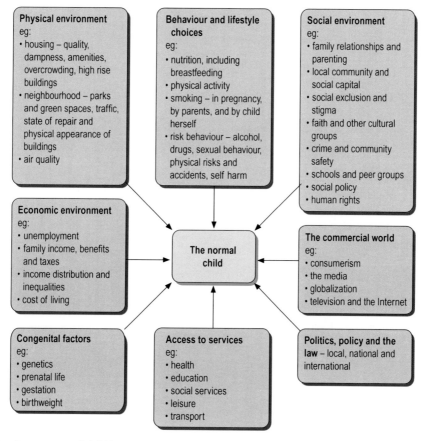

Figure 12.1   Key determinants of child health

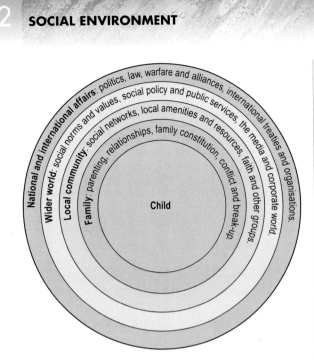

Figure 12.2 Layers of the social environment

Table 12.1 Components of the social environment
The child
The family environment
The economic environment
The effects of the social environment on lifestyle and behaviour
The local environment: communities and social capital
The physical environment
The policy environment and public services
The wider environment: media, marketing and the commercial world

Within each layer we can identify several different features of the child's social world: individuals; groups and organizations; and intangible collective factors such as policies, norms, social networks and interactions. Broadly speaking, at higher levels of social organization the latter two become more important and individuals less important, but this is not entirely true. Social norms and policies clearly have an impact at community level (partly through the mechanism of social capital, which will be examined later) and even at the level of a family or a parent (affecting, for example, decisions about breast or formula feeding) and particular individuals may have a profound influence at levels very remote from the child and family.

What are the important components of the child's social map (Table 12.1)? As well as those who have daily contact with the child (parents, grandparents, friends, childminders, nursery staff and school teachers) there are a range of professionals who have an interest in individual children and in how services and policy decisions affect children at large, including social workers, GPs, paediatricians, child psychiatrists and psychologists, therapists, midwives, health visitors, community nurses, police and probation officers. In the community there are others who play a role as stakeholders in society and

as part of the social environment, such as local residents, shopkeepers, leisure centre staff, bus drivers, religious leaders, youth workers and OFSTED inspectors. We might ask ourselves: what influence does each of these people have on children's lives? What does each see? What do they think about the influences on children's health and behaviour? What can they do to make a difference?

Social organizations range from the formal to the very informal; from groups based on collective worship to those, such as parent and toddler groups, based on common interest, mutual support and simply getting through the day. They include both statutory bodies and voluntary organizations: schools, youth groups, sports clubs and drop-in advice centres; peer-led and self-help groups; Brownie packs and music-making ensembles. Membership of constructive social organizations and networks has a positive influence on health, at an individual and a collective level, and for children they can enrich, safeguard, support growth and encourage exploration. The Early Years movement recognizes the vital importance of the health and wellbeing of children, and the adults they will become, and of the opportunities for learning and development in early childhood. Many interventions designed to improve child health and reduce inequalities (such as Surestart) focus on supporting early development and promoting a positive social environment for very young children. The biological basis for this approach, and the impact of the environment throughout a child's (and adult's) life course, is discussed later in the chapter.

LAYERS OF THE SOCIAL ENVIRONMENT

The first 'layer' is the child herself; but who is this 'normal child' whose world we are exploring? Just as there is a wide range of 'normality' in social circumstances and life experiences, so there is a vast range in terms of children themselves; indeed, with very limited exceptions (such as those with severe disabilities or life-limiting conditions whose experience of life is unavoidably different from that of other children) it might be argued that almost any child is as normal as any other. Increasingly, children across the country, and across many parts of the world, share values and cultural references, disseminated through the pervasive reach of modern media and information technology, and at a more fundamental level they share basic needs (for food, shelter and nurture), which reflect the unusually long period of dependence and immaturity that humans have compared with other mammals. Over the last century there has been an increasing recognition that children should also have in common basic rights- to life, identity, protection and education, for example- which are enshrined in the United Nations Convention on the Rights of the Child. These rights should extend to all children, whoever they are and wherever they live, including those who are excluded from many aspects of normal life. There is still a long way to go, however, before this goal is achieved. The vast majority of countries have signed the UN Convention on the Rights of the Child, but even so accidents of birth, geography and prejudice, and the selfishness and cruelty of adults, deny many children the most elementary of rights.

Children in Britain

According to the 2001 census, there are 14.8 million children and young people (aged under 20) in the UK, and 11.7 million dependent children (under 16 years, or 16–18 years and in full-time education)

Table 12.2   Social demography of children in the UK
Of the child population in the UK:
10% are from an ethnic minority group
19% of boys and 17% of girls have minor disabilities or long-standing illnesses (most commonly asthma)
11 per 10 000 boys and 5 per 10 000 girls have a severe disability (most commonly autism)
22% live in poverty
18% live in households where no adults work
12% live in overcrowded households
6% live in households with no central heating
149 000 provide unpaid care within the household
Over 58 000 children aged under 2 years live in homes two or more storeys above ground level
Data from Office for National Statistics website: www.statistics.gov.uk

(Table 12.2). The number of children in the population is declining (there are almost 2 million fewer under-20s now than in 1971) and for the first time ever, there are now more people aged over 60 than under 16 in the UK. Those under 16 years currently make up 20% of the UK population; down from 25% in 1971, and projected to fall to 17% by 2031. One-third of households in the UK have dependent children, and one household in nine has children under 5 years.

Different children and different circumstances

The determinants of health discussed in this chapter affect all children, but they do not affect all children equally. Children vary, and so do their social, economic and environmental circumstances: for some children the collective impact of these factors is positive, whereas for others they seriously threaten health and wellbeing. Do children's own intrinsic nature and characteristics affect their health? Clearly genetics has a direct impact but for many other factors (for example ethnicity, birthweight, disabilities and environmental factors) either have a role in causation or determine the extent of their impact. Nature plays a part, but so too do nurture and the way society shapes an individual child's experience. We now know a good deal about the way that environmental factors begin to influence health – setting the scene for adult health – before birth and during infancy.

Social inequalities A great deal of work has focused on exploring variations in health among children from different socio-economic backgrounds. There are clear patterns: children from lower social classes and from deprived areas tend to be less healthy and to have higher mortality rates then their peers from more affluent families. Socio-economic inequalities in health are discussed further in the section on poverty.

Geographical variation Where children are born and grow up affects their health. Rates of childhood poverty are much higher in inner cities than in suburban and rural areas, and in the worst wards up to three-quarters of children live in poverty. But there are pockets of rural poverty too, and isolation can be a real problem for poor families in rural areas with limited public transport. Statistical analysis shows that living in a deprived area adds to the disadvantage of individual families' poverty. Geographical comparisons at regional level also reveal inequalities: for example, rates of childhood obesity are highest in the North East and London, and lowest in the South East. Environmental factors account for many of these differences.

Ethnicity Ethnicity also has an impact on children's health. Babies born into black and minority ethnic group families are more likely to be breastfed, and those whose mothers were born in Africa or Asia are less likely to die of sudden infant death syndrome. However, overall infant mortality rates are higher for babies of mothers born in Pakistan, the Caribbean, and most parts of Africa. The social and physical environment is responsible for almost all of this variation, and we can unpick some of the relevant factors by examining data from health surveys and the census. Children of Indian, Pakistani and Bangladeshi ethnic origin are more likely to live with

both their natural parents than other UK children, but they are also more likely to live in low-income families. Sixteen per cent of white households are classified as low income, but all ethnic minority groups have a higher rate, reaching 60% for Pakistani and Bangladeshi families. Over 40% of Muslim children in the UK live in overcrowded housing (more than three times the average rate), over one-third live in households where no adult works (almost double the average rate), and one in eight live in housing without central heating (double the average rate). Patterns of social and environmental risk factors vary as much, if not more, *between* different black and minority ethnic groups as between the white population and all ethnic minority groups taken together, but they have in common the risk of racism, intolerance and stigma, and higher rates of social exclusion and poverty.

Asylum seekers Children seeking asylum in the UK have often experienced extreme social and environmental upset, including war and infrastructure breakdown, witnessing or suffering torture or other human rights abuses, separation from or death of friends and relatives, and the experience of flight and danger in transit. Once they have arrived in Britain, the problems associated with poverty and belonging to a minority ethnic group may be compounded by stigma and social exclusion.

Disability Despite the impact of legislation and of improvements in the acceptance of disability among the general public and providers of services, the social and physical environment still has a profound impact on the lives of children with disabilities, whether these are physical, intellectual or sensory. Children with physical disabilities may find it hard to use public transport or take part in sporting activities, for example, and discriminatory attitudes and stigma may affect access and participation for children with any kind of disability. There is a powerful school of thought that claims that disability, itself is socially determined: that the perceptions and reactions of society create the handicap associated with particular conditions, rather than the conditions per se. In an ideal environment, the lives of such children might not be substantially different from their peers'. At present, this is often not the case, and the impact of the child's difficulties may extend to the child's siblings, parents and even the extended family. Caring for a disabled child in the absence of adequate support from social care services can put an enormous strain on families. The family income may be reduced if one or both parents find it hard to combine employment with caring responsibilities, and the risk of conflict and family break-up may be increased as parents become increasingly worn down. Other siblings may resent the lack of time accorded to them, or feel guilty that life is easier for them. The practical, economic and psychological consequences may well rebound on the child herself, compounding the effect of her disability. Disabled children are also more likely to be abused by their parents or carers.

Vulnerable children Up to 20% of children in the UK face particular social difficulties that substantially affect their experience of life and limit their ability to exploit the opportunities other children take for granted. 'Vulnerable children' are those who would benefit from extra help from public agencies to

Table 12.3   Vulnerable children and 'children in need'
Vulnerable children include those: with disabilities
with behavioural and/or school attendance problems
with caring responsibilities – often for a parent with health (especially mental health or substance abuse) problems
with mental health problems of their own who misuse drugs who are teenage parents who are asylum seekers
'Children in need' are those vulnerable children who require specialist input and include: 'looked after children' – those in public care children in need of protection children in need of family support

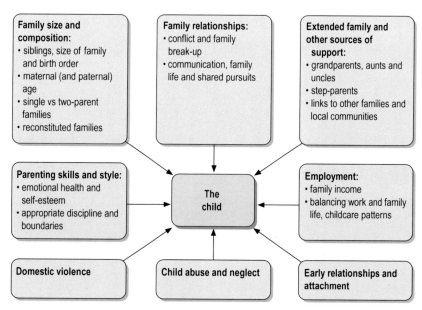

Figure 12.3   The family environment

improve their life chances and avert the risk of social exclusion. They include some of the children discussed above, as well as other groups (Table 12.3).

The family environment

Parents and families constitute the immediate social environment of most children and affect their health, wellbeing and development profoundly (Fig. 12.3).

Family life, and the kind of family in which the 'normal child' lives, have changed dramatically over the last few decades (Table 12.4).

Family composition Children can grow up healthily and happily in a wide variety of domestic settings:

single parents, step-parents and parents living apart can of course provide loving care and a secure environment. Nonetheless, disorder and disruption in their intimate social world can threaten children's wellbeing. Conflict between parents, family break-up and living with step-parents and step-siblings can all cause stress and vulnerability, and changes in circumstances (not least in economic circumstances) may complicate children's lives and have an adverse effect on their health and development. Domestic violence and family breakdown both increase the risk of child abuse and are associated with emotional and behavioural problems and poorer educational attainment. Children exposed to long-term unresolved conflict at home are more likely to have mental health problems and to find it difficult to establish healthy relationships in adult life, thus perpetuating the cycle of relationship failure and family breakdown.

Early mother–baby relationship The relationship between the baby and her mother (and father) in the

Table 12.4   Trends in family life and constitution
The number of children living in one-parent families has tripled since 1971, and now stands at 23% of children (and 27% of families – up from 8% in 1971)
Sixty-five per cent of children live with both natural parents and over 10% live in step–families
The average age of mothers has increased: in 2000, 46% of births were to mothers of 30 and over, compared to 32% a decade before
Teenage mothers account for 7.6% of births
As more women work, demand for 'wraparound childcare' has increased and children spend more time in daycare
The proportion of babies born outside marriage rose to 40% in 2001 (from 12% in 1980, and 6% in 1960), three-quarters of these births were jointly registered, however, mainly by cohabiting couples; 7.6% of births in 2000 were registered only by the mother (compared to 4.6% in 1975)
The proportion of babies whose mothers were born outside the UK is also rising – from 11.7% in 1991 to 15.5% in 2000
Forty per cent of first marriages now end in divorce

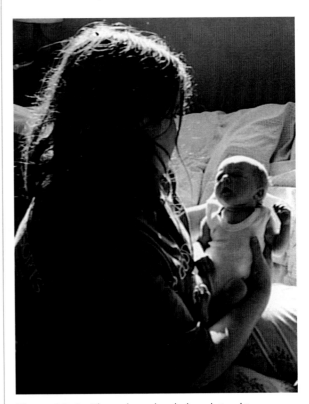

Figure 12.4   The early mother–baby relationship

first weeks and months of life is of vital importance for healthy growth and development (Fig. 12.4). Problems with mother–baby interaction may lead to insecure 'attachment' at the end of the first year (measured by the baby's response to temporary separation from the mother), which is associated with poor emotional and social outcomes. Insecurely attached babies tend, in later childhood and adult life, to have lower rates of self-confidence and self-efficacy, higher rates of anxiety and aggression, poorer ability to deal with stress and less success in forming relationships. Effective, empathetic nurture in the first year, by mothers (or others) who are able to 'read' and respond to their infants' needs, produces children who are more resilient in the face of stress and adversity and, importantly, seem less vulnerable to the effects of poverty and deprivation.

Many factors affect the early mother–baby relationship, including the mother's own experience of being parented, post-natal depression and socioeconomic deprivation. There are a number of successful intervention programmes that aim to promote attachment and, thus, improve babies' emotional and mental health, especially in mothers at high risk of encountering difficulties with parenting (such as very young mothers, those living in poverty and those with a history of mental health problems or drug abuse). These can make a significant difference to the environment of very young babies.

Parenting throughout childhood Relationships between parents and children continue to be important throughout childhood and adolescence: parenting style and, in particular, parents' approach to discipline, has a substantial impact on the child's predisposition to conduct disorder and antisocial behaviour. The balance between boundary-setting and supervision on the one hand, and punitive, cold and over-controlling discipline on the other, is a key factor at this stage. Children need clear and consistent discipline, but also warmth, encouragement and understanding. Baumrind has described the optimal style of parenting as *authoritative*, encompassing love, understanding and good communication, but with clear, agreed and appropriate boundaries for the child's behaviour. Children who grow up in family environments characterized by an authoritative approach to parenting tend to have higher self-esteem, better educational outcomes, more successful relationships with their peers and healthier lifestyles in adolescence. Less helpful parenting styles are either authoritarian (overly harsh and lacking warmth), neglectful (offering neither affection nor control) or permissive (warm and loving, but lacking boundaries). Again, interventions are available that can help parents modify their parenting style and improve the impact of this aspect of the child's environment on her development and wellbeing.

Abuse and neglect The most extreme form of poor parenting, which can have a profound effect on children's lives and health, is abuse (physical, emotional or sexual) and severe neglect. Abuse is not infrequently fatal; up to 100 deaths from abuse are identified every year in the UK and as many again may go undetected. Almost invariably abuse leads to serious physical and/or mental health problems. Abused children are also more likely to become abusive partners and parents in later life, once again illustrating the tragic transgenerational cycle of adverse events and circumstances. While abuse can take place in families from any background, some social and environmental factors play a part: physical abuse and neglect occur more frequently in those from lower socioeconomic groups; mental health problems and misuse of drugs or alcohol in the parents, and disability in the child, also increase the risk.

The economic environment

Poverty is still widely acknowledged to be the most powerful determinant of child health, even in the affluent UK, and income inequality accounts for much of the variation in morbidity and mortality in children across the country. Children are particularly susceptible to the negative effects of poverty and deprivation, which does measurable and serious harm to their health. The Joseph Rowntree Foundation has summarized its impact with the stark statement that 1400 children's lives would be saved per year in the UK if child poverty were eradicated. The UK government recognized the importance of concerted action to reverse the trend

Table 12.5   **Examples of social class gradients**
Infant mortality rate (age 0–1 year): social class V have double the rate of social class I, and the gap is rising despite the introduction of a national target to reduce it
Child mortality rate (age 1–15): social class IV and V have almost double the rate of social classes I and II
Deaths from road traffic accidents: class V five times higher than class I
Prevalence of mental health problems: class V three times higher than class I

of rising child poverty levels in the UK in the 1980s and 1990s and set a target of halving the extent of child poverty between 1998–99 and 2010, and eradicating it by 2020.

Impact of poverty One way in which the impact of poverty is apparent is in the differences in health between children at the top and bottom of the social ladder in the UK. There are social class gradients for almost all major causes of death and ill-health (Table 12.5).

Absolute and relative poverty It is significant that as the UK has become more prosperous, the distribution of wealth has become more unequal, with profound

Table 12.6   **Evidence for the importance of relative rather than absolute poverty includes:**
The existence of *gradients* for many health outcomes: mortality and morbidity decline gradually across social classes, or quintiles of deprivation, rather than dropping steeply below a certain level
The fact that countries with more equal distribution of wealth have better health (e.g. higher life expectancy) for a given level of national wealth (GDP); examples can be found in the developed world (notably in Scandinavia) and in less prosperous countries (such as Cuba, and the state of Kerala in India)

consequences for health and wellbeing. There is a key distinction to be drawn between *absolute* poverty, which has declined in prevalence over the last century in the UK (and is clearly less of a problem here than in those developing countries which are still riven by famine, drought and war) and *relative* poverty. The debate is of more than academic significance: absolute poverty can be alleviated by targeting the poorest in society with financial help and public services, while relative poverty can only be tackled by redistributing wealth within society (Table 12.6).

The European Union has adopted a measure of relative poverty that involves counting how many households have an income below 50% of the national average (median)— or how many children live in such households. The figures quoted in this chapter are based on this measure, which is widely used to compare countries or areas within countries. Measurements down to ward level allow very localized comparisons and the identification of small pockets of deprivation and 'hotspots' for child poverty. The UK compares very poorly to other Westernized countries, with more than one in five children living in poverty; around five times more than in Scandinavia. Child poverty levels in the UK have continued to grow in recent years, while the trend in many countries has been in the opposite direction.

Poverty and health inequalities A range of explanations has been put forward over time to explain how poverty causes differences in health between income groups. Although the theory that individuals at the lower end of the socioeconomic scale are intrinsically weaker and less healthy no longer holds any currency, the fact that unhealthy lifestyles are more common in low-income families still leads some commentators to point to socially and culturally determined differences in behaviour; in other words, to blame those affected for poor judgement and choice. However, lifestyle 'choices' are heavily affected by environmental factors, not least poverty, which constrain the choices available to individuals; and moreover, lifestyle risk factors alone cannot account for the level of health inequalities in the UK. It is now widely accepted that the connection between poverty and ill-health is a structural one:

that is, poverty and socioeconomic deprivation in themselves have an adverse effect on health.

The possible mechanisms linking poverty and health inequalities have been explored by Wilkinson. He suggests three possible explanations for the effect of unequal income distribution on health at population level:

1. It could simply reflect the aggregated effect of individual income levels: more poor people, worse health overall. Although individual income is important, careful analysis has shown that the differences in health between more-equal and less-equal countries are too great to be entirely explained in this way, suggesting that inequality (the unfair distribution of wealth) is bad for health in its own right.
2. It could reflect material deprivation: poor schools, damp and overcrowded housing, inability to afford healthy food or safety equipment, etc. These factors are certainly likely to play a part, affecting the environment in which families live and children grow up. Deprived neighbourhoods are less likely to have safe places for children to play, and poor families may find it harder to access health services, leisure facilities and other public amenities. The risk of accidents, respiratory infections, behavioural problems, obesity and poor educational attainment may all be increased.
3. It could be due to the psychosocial effects of poverty: awareness that others are better off, reinforcing the sense of being at the bottom of the pile. The psychological impact of marginalization and social exclusion (hopelessness, powerlessness, stress and low self-esteem) may precipitate domestic violence and crime, mental health problems, misuse of alcohol and drugs. We are beginning to unravel the mechanisms through which psychological factors can also have a direct impact on health; for example, by raising blood pressure and reducing the immune system's ability to fight infection. Together, these factors may provide part of the explanation for the impact of inequality per se. Uneven distribution of wealth affects health even at a local level: it is healthier to be poor in an area where everyone else is poor than in a generally prosperous area, which

illustrates the limitations of the material deprivation argument.

Recent progress in the UK As the first step on the path to eradicating child poverty in the UK, the government aimed to reduce the number of children in low-income households (defined as less than 60% of the average income) by one-quarter from 4.1 m to 3.1 m between 1998–99 and 2004–05, through a combination of financial support (for example tax credits and benefits) and public service changes to improve children's life chances. This initial target was not met, although significant progress was made, with a 700, 000 reduction in the number of children living in relative poverty by April 2005 – 300, 000 short of the target. The number of children living in absolute poverty fell further, from 4.3 million to 1.9 million between 1996–97 and 2004–05. The Joseph Rowntree Foundation and other independent organizations suggest that further action on tax credits and redistributive policies will be required.

The effects of the social environment on lifestyle and behaviour

It is now recognized that many 'lifestyle choices' about diet, exercise, smoking, alcohol and drug use, sexual behaviour and so on are substantially determined by aspects of the social environment. Since many habits and patterns of behaviour are established early in life, the effects of these environmental factors on young children can be powerful. Their parents' behaviour is important too: it can shape children's experience directly (by exposing them to cigarette smoke, or by determining what they eat) and, indirectly, by providing examples to follow (Fig. 12.5).

The notion of the 'obesogenic environment', for example, describes a world in which sedentary pursuits are the norm, active transport is on the wane and foods high in fat, sugar and salt are the most attractive and readily available. Indeed, the notion of 'lifestyle choice' may be misleading: people may make the only choices that are available to them, or those that are cheapest and easiest. There are often barriers of time, access and availability, skills, knowledge and, most significantly, cost, to making healthy choices. From a public health perspective,

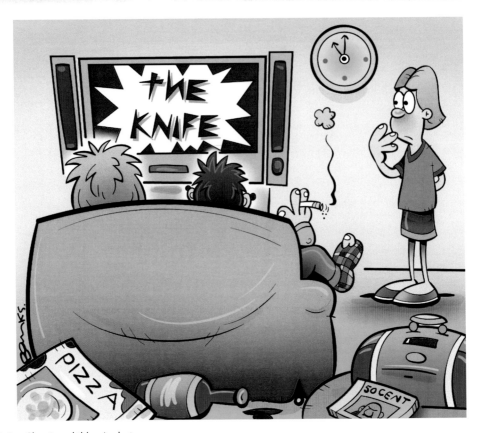

Figure 12.5 Shaping children's choices

what is amenable to change is the environment in which individuals act, rather than the actions of those individuals. There is a growing recognition that, while there are real concerns about the adoption of unhealthy lifestyles and risky behaviours, it is the environment that needs to change. The UK government's approach, outlined in the White Paper "Choosing Health", is to strive to 'make healthy choices easier'. It is important not to forget that healthy choices will always be more difficult for those living in poverty, however.

The importance of teenage and, indeed, pre-teen social norms in determining behaviour is evident not just in relation to collective pursuits such as smoking, alcohol and drug-use, but sometimes in 'epidemics' of self-harm or eating disorders. The power of peer role models can also be positively harnessed for health promotion initiatives to tackle, for example, smoking and drinking in young people.

Some important lifestyle factors are discussed in more detail below.

Diet and nutrition

Breast feeding The advantages of breast feeding were reviewed in Chapter 5. How to feed a baby is a highly personal decision, but the existence of social patterns in the uptake of breastfeeding make it clear that environmental factors play a part. Rates of breast feeding are increasing, and inequalities may be declining gradually, but they are still dramatic: in 2000, 91% of women in the highest social class started breast feeding, compared to 59% in the lowest social class and 53% of mothers with no partner. Rates were also higher among women with higher educational attainment. The differences between ethnic groups are interesting too: 95% of black women, 87% of Asian women and just 67% of white women started breast feeding. The rates declined in all ethnic groups with birth order, but most dramatically for white

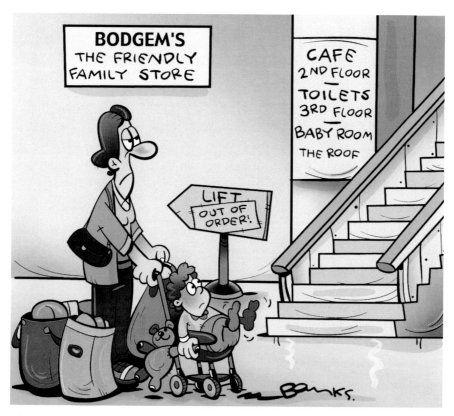

Figure 12.6   The environment can encourage or deter breast feeding

women: from 72% for first babies to 50% for third babies and 23% for fourth or subsequent babies.

In this instance, social and cultural norms affecting different groups of women clearly affect individual behaviour and hence the health and development of the child, but there is also scope for change in society at large to raise the overall proportion of mothers who choose to breast feed, and who manage to sustain it. Recent legislation in Scotland gives women the right to breast feed in all public places, a laudable step forwards in changing the social environment to the advantage of child health (Fig. 12.6).

Nutrition in later childhood After weaning, differences in cost, availability, convenience and attractiveness of foods play a significant role in shaping children's diet, whether it is bought for them by their parents, provided by their school or chosen by older children for themselves. The quality of school food is an important area of policy and local

practice which can make a particular difference to the diet of children from less well-off families who are entitled to free school meals. The potential benefits can be extended where breakfast clubs and afterschool clubs offer food at other times of day. But families' food purchasing and consumption habits are the most important influence, especially for younger children. Some of the factors affecting the kind of food people buy and eat, many of which reflect the social environment, are illustrated in Figure 12.7.

Parents are often short of time and may lack the skills needed to identify and prepare healthy foods: the contents of their shopping basket owe a great deal to marketing pressure, aimed both at them and at their children. They do not want to waste money on food their children won't like, and even if they aim for healthier options, food labelling can be very confusing and processed foods often contain large

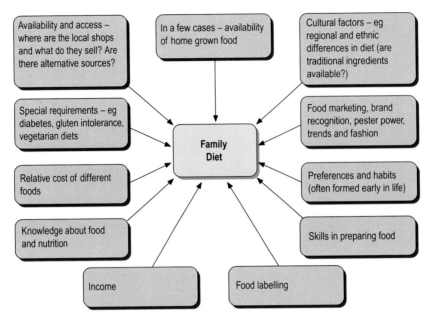

Figure 12.7   Environmental factors affecting food people buy and eat

amounts of 'hidden' fat, salt and sugar even if they carry a 'healthy' brand name. It has been repeatedly shown that healthy food (such as fruit and vegetables, fish and wholegrain bread) costs more than unhealthy food (such as processed meat, chips, biscuits and sliced white bread). Pressure from out-of-town supermarkets often squeezes out local shops that people can walk to, and where they remain the prices are often higher and the range of goods less wide, penalizing those without a car. Initiatives such as local food cooperatives and farmers' markets can help make fresh, healthy, sustainable food available to the local population.

Food poverty Despite government initiatives to promote '5 A DAY' fruit and vegetable consumption, which could have a dramatic impact on the population's health, we are a long way off this target, and children (and adults) from lower social classes eat half as many portions of fruit and vegetables as those from professional classes. The recent white paper, *Choosing health: making healthy choices easier,* puts forward a raft of proposals to improve children's diets, including higher standards for school meals, better labelling, action to reduce marketing of unhealthy food to children, extending the School Fruit and Vegetable Scheme and teaching children

Table 12.7   How is diet affected by income?
Low-income families:
spend substantially less on food in absolute terms
spend a higher proportion of their budget on food (up to 25%, as opposed to around 15% for those in higher income brackets)
consume more calories overall
get more of their calories from unhealthy sources (saturated fat and sugar)
eat around half the quantities of fruit and vegetables
eat fewer breakfast cereals and more bread and biscuits
drink more whole milk and less skimmed milk than **higher income families**

and parents about food preparation. Again, however, it is clear that poverty is a critical issue in shaping the choices available to some groups of people. The notion of 'food poverty' is defined as follows by *Sustain*:

Lack of money, inadequate shopping facilities, conflicting information about food and health, and poor transport mean that many people are denied healthy food choices. This has become known as food poverty.

An estimated 14 million people, including one-third of the child population, live in food poverty in the UK. National surveys show significant differences in shopping patterns between different income groups, and these are reflected in the nutritional value of the food they eat. The main differences are summarized in Table 12.7.

Physical activity Nutrition and physical activity represent two sides of the 'energy equation' that controls the development of overweight and obesity. Changes in both diet and exercise have contributed to the huge rise in obesity levels in children in the last 20 years and to the recognition that it now poses a serious threat to health and wellbeing (Tables 12.8 & 12.9).

Like nutrition, physical activity is a complex area involving many different factors. But physical activity is important not just because of the calories it burns or the cardiovascular fitness it helps to foster. There is considerable evidence that exercise has psychological benefits for people of all ages, but for

Table 12.8   Childhood obesity: facts and figures
Rates of obesity have doubled in 6-year olds (to 8.5%) and trebled in 15-year olds (to 15%) in the last 10 years: obesity is increasing more rapidly in the UK than any other part of Europe
Obesity could soon be the biggest cause of premature death, with the longevity gains of the last century being reversed and parents outliving their children
Changes in both diet and physical activity account for the increase: on average, children in England eat twice the amounts of saturated fat, salt and sugar that they need; 40% of boys and 60% of girls do not get the recommended one hour of physical activity a day

Table 12.9   The impact of childhood obesity
Psychosocial effects – social isolation, bullying, low self-esteem, depression
Poor mobility (thus vicious circle)
Lower levels of educational achievement
Two-thirds of obese children have one or more risk factors for heart disease (e.g. high blood pressure) and type 2 ('maturity onset') diabetes is now being seen in children
Other medical problems: e.g. sleep apnoea, orthopaedic problems, benign intracranial hypertension
Twenty-five per cent risk of becoming obese adults (especially if parents are overweight) rising to 70% for obese adolescents

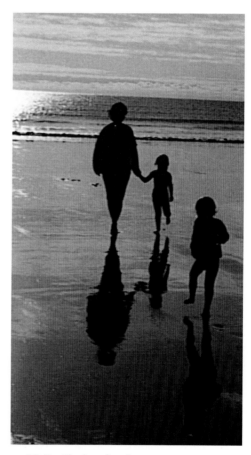

Figure 12.8 The benefits of exercise

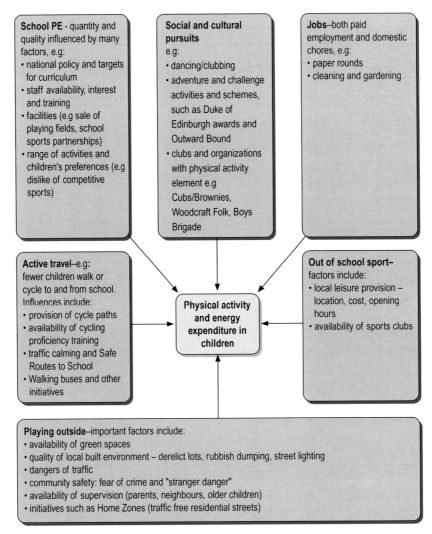

Figure 12.9 Social, economic, and policy factors affecting exercise

children the freedom to play outside, interacting with other children and allowing their creativity free rein, is vital for healthy development (Fig. 12.8). Lack of opportunity to venture beyond the television screen or the sofa is damaging emotionally and psychologically as well as physically. Even walking to school can be an important social ritual: a time for younger children to enjoy the company of parents, and a time without adults for older children.

The environment plays a significant role in shaping the amount and type of physical activity children and young people engage in: educational policy, local planning and transport policy, leisure provision,

youth culture and fashion, community safety and employment prospects are all important. Figure 12.9 illustrates some ways in which children take exercise and the social, economic and policy factors that may have an influence on physical activity.

Smoking Smoking in pregnancy increases the risk of low birth weight, stillbirth and infant death. Overall, smoking rates in pregnant women are falling (from 23% in 1998 to 20% in 2000), but there are still significant differences between social classes. According to the Infant Feeding Survey, 4% and 8% of women in social classes I and II respectively smoked during pregnancy in 2000, compared to 21% and 26% in social classes IV and V. Smokers in the household also increase the risk of sudden infant death and respiratory problems in children. Maternal (and paternal) behaviour thus affects the baby's intra-uterine and early postnatal environment and subsequent health, and, as for other aspects of behaviour, the inequalities in smoking rates reflect, at least in part, the impact of the mother's social environment. Several studies have shown the complexity of the factors that predispose to 'choosing' to smoke; for many women living in very deprived circumstances it is one of the few pleasures available and, moreover, an addictive pleasure. The fact that raising taxes on cigarettes does more to deter richer smokers than those who can least afford it illustrates the elusiveness of easy solutions, but for

the sake of children's health it is important that solutions are pursued. Smoking in childhood is discussed below.

Risk behaviour and adolescent health (Fig. 12.10) As they approach adolescence, children begin to make more lifestyle choices for themselves, adopting patterns of behaviour and experimenting with risks that can affect their health substantially and may contribute to premature mortality. As well as diet and exercise, substance misuse (for example smoking, alcohol and drugs), risky sexual behaviour and taking physical risks are common, and becoming more so as young people of this age have more money and the opportunities open to them increase. Parental behaviour may provide a model for children, and many elements of unhealthy lifestyle

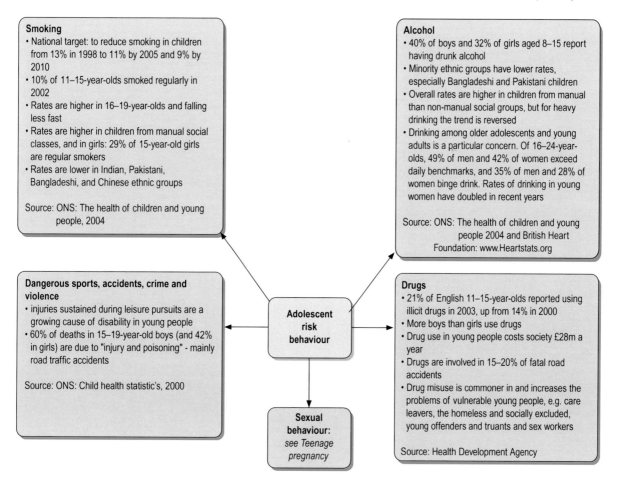

Figure 12.10 Adolescent lifestyle factors affecting health

are more common in low-income families. Marketing strategies aimed at adolescents, peer pressure and lack of perceived opportunities for employment and advancement also play a part. Although young people from all social classes experiment and take risks in their teens, those from more affluent backgrounds are more likely to leave these patterns of behaviour behind as they enter adulthood.

Teenage pregnancy Sexual experimentation in adolescence may be a positive experience, but it can also lead to emotional distress, sexually transmitted diseases (chlamydia is a particular problem in this age group, and may lead to fertility problems later) and unwanted pregnancy. Teenage pregnancy is a public health priority in the UK and the focus of a national strategy driven by targets supported by the Public Service Agreement for the NHS. The UK has the highest rate of teenage pregnancy in Western Europe: our rate is three times higher than Germany, four times higher than France and seven times higher than Holland. One in ten births in England is to a teenage mother. In 2000, there were 38 700 conceptions in young women under 18 in England, of which one-fifth

(7600) were to girls under 16 years. Just under one-half of these pregnancies were terminated.

Environmental factors, particularly socioeconomic disadvantage, strongly influence the risk of teenage pregnancy, which in its turn fuels the cycle of deprivation by increasing the risk of poor social, economic and health outcomes for both the young mother and her child (Table 12.10). Low self-esteem, lack of employment opportunities and the hope of higher status and independence as a mother are all important risk factors. Rates of teenage conception are almost ten times higher among young women in social class V than among those in social class I. In 2000, under 1% of births to women with partners in social class I was to teenage mothers, compared with 15% in social class V. The daughters of teenage mothers also have a higher chance of becoming teenage mothers themselves.

Other groups at high risk of teenage pregnancy include young people looked after by the local authority ('in care'); those excluded from school, regularly playing truant or with low educational attainment; victims of childhood sexual abuse; and young offenders. Studies have found that:

- one-quarter of girls in care have a baby before the age of 16 and nearly one-half become teenage mothers within 2 years of leaving care
- in one small study, 14% of girls excluded from school became pregnant while excluded

Table 12.10	The impact of teenage pregnancy
Social impact	Increased risk of: • low educational attainment • social isolation
Economic impact	Increased risk of: • poverty • unemployment
Health impact	• higher risk of complications in pregnancy: pre-eclampsia and anaemia • higher rates of smoking in pregnancy • lower average birth weight • higher rates of some congenital malformations • infant mortality rate more than double the national average • higher maternal mortality rate • lower rates of breast feeding

Table 12.11   National Teenage Pregnancy Strategy Targets for England
Reduce the under-18 conception rate by 50% by 2010 against a baseline in 1998, with an interim target of a 15% reduction by 2004
Achieve a well-established downward trend in the under-16 conception rate by 2010
Reduce the inequality in rates between the fifth of wards with the highest under-18 conception rate and the average ward rate by at least 25% by 2010
Increase to 60% the participation of teenage parents in education, training or employment to reduce their risk of long-term social exclusion by 2010

- teenage mothers are six times more likely to have no academic qualifications than the general population
- young people who have been in trouble with the police are twice as likely to become teenage parents
- up to one-third of male young offenders have fathered a child.

The National Teenage Pregnancy Strategy (Table 12.11) aims to help young people resist peer pressure to have early sex and to use contraception if and when they decide to become sexually active.

The local environment

Communities Understanding of the way in which community life influences health has developed significantly in recent years. Do people in a road, an estate, a neighbourhood know each other? Would someone notice a child alone on the streets and feel she was their responsibility? Do neighbours look after each other's children in an emergency or other circumstance? Are there sources of informal advice and help for young and not so young mothers? The answers to questions such as these have important implications for the existence of social support or social isolation, for the fear (and the prevalence) of crime, and for the quality of everyday life. They can affect children directly, by including them in social networks that extend beyond the family, offering alternative role models and authority figures and giving them greater independence to play and explore their world within the security of collective responsibility. They can also affect children indirectly via an impact on their parents' emotional wellbeing, parenting capacity and perhaps opportunities for employment.

Inclusion and exclusion The opposite of social inclusion, where people feel part of the local community, is social exclusion. Even in areas where social networks are strong, some individuals or families may be excluded, often due to their difference from the local norm in terms of income, behaviour or lifestyle, health (especially mental health or dependence on drugs or alcohol), race, religion, gender or sexual orientation. Many children who are vulnerable or in need, such as asylum seekers, minority ethnic groups, travellers, children with disabilities, children with caring responsibilities and children looked after by the local authority, are also socially excluded as a result of intolerance and stigma.

Social capital The term social capital describes the effects of social cohesion, mutual co-operation, trust and participation within a community. It is generated by complex interrelationships and social networks, what has been described as the 'invisible glue' that binds people together, and is associated with a sense of belonging and shared identity, civic pride and the desire and ability to work together for the collective good. There are measurable benefits for health associated with living in communities with high social capital, including higher life expectancy and lower crime rates. While lower crime rates may be explicable through the mechanism of informal social control, the benefits of higher life expectancy and lower incidence of cancer and heart disease are more surprising and require a more subtle explanation.

The relationship between poverty and social capital is an interesting one. Although poorer communities tend to have lower levels of social capital, in some cases, such as long-established immigrant communities, the opposite is true. In these cases, social capital may offer some protection against the negative health effects of poverty.

The physical environment

The physical environment is included here partly because social values and social policy affect the quality and appearance of children's surroundings – the house, flat, street or neighbourhood where they live, the air they breathe, the open spaces available for them to play in – but also because it is often hard to distinguish the impact of physical and social aspects of children's surroundings. Is a child's home, for example, a matter of bricks, mortar, plasterboard and mould, or of people and their actions: secondhand smoke, a television permanently on, chips rather than green vegetables for dinner? Are the graffiti on the walls, the broken lift, the dark street corners and the smashed windows simply concrete facts, or does their impact have more to do with the social deprivation and despair they reflect?

Housing, air quality and the built environment The statutory minimum standard for housing incorporates nine criteria that define whether properties are fit for human habitation, including structural stability, adequate lighting, heating and ventilation, and disrepair and damp. Many children in low-income families live in poor accommodation that may be damp, poorly heated and overcrowded. Such children are more likely to suffer from asthma and infectious diseases. Pollution and poor air quality in inner city areas is also associated with worsening of respiratory conditions. 'Poor neighbourhoods' are those in which more than one in ten buildings are defective or derelict, or where there are vacant lots, litter dumping, vandalism, graffiti and so on: areas in which parents may not want their children to play outside, and where they may suffer injuries if they do. The physical environment also has a powerful impact on active travel, encouraging or deterring walking and cycling. Research by the charity Sustrans shows that the built environment and travel patterns are closely linked to levels of obesity, and that traffic calming in deprived urban areas can significantly increase the numbers of people willing to walk.

Sustainability and the global environment Our interaction with the physical environment – depleting natural resources, generating pollution and greenhouse gases – has serious implications for the health and, indeed, the existence of future generations of children. Sustainable development involves working towards an environmental status quo across the globe, with resources being conserved and the accumulation of waste being kept to a minimum. Public policy and social attitudes have an enormous impact on the global physical environment, for example, through lifestyles that involve the use of gas-guzzling cars and pre-prepared, packaged food, and through governments' willingness to commit to emissions standards or promote recycling. As we consider the environments in which children live, it is important that we continue to look outwards to the world's ecosystem and recognize our role in preserving it for the future.

The policy environment and public services

Social policy may operate on a level far removed from the individual child, but its effects are pervasive. At an international level, Human Rights law, and specifically the United Nations Convention on the Rights of the Child, offer a safeguard to all children whose countries are signatories to it, although loopholes left for those without a long-term right to remain may undermine the security of already vulnerable children. European legislation on, for example, employment conditions and food safety provide further examples enacted at supranational level.

Laws and policy directives at national level determine the availability of the public services that are part of the 'social fabric' of the country, and local government makes important policy decisions too, shaping local schools, facilities and services. Recent government policy initiatives in the UK recognize the connections between different areas of public life, and the need for action across a wide spectrum to improve the health and wellbeing of the population. Much that concerns the child population now comes under the remit of the Minister for Children, but almost every government department, local service or aspect of policy has an impact on child health and wellbeing. Examples include access to childcare, the availability of social support and the effectiveness of child protection arrangements; the availability and quality of education, the success of inclusion policies and action to reduce truancy; the availability, opening hours, appeal and cost of leisure and sporting facilities; the way transport policy shapes people's lives, encouraging walking and cycling and enabling easy access to shops and other facilities; access to training and support for those seeking employment; and the availability and appropriateness of healthcare, especially for hard-to-reach or socially excluded groups, those with special needs, or those who are suspicious of mainstream services (which includes many adolescents).

Education Educational attainment has a significant impact on health, even when related factors such as social class and employment are taken into account.

Much attention has been focused recently on the provision of early education, which has a powerful influence on children's development and their subsequent progress and health, but educational inequalities in later childhood and adolescence are important too. A recent report by the London Health Commission showed that the gap in educational attainment at GCSE between Inner London and Outer London is decreasing, but there is still a 10% difference in the proportion of pupils reaching the target of five GCSEs at grades A* to C (51.9% compared to 41.1%). Only 25% of London children eligible for free school meals met the target. There are large variations in attainment between ethnic groups too: according to 2002 data from the Department for Education and Skills, the national average for white pupils is 51%, for black Caribbeans 30%, for Pakistanis 40%, for Indians 64% and for Chinese 73%. It is suggested that factors that may play a part include social class and neighbourhood, the influence of peers and teachers, school effectiveness (the best schools do not tend to be found in the most needy areas), language proficiency, recency of migration and social inclusion and integration.

Some children miss a significant amount of schooling, for a variety of reasons:

- because of chronic illness or conduct disorder
- because of frequent moves (e.g. those from traveller communities, or those whose families have suffered break-up and instability)
- because they feel unsafe in school, e.g., as a result of bullying (which may be racist, homophobic or otherwise discriminatory and stigmatizing)
- because of caring responsibilities at home.

For these children, who are often already at a disadvantage compared to their peers, poor educational attainment may contribute to another vicious cycle of poor employment prospects and life chances, social exclusion and poverty.

Schools play another significant role too: the social and physical environment that surrounds children in school can have a powerful influence on health and wellbeing. The national Healthy Schools Programme recognizes this, and supports the promotion of physical, mental and emotional health throughout the school community, including staff. School initiatives may incorporate such diverse elements as fostering a positive school ethos, which can boost children's mental health and self-esteem; participation and community development, through school councils, etc.; modifications to playgrounds and lunchtime activities to encourage exercise, tackle bullying and perhaps even allow children to grow vegetables; breakfast clubs, healthy snack bars and cooking clubs to promote healthy eating.

Health services Inequalities in health do not directly reflect health service provision, but inequitable access to health care can certainly exacerbate them. Many of those who most need health services find it hardest to obtain them. Several factors contribute to this:

- geographical skewing of provision (the 'inverse care law' describes the way high-quality services have tended to be clustered in more prosperous and healthy areas at the expense of deprived neighbourhoods)
- a tendency to focus on 'high tech' interventions rather than long-term care (for children with severe disabilities, e.g.) or health promotion
- the barriers created by, e.g., language and lack of interpreting provision; limited clinic hours; poor provision of public transport; and 'gatekeepers' (such as receptionists) whom the more articulate and empowered are more likely to get past.

Preventive and screening services in primary care, such as immunization, antenatal care, child health surveillance and preventive dentistry, play an important role in ensuring a healthy start in life for all children. The health-promoting potential of public health professionals such as midwives, health visitors and school nurses is being increasingly recognized. Universal services such as these may also offer a vital 'way in' to families who are experiencing difficulties, and children who may be at risk of failure to thrive, neglect or abuse. The NHS has a responsibility to promote equity in health. As the Children's National Service Framework is implemented; as the NHS follows the direction set by the White Paper *Choosing health: making healthy choices easier* and moves further towards the realm of preventive medicine and health promotion; and as integration of health and social services is pursued through Children's Trusts and other initiatives, there will be real opportunities to make a difference. It is important that the voices of children and young people themselves continue to be heard, and that the health service evolves in a way that meets their needs.

Transport Transport policy has been mentioned in passing several times in this chapter. Its effects on health are manifold. Families on a low income, especially those living far from shops and amenities, may depend on public transport and their choices and opportunities may be heavily constrained by the availability of cheap, convenient bus or train services. As well as day-to-day necessities, their access to relatives, leisure and cultural facilities and the countryside may also be limited. How children travel to and from school and how they get about at other times depends to a large degree on the attractiveness, safety and ease of cycling or walking and, again, on the availability of public transport. Poor provision of buses and safe cycle lanes (and cycle training), and road safety concerns, increase the use of cars for frequent short journeys, contributing to pollution, obesity and traffic danger. Road traffic accidents remain a major cause of injury and death in children, and child pedestrians from lower social classes are at very much higher risk of being involved in accidents. Traffic calming measures, Safe Routes to School and enforcing local speed limits can reduce the number and severity of accidents. The likelihood of death or serious injury rises dramatically with every 10 miles-an-hour increase in speed.

The wider environment: media, marketing and the commercial world

Retailing and commerce Like the rest of the population, children are exposed every day to products, images and ideas from across the globe. These reach us through television, video, DVD, computers and the Internet; in advertisements on billboards, buses, screens and magazines; and on packaging for food, toys, toiletries, gadgets and accessories. They are generated by multinational corporations whose tentacles reach into almost every corner of the globe, and by marketing and advertising companies who are increasingly wise to the purchasing power of younger and younger

children, and increasingly cunning about how to exploit their young target audience. The House of Commons Select Committee Report on Obesity, published in March 2004, set out alarming evidence of marketing campaigns for junk food aimed at children that deliberately set out to exclude parents, bypassing traditional media altogether and instead passing 'secret messages' through networks of children. The same report presented a stark comparison between the amount of money spent every year on advertising confectionery, cakes and crisps and the paltry sums devoted to promoting fruit and vegetables and other healthy products.

Developing effective strategies for altering consumer behaviour is the *raison d'etre* of the advertising agencies, and the increased sales they deliver ensure that the power of multinational corporations and their brandnames grows ever greater. In addition to the effects on children in the UK, the trading giants have a substantial impact on children in the developing world: for example, those whose labour goes into the products, and those who are fed expensive formula milk which may be made up with contaminated water. There are examples of responsible behaviour within the food industry, such as the 'fair trade' movement and recent moves to shrink portion sizes and to seek ways of reducing the fat and sugar content of processed food. However, it is worth remembering that food producers and retailers are only likely to take account of public health issues insofar as they offer a way to boost sales by cashing in on popular concern (Fig. 12.11).

The media and communication Modern communication – mobile phones, with text, photo and even video messaging; e-mail and chatrooms; the messages conveyed by fashion choices and designer labels – is powerful and pervasive, changing the patterns of social interaction between young people dramatically. Camera phones can be used to flash images across the classroom out of sight of the teacher, offering the potential for bullying and invasion of privacy; paedophiles can 'meet' children in unpoliced chatrooms. On a more mundane level, young people can communicate both instantly and at one remove, enabling plans to be infinitely flexible and the constraints of face-to-face contact to be removed. This has its benefits, giving children greater

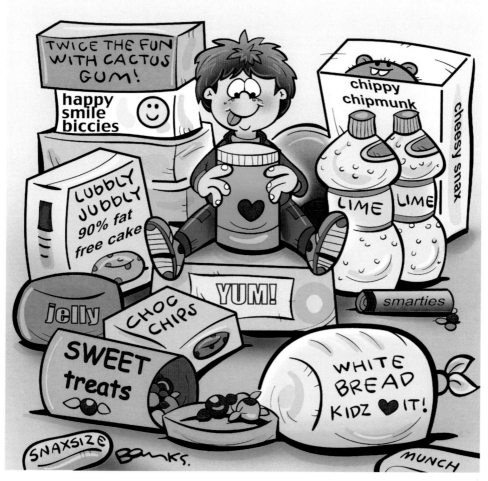

Figure 12.11   Media influence

freedom and allowing parents to keep in touch with them while they are out and about; but it also has its disadvantages, allowing young people to hide behind the shield of technology and to say things that they might not feel comfortable with if they were communicating on a more direct and personal level.

The impact of new technology on children's health is not yet known, but we do know a considerable amount about the effects of television. Television may be a godsend to stressed parents as a source of cheap and absorbing entertainment: safer, they may feel, than having their children roaming the streets, and more palatable than having them under their feet all day long. However, watching TV is a very sedentary pursuit, often accompanied by a packet of crisps or biscuits, and it can reduce conversation and interaction within the family. There are potential educational benefits (from schools programmes, for example, and the many high-quality documentaries, dramas and news programmes for young people), but as with food and nutrition the balance of benefit and harm depends on both quantity and quality, and many children's TV diet is both excessive in volume and rich in junk, including frequent advertising breaks on most channels. Children may not even focus on a particular programme, but flick from channel to channel through the bewildering array on offer as their concentration span flags.

Reducing the amount of time children spend watching television has been shown to have a positive impact on both obesity and aggressive behaviour (see also Chapter 9). It is also important to ensure that children are not exposed to inappropriately violent or sexualized behaviour on screen: the evening 'watershed' may not be effective in preventing this, since many children do a substantial amount of their watching late into the evening, often alone in their own bedrooms rather than as part of the cosy family group around the set that advertisers are fond of portraying. Watching television carries opportunity costs too: in 1999, children spent on average 11.4 hours a week watching television and videos compared with 7.5 hours on physical activity out of school.

The growing child

One way of visualizing a child's journey through life is to imagine the child moving gradually outwards through the different layers of the social environment that have been discussed in the preceding sections and that have surrounded the child from birth. As the child grows up, the boundaries of the world shift, and so too do important factors such as what matters most to the child or where he or she turns for information, advice and comfort. For the newborn, the social world does not extend much beyond the mother, but as the baby gets older the rest of the family has a growing role. For the toddler, the local community becomes increasingly important, offering play facilities, encounters with other children and families, perhaps childminders or crèches. The preschool child's world may extend to include nurseries or other early learning opportunities, and greater awareness of other children and adults (friends, professionals, members of the local community). At school entry there is a quantum leap – the first of several – towards independence from the family, while teachers and the child's peer group become more important influences. Gradually the child becomes aware of the wider world, the whole country and the whole globe, and national and international factors come to have more relevance. The child's social and emotional development mirrors this progress out into the world, and the important outcomes at each stage reflect the sphere

in which he or she operates: for example, attachment to the mother for the infant; ability to relate to peers and share toys for the pre-school child; ability to participate in and benefit from mainstream education; emerging individuality and self-image in the adolescent; and the ability to make healthy choices throughout life.

The impact of prenatal life and infancy on later health

A child's early environment and experiences not only affect health and wellbeing in childhood, but they cast a shadow into later life too. There is growing evidence that factors operating in infancy - and indeed in fetal life-affect adult health.

- *Socioeconomic circumstances* in early life have been shown to have an impact on adult health as well as child health. This is believed to be due in part to the direct, long-term effects of childhood poverty and deprivation, and in part to the fact that poor socioeconomic circumstances in childhood tend to persist into adulthood, through the cycle of poor health and educational attainment, poor employment prospects and low income.

- The importance of *early care, mother–baby attachment and parenting* is demonstrated by studies showing that nurture in infancy affects the ability to form positive, supportive relationships in adulthood, and that such relationships in turn help protect individuals against physical and mental ill-health. Research on brain development, summarized in the next section, offers a neurological explanation for this causal chain.

- Barker is one of the key exponents of *biological programming*, which points to direct links between specific events and circumstances at critical periods in early life and later consequences for health. The devastating effect of certain drugs (e.g. thalidomide) and infective agents (e.g. rubella or toxoplasma) on fetal development is well known, but the 'Barker Hypothesis' takes a broader view. Barker first suggested that environmental factors operating before birth and in infancy might be responsible for variation in adult health after observing the association between low birth weight and below average weight at 1 year of age, and coronary heart disease later in life. Several studies have subsequently supported his findings and confirmed the link between impaired fetal and infant growth and higher risk of high blood pressure, heart disease, stroke and diabetes in adulthood, especially when small babies become overweight adults. Barker coined the term 'the thrifty phenotype' to explain these findings, suggesting that the body responds to early undernutrition with metabolic and endocrine changes that are designed to cope with hardship and poor availability of food, but that predispose the individual to obesity and other adverse health outcomes if food subsequently becomes more plentiful.

Birth weight

Birth weight is an important predictor of health in infancy and beyond, and is heavily influenced by environmental factors (Table 12.12)

Brain development in early life

Bronson summarizes advances in our understanding of brain growth that underline the importance of a child's experience and environment in the early years in shaping the way the brain develops. During the first 3 years of life, the number of brain cells (neurones) and connections between them (synapses) increase rapidly, reaching double the final adult level: a phenomenon known as 'overwiring', which means the young child's brain has enormous potential and the flexibility for patterns of connections within the brain to be shaped in many different ways. The number of neurones and synapses then gradually dwindles during childhood and adolescence. Neuronal connections and communication routes that are frequently used are stimulated and strenthened, while unused connections are lost through a process known as 'synaptic pruning'. The brain moves from being 'softwired' (the early, flexible state) to being 'hardwired'. Brain activity that is encouraged by environment becomes more effective and efficient as frequently used patterns are learned, but the 'architecture' of the brain becomes more fixed, establishing patterns for the future and restricting the potential to change the way the brain responds to stimuli.

Research is illuminating the way nature and nurture interact during early life, with both positive

Table 12.12 Environmental factors affecting birth weight	
Smoking	Mothers who smoke in pregnancy are more likely to have small babies
Social class	Babies with fathers in non-manual occupations are heavier on average than those with fathers in manual occupations
Partner	Babies whose birth is registered only by the mother (i.e. without a father mentioned on the birth certificate) are on average lighter than jointly registered babies in any social class
Ethnic group	There are substantial differences in the birth weight of babies born to mothers in different ethnic groups: Asian babies are the lightest, black babies the next lightest and white babies the heaviest
Mother's Country of birth	The percentage of low-birth-weight babies is much higher among women born in the Caribbean Commonwealth, India, Pakistan, Bangladesh and Africa (excluding Southern Africa)
Maternal age	Teenage mothers and those in their 40s are most likely to have low birth weight babies and mothers aged 25–34 years are least likely
Social deprivation	More low birth weight babies are born in deprived areas
From: The health of children and young people, National Statistics	

and negative aspects of the child's environment helping to shape brain development. Negative early experiences such as sensory deprivation, maternal depression, trauma and neglect, institutionalization and the impact of poverty have been shown to affect brain activity, growth and development adversely. Appropriate, attuned care and nurture are beneficial, and early interventions that improve a child's social environment and care have the potential to alter the course of brain development.

Although the environment plays a role throughout childhood, the brain is most susceptible during certain sensitive periods of development. In general, the first years of life are the most critical, but the timing varies for different parts of the brain. Visual and auditory stimuli, for example, are especially important very early in life: at 2 or 3 months of age. The frontal lobes are responsible for many cognitive and social functions, such as problem-solving, understanding, empathy, communication, motivation, control of emotions and behaviour and establishing a sense of self. The process of growth and reduction of synapses in this area of the brain occurs more slowly than in other areas, with most of the 'pruning' taking place between about 7 and 16 years of age. Thus, the social environment continues to affect social and cognitive development throughout later childhood and adolescence.

The life course approach

There are therefore sensitive periods in a child's life when environmental factors can have a critical influence on health and development – through an effect on birth weight, or synaptic pruning, for example. But do these mechanisms fully explain the impact of early environmental factors on health? How can sense be made of the complex web of causation and influence in order to understand how environmental influences throughout life interact to shape an individual's responses, resilience and risk of disease? Kuh and Ben-Shlomo offer an integrating framework that takes account of the multitude of social and environmental factors operating at different stages of life, outlining what is known as the *life course approach* to epidemiology. This model sees causation in terms of the cumulative effects of environmental and other factors throughout life,

recognizing that early events and circumstances interact with later ones in shaping individuals' overall risk of disease. Exposures in childhood are seen, therefore, as a vital part of the overall picture. It is important to remember, too, that childhood experience is valid and important in its own right, and not simply as a precursor to adult life.

CONCLUSIONS

This chapter has considered many aspects of the child's environment, outlining the importance of a wide range of social factors as determinants of child health. But which are the *most* important? How can factors operating close to the child be compared with those that exert their effects from a distance?

There is a continuing debate in public health circles as to the relative importance for child health of 'micro' level socioenvironmental factors, such as family relationships and parenting, and 'macro' level factors, such as poverty and social policy. The young child's immediate environment has a powerful influence on development and wellbeing, and interventions that support parents and families and promote emotional wellbeing can do much to mitigate the impact of adverse socioeconomic circumstances in individual cases and, indeed, to break the intergenerational cycle of poor parenting and emotional deprivation in early life. But there is a strong argument that solutions which focus on individuals will never improve the general lot of children in the UK while the stark economic inequalities that shape our society remain. It is true that neither suboptimal parenting nor family break-up, domestic violence nor child abuse are uniquely the preserve of low-income families, but it is the case that poverty, deprivation and the deadening effects of living in a depressed environment make it much harder to be a good and effective parent. In other words, macro level economic inequity accounts for much of the variation in micro level environmental determinants of health such as the family environment. Similarly, individual 'choices' about lifestyle and behaviour are heavily affected by social and environmental cues, and poverty and deprivation are associated with a higher prevalence of unhealthy lifestyles in lower socioeconomic groups.

The primary purpose of this chapter is not to propose child health policy, but rather to explore the powerful impact which the social environment has on child health, and to illuminate the complex interactions and connections between different layers of the environment. Nonetheless, it is difficult to resist the small step from 'How does the social environment affect children?' to 'What can we do to make things better?' Unlike earthquakes or newly emerging killer bugs, many of the factors discussed in this chapter are within our collective control. Improvements in children's social and physical environments can be achieved through action at several different levels: by international organizations, governments, communities and individuals. Public health professionals and bodies can provide an organizing force, and can offer expert skills such as health needs assessment and health impact assessment to help target action where it is most needed, but they can do little on their own. All those who are interested enough to have read this far have an important role to play in tackling the problems this chapter has set out; as advocates, role models, parents, professionals and global citizens.

Further reading

Barker D (ed.) 2001 Fetal and Infant Origins of Adult Disease. BMJ Books, London (see also articles collected at www.bmj.com under 'Barker Hypothesis')

Baumrind D 1991 Parenting styles and adolescent development. In: Learner R, Petersen AC, Brooks-Gunn J (eds) The Encyclopedia on Adolescence. Garland, New York

Blair M, Stewart-Brown S, Waterston T, Crowther R 2003 Child Public Health. Oxford University Press, Oxford

British Medical Association 1999 Growing up in Britain: ensuring a healthy future for our children. A study of 0–5–year-olds. British Medical Association, London

Bronson M 2000 Self-regulation in Early Childhood. Guilford, New York, chapter 6

Hall D, Elliman D 2003 Health for all Children: a programme for child health surveillance, 4th edn. Oxford University Press, Oxford

Kawachi I, Berkman L 2000 Social cohesion, social capital and health. In: Berman L, Kawachi I (eds) Social Epidemiology. Oxford University Press, Oxford

Kuh D and Ben-Shlomo Y 2004 A Life Course Approach to Chronic Disease epidemiology, 2nd edn. Oxford University Press, Oxford

Lynch JW, Davey Smith G, Kaplan GA, House JS 2000 Income inequality and mortality: importance to health of individual income, psychosocial environment, or material conditions. British Medical Journal 320: 1200–1204

Macfarlane A, Stafford M and Moser K 2004 The health of Children and Young People. National Statistics, London

Meltzer H, Gatward R, Goodman R, Ford T 1999 The Mental Health of Children and Adolescents in Britain. National Statistics, London

Office for National Statistics 2000 Child Health Statistics. National Statistics, London

Spencer NJ 2000 Poverty and Child Health. Radcliffe Press, Oxford

Weare K 2000 Promoting Mental, Emotional and Social Health: a whole school approach. Routledge, London

Wilkinson R 1992 Income distribution and life expectancy. British Medical Journal 304: 210–213

Websites

www.statistics.gov.uk (access to information from UK Census and other publications)

www.sustainweb.org (campaign for sustainable food and agriculture)

www.sustrans.org.uk (charity supporting active travel)

www.jrf.org.uk (Joseph Rowntree Foundation – charity concerned with social policy research and development, covering topics such as child poverty)

13 Boundaries of normal in health

N. Kennedy

▼ OVERVIEW

The boundaries between normality and abnormality when dealing with infants and children are seldom precise. Normality is a relatively broad-based situation, with a fair degree of variability. This chapter seeks to outline some of the common symptoms and signs that parents consult their doctors about and tries to outline where these symptoms may fall within the bounds of normality and the reasons why sometimes they fall outside and require further investigation. It is important, clearly, not to miss or delay diagnosis of a condition that requires treatment. It is equally important not to over-investigate, when this is not necessary or appropriate. The 'art' of the good children's advisor involves knowing when to reassure and when to embark on further assessment, which inevitably will aggravate the anxiety that the child's parents already have. It can be a very delicate balancing act indeed.

INTRODUCTION: NORMAL DEVELOPMENTAL VARIATION

Many factors are known to affect the rate of developmental progress (Table 13.1).

Common orthopaedic variations of normal

Postural deformities of the legs and feet

Flat feet (Fig. 13.1) The foot of a normal toddler is 'chubby', and the fat pad on its medial aspect gives the impression that the foot is flat. Usually, by the age of $2^{1}/_{2}$ to 3 years, with increasing weight-bearing activity, the normal foot arch develops and the 'flat footedness' resolves spontaneously.

In-toeing (Fig. 13.2) This is another postural problem of the feet noted by parents and referred to GPs. It can be caused by medial rotation of the forefoot (metatarsus varus), tibial torsion or anterior rotation of the femoral neck causing the foot to turn inwards. It may be unilateral or bilateral. The gait may appear cumbersome and it may cause falling through tripping. It usually resolves spontaneously and orthopaedic surgery is rarely required.

Out-toeing (*external rotation*) This is less common and is caused by femoral retroversion. The child walks with the feet pointing outwards; spontaneous resolution is the norm.

Bow legs (*genu varum*) and knock-knees (*genu valgum*) (Fig. 13.3) These are both variants of tibial posture and growth that rarely require any further investigations. These problems are benign, postural in origin and resolve as the children grow. They do not require orthopaedic intervention. A physiotherapist may offer reassuring advice.

Table 13.1   Factors to be considered in assessing developmental progress

Race	Black children tend to have more advanced motor development than Caucasian children
Genetic endowment	Children of parents with learning difficulties are more likely than other children to show slow development In general, there is a 'regression to the mean' and parents with superior intellectual ability sometimes have unrealistic expectations of their children and have to be gently reminded of this A useful question is to ask parents about their academic attainments
Locomotion	Bottom shufflers are invariably late walkers (often familial)
Sex	Females tend to be more advanced than males in language and social skills
Siblings	Twins often appear to have slow speech development, although communication with each other may be good but idiosyncratic
Bilingual home	English language may be relatively delayed if the first language spoken in the family is not English Most normal children manage very well and become fluent in both languages, especially after exposure to an intense English environment at nursery or school
Nutrition	Mild undernourishment, particularly iron deficiency, may cause developmental delay, which is reversible when the nutritional intake is corrected Prolonged or severe undernutrition may cause irreversible damage
Environmental stimulation	Children learn by an operant process and if they do not have the opportunity for developing through play and social interaction they may be delayed Some parents do not understand the need to interact (play) with their child and it must be explained to them This reversible type of benign understimulation should be distinguished from neglect, which is malignant and must be dealt with as quickly as possible

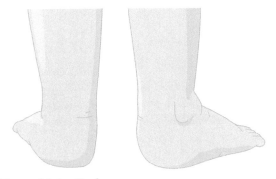

Figure 13.1   Flat feet

An exception is in-toeing or out-toeing associated with abnormal posture of the feet that may be due to talipes (Fig. 13.4). This can be associated with other abnormalities and requires orthopaedic assessment.

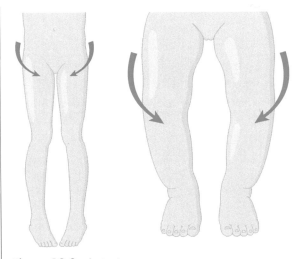

Figure 13.2   In-toeing

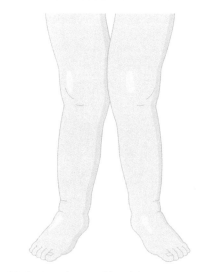

Figure 13.3 Bow legs and knock-knees

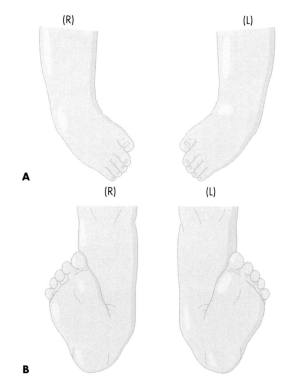

Figure 13.4 (A)Talipes equinovarus and (B) talipes calcaneovalgus.

Other serious conditions that require further hospital investigation for their diagnosis and treatment include congenitally dislocated hips, cerebral palsy and rickets due to vitamin D deficiency.

Growing pains

These are very common especially in children aged 4–9 years, when the incidence is 10–20%; although this is probably an underestimate as many cases do not present to health professionals. The child complains of pain/ache in the *muscles* (not joints or bones) in the legs (front of thighs and calves) and, less often, the arms. The distribution is usually bilateral and symmetrical. They tend to occur towards the end of the day when the child is tired and rarely at night. The child must be carefully examined to exclude pathology such as abnormal posture and bone or joint disease, when tenderness and restriction of movement is a cardinal sign that is absent in growing pains. In fact, the child often welcomes palpation and muscle massage can be helpful.

Rashes and skin problems

Napkin rashes

These are common, although less of a problem with the use of disposable napkins. The commonest cause is a chemical irritant dermatitis caused by ammonia produced by the mixing of urine and faeces on the skin. This responds to frequent napkin changes, often in association with leaving the skin exposed to the air. Milder forms are usually associated with a red skin rash, which may develop small ulcers and become secondarily infected. This usually responds to a barrier cream such as zinc and castor oil, but may require treatment for fungal infections (thrush) or bacterial infections (*Staphylococcus aureus*). Other causes of napkin dermatitis include seborrhoeic dermatitis and atopic eczema.

Seborrhoeic dermatitis (cradle cap)

This rash often starts in the first few months of life, commonly appearing on the scalp as a scaly eruption that may then spread onto the face, ears, elbows and knees, and to the napkin area. Mild cases respond to moisturizers (emollients), but moderate or severe forms require Hydrocortisone 1%. Secondary infection with fungal infections (thrush) or bacterial infections (*Staphylococcus aureus*) may occur and require appropriate treatment.

Atopic eczema

Eczema affects up to 10% of children. There is often a family history of atopy (eczema, asthma and hay fever). Breast feeding is considered to delay the onset of eczema in those who are susceptible. Many cases resolve by the age of 5 years, and the majority by the age of 12. The onset of eczema is a red, wet and sometimes crusted rash, with dry skin causing the infant to itch in affected areas. In children under 1 year, it often appears first on the face, neck and trunk, while in older children it affects mainly the elbows and knees. The napkin area is commonly affected. The treatment of mild cases consists of moisturizers (emollients) to the skin, to prevent the skin from becoming dry and thereby reducing the irritation. It is also advisable not to use soap or detergents on the skin, and cotton clothing is advised; avoiding, in particular, wool and nylon. Treatments with emollients on the skin and in the bath are recommended and topical Hydrocortisone for moderate or severe cases. Antibiotic or antifungal treatment is used for secondary infection, and antihistamines are used to suppress the irritation.

In some children who are not responsive to the above treatment, the possibility of food allergy should be considered. The main food allergens are cows' milk, egg and wheat. Dietary elimination of these under the supervision of a dietician may cause a resolution of the eczema.

Warts and molluscum contagiosum

These are both very common and probably one or other will occur in most children at some time, as they are highly contagious. Warts are small fleshy tumours caused by infection with human papilloma virus. They are unsightly and can be a nuisance if in a site prone to trauma (where they often occur), for example arms and legs, as they bleed easily. They are not painful unless they are on the soles of the feet (verruca), when they are compressed and invade the deep skin layers.

Molluscum contagiosusm is caused by a pox virus. Lesions are circular shiny papules (sometimes described as 'pearls') with a depressed centre (umbilication). Eczema may develop around the molluscum and they can spread along lines of trauma, for example if scratched, and become secondarily infected.

Warts and molluscum are self-limiting and will resolve spontaneously over 6–12 months. Thus, treatment is often not required unless there are complications. In that case they can be painted with keratolytic agents, surgically excised or frozen with cryotherapy, which is also used for verrucae.

Milia

These occur in newborn babies as small cysts in the epidermis, often pale yellow, occurring around the nose and cheeks. They resolve, often in the first month of life.

'Stork marks'

These are pink areas, often over the upper eyelids, central forehead and nape of the neck. They generally fade within the course of the first year and are of no clinical importance.

Strawberry naevi (capilliary haemangioma)

These are raised red lesions occasionally seen in the newborn, but often not visible until 4–6 weeks. They generally enlarge over the first 6 months or so and then regress to disappear by the age of 12–18 months. Central blanching of these lesions is often the prelude to their spontaneous involution. They do not require referral. Parents can be reassured that they will not persist.

Port wine stains

These are more permanent lesions, often occurring on the face. They are purply red in colour, flat and well defined, and require referral to a paediatrician or dermatologist for specialist advice; treatment is now available using laser therapy. There is a rare form of port wine stain called the Sturge–Weber syndrome associated with epilepsy.

Mongolian blue spots

These are dark blue, macular discolourations of the skin at the base of the spine and on the buttocks, often found in Afro–Caribbean or Asian infants. They fade slowly over the first few years and are of no clinical significance. The importance is that they may be confused with a bruise.

Café-au-lait patches

These are light brown irregular patches varying in size from a few millimetres to several centimetres found anywhere on the body. Isolated patches are normal, but a total of more than six is an indicator of neurofibromatosis, which is a serious neurological disorder that needs specialist investigation.

Infestations

Scabies

This is a disorder caused by a mite and can occur in young children. It presents with itchy papules, often between the fingers, on the wrists, genitalia and around the axillae. It may also occur with an eczematous rash on the face and trunk. The itching is particularly worse at night and if other members of the family are affected it makes it more likely that the rash is scabies in the child. Various preparations are available, including permethrin, and for younger children, malathion.

Head lice

A child who presents with an itchy scalp, which otherwise looks healthy, may be suffering from head lice. The female louse lays many eggs, which may be visibly fixed to the hair shafts close to the surface of the skull. Unlike dandruff, they cannot easily be brushed or blown off. There are various treatments including malathion, carbaryl or pyrethroid/shampoos. Lice develop resistance quickly and most areas have a locally recommended schedule. Treatment may have to be repeated and, particularly in school children, recurrent head lice may all originate from a single untreated source. The heads of classmates of those affected should also be inspected. Head lice can be controlled by regular use of a fine 'nit comb' after shampooing ('bug-busting'). This, however, cannot eliminate lice completely without chemical treatment.

Threadworms

This is a common problem in young children. They can often be asymptomatic, but may cause intense itching in the anus, particularly at night. In a girl there may be inflammation of the vulva. Parents often notice 1 cm long, white, thread-like worms in the child's faeces or around the anus. Treatment with piperazine or mebendazole is very effective and should be taken by all members of the family at the same time to prevent reinfection within a family group.

Systemic infections

Normal children inevitably suffer from feverish illnesses from time to time. Most are due to minor infection of the upper respiratory tract, skin, eyes or intestinal system and are often caused by viruses. The usual course of the illness is to cause irritability, loss of appetite and lethargy and to resolve over 2–5 days. Most cases are managed completely at home and professional advice is not sought or needed.

There are a number of specific viral infections that cause a skin rash (exanthema) and are well recognized by parents. They are becoming rarer as several are covered now by routine immunization–(measles/mumps/rubella [German measles]). A vaccine is also under consideration for chicken pox. The reason for this immunization programme is that, on rare occasions, these infectious diseases can cause serious complications, such as meningitis. Others, including roseola infantum and fifth disease (erythema infectiosum), do not cause serious problems and there are no plans to prevent them by immunization.

These infections will not be described in detail in this book as information on them is readily available elsewhere. For basic information see Table 13.2. Many are notifiable to the local health authority in order to keep up epidemiological surveillance and to ensure that infectious disease controls are in place. In general, no treatment is required for individual children (unless they are immunocompromised) and

Table 13.2	Childhood infections					
	Measles	**Rubella**	**Chickenpox**	**Roseola**	**Fifth disease**	**Mumps**
Typical age	1–4 years	Throughout childhood	5–10 years	7–18 months	5–10 years	5–10 years, young adults since vaccination
Cause	Measles virus	Rubella virus	Herpes varicella zoster virus	Herpes virus 6 and 7	Parvovirus	Mumps virus
Spread	Droplets	Droplets	Contact	Droplets	Droplets	Droplets
Incubation period (days)	8–12	15–21	14–21	8–10	4–18	14–24
Typical features	Coryza, cough, earache, blotchy rash	Maculo-papular rash, lymph-adenopathy	Itchy rash in crops – papule-vesicle scab	High fever – rash	Rash on face (slapped cheek)	Pain and swelling of parotid gland
Infectivity (days) in relation to rash onset	3 days before to 4 days after	7 days before to 4 days after	2 days before to 5 days after	Unknown Low infectivity	7 days before	6 days before to 7 days after onset of swelling
Exclusion from nursery/ school	Until 4 days after rash appeared	Until 4 days after rash appeared	Until all vesicles have crusted over	Not necessary	Not necessary	Until 7 days after onset of swelling

appropriate advice is to keep them comfortable with plenty of fluids and, if necessary, an anti-inflammatory analgesic such as paracetamol or ibuprofen. Affected children should be kept out of nursery or school while they are infectious.

The crying child

All infants cry at times, for example when uncomfortable, hungry, on waking, or when requiring a napkin change. In these situations, feeding, picking up and reassuring or changing the child is usually sufficient.

Crying that persists despite these measures may suggest an illness such as an infection of the ears (otitis media), the urine (urinary tract infection [UTI]) or, very rarely, meninges (meningitis). In these situations it is important that the child is taken to the GP or hospital for assessment, diagnosis and management of the underlying problem. NHS Direct can be consulted by telephone or Internet to give advice.

However, in the vast majority of occasions the situation can be managed by the parent alone.

Teething

Teeth start to form from approximately 16 weeks of gestation and all 20 of the primary dentition are present by 6 months of prenatal life. On rare occasions a baby is born with erupted teeth, but usually the first tooth (normally a central lower incisor) appears around 6 months of age. The upper central incisors erupt within a few weeks, followed by the lateral incisors (usually upper then lower). In the 2nd year the first molars and canines appear and, finally, the canines early in the 3rd year, so that most children have a full set of 20 primary dentition before their 3rd birthday.

'Appear' is the operative word and in the majority of children the first indication of tooth eruption is a white line on the gum where the mucous membrane is stretched and avascular. This is followed soon afterwards by the appearance of a razor sharp tooth crown, which comes through the gum 'like a mushroom' with no warning or symptoms. Many disorders are blamed on 'teething' and, although it may cause some discomfort and redness of the gum as the mucous membrane is stretched, undergoes avascular necrosis and is compressed as the tooth pushes through, it does not cause systemic illness such as fever, rash, lethargy, excessive irritability, diarrhoea or vomiting. Any discomfort can be relieved by chewing and the baby may be given a soft object such as a wet cloth or rubber ring or the gums can be rubbed with a finger. Paracetamol or ibuprofen liquid can be administered if necessary. Exposed teeth should be gently brushed with water at first and then children's fluoride toothpaste when the child can spit it out (around 2 years). Sugary food and drink should be avoided.

Dummies are controversial, but temporary use as a pacifier at sleep times is not thought to be harmful. However, they should never be laced with sweet liquid.

At approximately 6 years, the roots of the primary teeth are reabsorbed into the surrounding bone and the crowns exfoliate. The permanent teeth appear in a set order (Table 13.3) starting with the first molars and ending with the third molars (wisdom teeth), which do not appear until young adulthood. This process is usually as trouble–free as the primary dentition and the main worry for most children is whether the tooth fairy will come when the primary teeth fall out!

There is considerable variation in the timing of dentition, but the order is usually constant. Occasionally, a permanent tooth appears before its corresponding primary tooth is shed. If the latter is mobile (wobbly tooth) it should be removed as quickly as possible, if necessary by a dentist. The teeth are sometimes irregular at first, but they will normally straighten up and become well spaced without intervention. Minor variations in colour

Table 13.3   Dentition in childhood

Teeth type	Eruption age
Deciduous teeth	
Central incisors	6–7 months
Lateral incisors	7–8 months
First molars	1 year
Canines	18 months
Second molars	2 years
Permanent teeth	
First molars	6 years
Central incisors	6–7 years
Lateral incisors	7–8 years
Canines	10–11 years
First premolars	10–11 years
Second premolars	11–12 years
Second molars	11–12 years
Third molars	18–21 years

occur: teeth can be stained by liquid iron medication or drinks including tea and coffee. This is temporary, but permanent yellow/brown discolouration can occur after tetracycline ingestion, including maternal treatment in pregnancy.

Atopy/allergy

This is a complex area, but an important problem in childhood that seems to have become more common over the last 20 years. Allergy and hypersensitivity are used interchangeably to describe an immediate (Type 1) reaction after exposure to an allergen, leading to conditions such as hay fever, wheezing and asthma, eczema, abdominal pain or diarrhoea, rash and, very rarely, anaphylaxis with swelling of the lips, tongue and airway.

In many cases it is not possible to confirm the diagnosis of allergy, particularly with foods, as the symptoms the children have, which include diarrhoea, abdominal pain and poor appetite, may also occur in normal children and not be associated with an allergic cause at all. Important features are the wellbeing of the child and, in particular, growth prior to the start of the problems. Children growing normally are less likely to be suffering from long-term problems. First-line treatment is to identify and eliminate the allergen, which is often difficult as children are frequently allergic to many common substances that cannot be avoided, for example house dust, animals, pollen. Second line is medication with antihistamines or steroids.

Referral to a paediatrician may be appropriate if the child appears not to be thriving, is generally unwell or has intolerable symptoms.

Atopy

This is the term given to a number of disorders that tend to occur in certain children and their families. These are hay fever, allergic rhinitis, eczema, asthma and urticaria. Many of these atopic children have positive skin tests to allergens such as house dust mite, pollen and animal danders, and on investigation are found to have a raised level of eosinophils in the blood and raised serum levels of IgE.

The history is most important in diagnosing these children and often the diagnosis can be made from both the history of the child's complaint and a positive family history. Skin testing and RAST tests can be helpful in identifying specific allergenic factors.

Hayfever/allergic (perennial) rhinitis The child has a blocked nose associated with a watery nasal discharge usually from May to August. Sneezing is also a common complaint. The allergen is usually grass pollen, but occasionally also pollen from trees shrubs and flowers. The swollen mucous membrane in the nasopharynx may block the meatus of the Eustachian tube causing secretory otitis media (glue ear) and conductive deafness. Treatment includes non-sedative antihistamines and intranasal steroids.

Urticaria

These are demarcated itchy wheals and can appear suddenly. They are a reaction to, for example drugs, food, insect bites and viral infections. Treatment consists of exclusion of known triggers, antihistamines and, if severe, corticosteroids.

Food allergy

Common foods include wheat, fish, shell fish, eggs and cow's milk. Allergy to these foods may produce mild or severe urticaria and, in rare cases, anaphylaxis. However, the link between possible allergy and foods is usually more vague. Cow's milk allergy can be associated with vomiting, diarrhoea, constipation, eczema and, rarely, anaphylaxis (see also Chapter 5).

Peanut allergy This is an increasing problem possibly due to the use of peanut derivatives in manufactured foods. The incidence is between 0.5 and 7.5% and is more common in atopic children. Fatal reactions can occur in asthmatics. Diagnosis can be made by skin and RAST tests. Treatment is exclusion of peanut additives from diet and an adrenaline spring-loaded pen (Epipen) can be carried to be used if anaphylaxis occurs.

Ear, nose and throat symptoms

Snuffles/blocked nose

It is a common symptom occurring in children under 5 years and is associated most commonly with viral upper respiratory tract infections (URTI/coryza), which leads to excess nasal mucus and catarrh. This leads to a blocked nose, which particularly affects small children due to the small aperture of the nostrils and may lead to feeding difficulties as they particularly rely on nasal breathing during bottle or breast feeding. The discharge may become discoloured and thick due to secondary bacterial infection, but this may also occur with ongoing viral infection and generally antibiotics are not required. Treatment options include saline nasal drops, steam inhalation and postural tilting. Other causes of nasal blockage include enlarged adenoids, nasal polyps and, importantly, inserted foreign bodies such as beads. Snuffles without systemic upset do not contraindicate routine immunizations.

Cough

This is a common symptom in childhood, distressing to both child and parent, but often self-limiting and not requiring active intervention. Causes and management for acute and chronic cough are different.

When excess mucus or foreign or irritable matter is present in the bronchial tree, the cough reflex is initiated. This produces a rapid movement of air, carrying with it foreign matter (dust, mucus or sputum). Cough is not usually serious, but if the child appears systemically unwell then investigations should be undertaken.

Common causes include tonsillitis and pharyngitis, the majority being caused by viral infections. The commonest bacterial cause is beta haemolytic streptococcus. Other causes include, sinus infection, post-nasal drip, diphtheria and as part of an infectious disease such as measles or chickenpox. In these, the cough tends to be associated with excessive mucus and resolves spontaneously within a week or so.

Cough in the child who is unwell Examination by the doctor (GP or hospital doctor) in these cases, is very important in establishing whether:

a. treatment is required
b. hospital investigations are necessary.

Other causes of cough to consider are foreign body (inhaled peanut or bead), asthma (where the cough is chiefly at night in the early stages) and post-nasal drip (when catarrh from the sinuses causes irritation, producing a persistent cough). The examining doctor must examine the throat, ears and chest, and further examinations such as sputum analysis and a chest X-ray may also be required.

Chronic cough Cough that has persisted for more than a few weeks requires more detailed examination and should be investigated to exclude other conditions such as cystic fibrosis, recurrent lung infection, pulmonary TB, HIV or a foreign body. There is more likely to be constitutional upset in the child, with recurrent fever and possibly weight loss with poor appetite and referral will be necessary to identify specific causes.

Wheezing

This common childhood symptom is produced by airway constriction in the lung, the constriction associated with muscle spasm, mucosal swelling (oedema) and increased secretions. The triggers of these are generally threefold: allergy, infection and emotional factors. Causes to consider with a wheezy child under the age of 5 years include:

- a viral-induced wheeze with an upper respiratory tract infection
- asthma
- bronchiolitis
- a foreign body, e.g. inhaled peanut or bead
- food allergy
- rarer causes-cystic fibrosis and gastro-oesophageal reflux.

Children may wheeze with viral infections and yet remain quite happy and be able to feed and sleep without difficulty, but in general wheezing tends to cause them to be short of breath and have difficulty feeding and exercising, and the noise produced can be very frightening to parents. Management is aimed at identifying first the cause of the problem and, secondly, the appropriate treatment. Medication designed to dilate the airways (bronchodilators) are available, but tend to be less effective in children under 18 months or so, and antibiotics are available for specific infections. Inhaled steroids can effectively prevent wheezing as well as being used during acute episodes.

Sore throat

Children under the age of 2 years have difficulty locating pain to specific sites and sore throat may be suspected by the mother from other clues such as the child being irritable and crying or going off feeds or fluids. The majority of sore throats are caused by viral infections and do not require antibiotics. Fluids and analgesics such as paracetamol are sufficient and the infection resolves spontaneously over 5–7 days. Bacterial infections tend not to respond so quickly to simple measures. Beta haemolytic streptococcus is the commonest infecting organism and is usually sensitive to penicillin.

In older children glandular fever (infectious mononucleosis) commonly presents with a sore throat and painful enlarged neck glands. While the condition may be suspected on clinical grounds, a blood test (monospot) is required to confirm the condition. Antibiotics are not required and the parents should be warned that the child may suffer from more protracted symptoms after the sore throat has improved, such as fatigue and lethargy for several weeks.

Earache (otalgia)

Children can generally localize pain to either ear from around the age of 2 years. It can be a very sharp, piercing pain, often spasmodic, but also continuous and may be associated with high fever and vomiting. Occasionally, the child complains of feeling giddy or has an unsteady gait with ear infections. There are two main causes of earache.

Otitis externa This is an infection of the pinna and ear canal. There may be a discharge from the ear, often green and sometimes bloodstained, and swelling around the external ear. Causes include viral, bacterial and fungal infection, but bacteriological swabs need to be taken to identify the infecting organism, particularly if antibiotic or antifungal drops are to be used. Analgesics and aural toilet remain important parts of management of the condition.

Acute otitis media (AOM) In middle-ear disease the child complains of pain associated with fever. This is often caused by viral infections, but secondary bacterial infections also occur. The chief problem is a blocked drainage system from the middle ear via the eustachian tube to the nose. This blockage can be caused by excessive mucus or fluid in the middle ear or enlarged adenoids. Treatment consists of analgesics, which are very important and antibiotics are now considered as less important. Studies suggest that viral infections predominate as the causative agent of AOM and antibiotics are unnecessary. Recurrent episodes may require removal of the adenoids that obstruct the Eustachian tube or the insertion of grommets (a small tube in the ear drum) that acts as an artificial Eustachian tube and helps to ventilate the middle ear (keeping the pressure either side of the ear drum equal to atmospheric pressure).

Glue ear (SOM/OME)

This is poorly understood, but implies the accumulation of fluid in the middle ear. It may become very viscous (glue) and compromise the mechanical transmission of sound waves by the ossicles. Glue ear commonly causes a mild-to-moderate hearing loss (40–50 Db). In most children this is intermittent and does not interfere with language and educational development. However, if hearing remains impaired longer than 2 months there is a risk of language difficulty. Treatment with myringotomy and grommets is used. Some allergic children respond to medical treatment with topical intranasal steroids.

Nose bleeds (epistaxes)

Nosebleeds are very common in childhood, but rare in infancy and less common after puberty. They occur usually from bleeding from the front part of each nostril (Little's area) where there is a large collection of small veins.

Trauma from nose picking or an infection of this area (vestibulitis) leads to bleeding. Other causes include a foreign body, for example a bead, and rarer causes include bleeding disorders. Recurrent nosebleeds require to be checked by a doctor and may require hospital attention. Simple first aid measures such as pinching the nose often suffices, but prolonged nosebleeds of greater than half an hour should be seen and may need to be treated in hospital. Nasal packing and cautery to the affected part of the nasal septum are sometimes required.

Gastrointestinal tract symptoms

Nausea and vomiting

Nausea and vomiting often go together in young children and, whilst vomiting associated with diarrhoea is usually due to gastroenteritis, it may also occur with other illnesses such as ear infections, UTI, meningitis and other conditions. Vomiting alone can also occur in bowel obstruction and this needs careful consideration by history and examination. *Pyloric stenosis* occurs in the first 3–6 weeks of life and causes projectile vomiting. If not treated, dehydration can occur. The condition, which has a male prevalence (6:1), is caused by hypertrophy of the circular muscle of the pylorus and leads to a blockage at the gastric outlet. A simple operation (Ramsted's procedure) is curative.

Reflux

All young babies regurgitate small amounts of feed at first (posseting) and this is due to a lax gastro-oesophageal sphincter. Fifty per cent of babies at the age of 2 months possett, but by the age of 6–12 months it has usually resolved. More extreme varieties of this condition lead to reflux disease and require medication with Gaviscon or the use of milk thickeners, such as Carobel and, more recently, drugs to reduce the acidity of the stomach contents and improve motility of gastric contents from the stomach into the small bowel. This condition is known as gastro-oesophageal reflux disease (GORD). This is more common in low birth weight babies, those with cow's milk allergy, respiratory disease and some central nervous system disorders. Owing to poor intake growth failure may occur. Surgical correction is rarely required.

Acute diarrhoea and sickness (gastroenteritis)

The commonest causes of this condition are viral, for example rotavirus, adenovirus and echovirus. These lead to a short-lasting illness of 2–3 days of acute vomiting followed 12–24 h later by diarrhoea. It is now advised that feeding (especially breast milk) should continue in small frequent amounts, if necessary, by spoon. Fluids may be augmented by the use of glucose electrolyte solutions, for example Diarolyte. The risk of this condition is dehydration and it is important that the baby or toddler is checked if the vomiting or diarrhoea persists for greater than 24 h. Dehydration can be recognized by finding a dry tongue, sunken eyes and loss of skin elasticity (turgor). If there are signs of tiredness, unwillingness to feed or drowsiness, the child may be >10% dehydrated and require hospitalization for I.V. fluids.

Bacterial causes of gastroenteritis include Salmonella and Shigella, which may cause food poisoning. *Escherichia Coli* and Campylobacter is often associated in older children with abdominal pain and blood stained diarrhoea, particularly after foreign travel.

Admission to hospital nowadays is rarely required for gastroenteritis, but some children do, however, still require I.V. fluids or investigation of prolonged diarrhoea, for example stool culture. If the diarrhoea persists for more than 2 weeks, the child should be investigated for causes such as lactose or cow's milk protein intolerance, which requires milk to be excluded for a longer period from the diet and sometimes milk substitutes, for example soya milk, for a temporary period.

Chronic diarrhoea

Persistent diarrhoea for greater than 2 weeks has a number of causes. Probably the commonest cause is toddler diarrhoea. The exact cause of this is not known, but it may result from the inability of the colon to handle the fluid load. The stools contain undigested food and are loose. The child clinically is thriving. Treatment is by explanation that it is a very common but temporary problem.

Lactose intolerance

Lack of the enzyme lactase in the small bowel lining leads to diarrhoea with the undigested lactose (milk sugar) being degraded to lactic acid and CO_2. It can be an inherited condition, although is often a temporary one after an acute episode of diarrhoea and vomiting. Avoidance of milk for a time may help resolve the problem or the use of a lactose-free milk.

Abdominal pain

This is a very common symptom of childhood and has many different and varying causes. Recurrent abdominal pain occurs in approximately 10% of school age children, but more than 90% of these have no organic cause. Psychosomatic abdominal pain has certain characteristics that include: the site of the pain being around the umbilicus (periumbilical), the timing of the pain often being in the morning, an association with a family history of travel sickness, irritable bowel or migraine, and a lack of other serious features to suggest organic disease. Emotional factors certainly play a part and a full history and examination by a GP or paediatrician and reassurance are essential for management.

Infantile colic

This condition, also called 3-month colic, is well known to mothers. The infant has bouts of screaming associated with crying and drawing up of the legs. This tends to resolve by the age of 3–4 months and many causes have been suggested including cow's milk allergy and maternal anxiety, but no definite single cause has been found. Cuddling the baby may bring about resolution, but illness in the child needs exclusion if the colic continues. This will require a thorough examination by the GP. Remedies such as gripe water and Infacol help, but time and age (3–4 months) seem to be the best solutions to the problems. Abdominal pain lasting for longer than 1–2 h, particularly associated with vomiting without diarrhoea, will usually alert the parent or carer to seek medical advice and the doctor must assess to identify a cause, treat or refer for further investigation.

Constipation

Constipation is a common symptom of childhood. Parents are often worried if their baby or toddler passes only small, hard motions or goes several days without opening his bowels. However, this may be quite normal and some breast–fed babies may go several days without a motion. If the child is healthy and thriving the parents can be reassured that there is no specific problem, but there are certain situations where the problem merits further investigation. The help of the health visitor in this situation can be invaluable and simple measures such as increasing fluid intake may suffice and in older children increasing the roughage in the diet can produce a more satisfactory bowel motion with increased frequency. However, on some occasions softeners such as lactulose can be used and, rarely, a glycerine suppository may be appropriate, but not on a regular basis. An anal fissure may inhibit the child from passing a motion because of the pain, which occurs when the anus is stretched. A history of bleeding or the child crying on the passage of stool may be a clue to this condition.

Soiling

Soiling is a phenomenon that occurs in children with constipation when the rectum becomes full of hard faeces that are difficult or impossible to pass and liquid motion above these seeps out and the child soils his pants. Treatment consists of ensuring that the rectum is emptied of the hard motion by the use of a stool softener or laxative or in some children a micro-enema. Exploration of other associated factors, such as anxieties about using the toilet or fear of passing a motion because of pain from a fissure, need to be explored thoroughly with the child in a sympathetic manner to ensure a more regular pattern to their bowel motions and correction of the problem. The anus should be examined gently. A very small number of children have a neurological problem of the bowel due to spinal abnormality, usually associated with urinary incontinence or infection. This requires further investigation and referral to a hospital paediatric department.

Encopresis

This may be associated with soiling, but is often associated with passing of motions in unusual places and unacceptable places. It is more common in boys than girls and requires a detailed history, examination and correction of problems such as chronic constipation, adequate toilet training and exploration of possible trigger factors, such as anxieties regarding school, toileting at home and parental demands. As well as medical therapies with laxatives and softeners, family therapy and help from clinical psychologists may be indicated.

Blood in the stool

Blood in the stool in childhood invariably has a benign cause in contrast to blood in urine (haematuria), which is usually serious and requires investigation. In the newborn period, swallowed maternal blood from the nipple may occur in the stool of breast–fed babies and may be distinguished biochemically. In toddlers, bleeding may occur with severe gastroenteritis, from an anal fissure and anal polyp. Once noted the child should be seen by the GP in the first instance. A hospital referral is appropriate only if the bleeding is heavy or recurrent.

Urinary tract symptoms

Dysuria

Dysuria – pain on passing urine – often described as a warm or burning feeling, in the urethra or lower abdomen, is an unusual symptom for a child to complain of and must be taken seriously. This is because it often indicates the presence of an infection in the urinary tract and identification of the causative organism and correct antibiotic treatment is very important to prevent later complications. In infants under 2 years of age the symptoms of UTI are notoriously difficult to identify and are non-specific, for example the child may just appear unwell, be febrile, or vomit. Simple measures, such as increasing fluid intake and analgesics such as paracetamol, will help, but the most important action for parents is to seek medical advice and have the infant examined and the urine cultured.

Blood in urine (haematuria)

This can be an alarming symptom both for parents and child who notice a red, pink or brown discolouration in the urine. It must be treated seriously and investigated, but there are non-medical causes and these include: beetroot, causing red discoloration of the urine, and certain dyes in sweets. However, these are rare and a child presenting with blood in the urine must be fully investigated.

Polyuria

This describes the passing of excess amounts of urine and is usually noted by the parent. Causes include the child drinking an excessive amount of fluid (habitual polydypsia) and diabetes mellitus. The commonest cause is habitual polydypsia and can usually be managed by the GP and reassurance given.

Enuresis

Children develop urinary incontinence from around the age of 3 and the term enuresis has become synonymous with bed-wetting (nocturnal enuresis). However, it may occur in the day as well due to a maturational delay of the urinary sphincter mechanism and is more common in boys than girls. There is also often a strong family history with two-thirds of children having a first-degree relative affected. It is not just a problem of 3–4–year olds, 15% of 5–year–olds and 3% of 10–year–olds suffer from enuresis.

With age, urinary continence is developed and the problem resolves spontaneously, but certain conditions need to be excluded. These include constipation, where the loaded bowel presses on the bladder, UTIs and polyuria. Full history and examination of the child is necessary plus a urine dipstick test to exclude sugar in the urine (diabetes mellitus) and bacteriology (to exclude infection). A star chart can be used to give positive encouragement. A buzzer alarm is also available for children around the age of 7 onwards, where the child is woken at the moment of passing urine at night. After a short period of using the alarm the child often becomes dry. In certain cases drugs, for example Desmopressin, which can be taken as a spray or tablet, can be used both in the short term and longer term, if necessary.

Neurological symptoms

Funny turns, fits and faints

Parents who witness their child having a fit will often describe it as the most frightening experience they have had and frequently say that they thought the child had died. Often the child is taken immediately to hospital or the GP called immediately. In young children, the commonest cause is a febrile convulsion with a prevalence of approximately 5% in children under 6 years. These fits occur with a sudden rise in temperature, the child often being quite well before the onset of the fit and often not noticeably hot. They are usually generalized in that the body stiffens and is followed by shaking of the limbs, which usually lasts for less than 5 min. This is followed by a period of sleep.

The best advice for a parent at this stage is to ensure that the child is lying on their side, slightly head down to prevent inhalation of vomit. Children (especially if less than 2 years old) are usually admitted to hospital after the first febrile fit, although often the cause may be discovered by an examination of the throat, ears and chest. Once other causes, such as meningitis and UTI have been excluded, parents can be reassured that the prognosis following febrile convulsions is excellent and the child will be normal. The only exceptions to this general rule are when the convulsions are prolonged, not generalized, where there is a family history of epilepsy and the child is less than 1 year old. In these cases the risk of subsequent epilepsy is around 10%.

A vasovagal attack (faint/syncope) may be mistaken for a seizure. It often occurs in older children when they have been standing for a long period or after anxiety or fright. They feel giddy and then collapse. They may twitch, but recover once they have fallen. Breath-holding (Blue) attacks, which occur in toddlers, are usually brought on by a painful stimulus or when they have been scolded. The child screams, holds his breath and then goes blue around his face. Should he continue to hold his breath for more than a few seconds he becomes limp, loses consciousness, occasionally even twitching. Reflex anoxic seizures (during breath–holding attacks) are episodes that are precipitated by fright or painful stimuli and the hallmark is that the child becomes deathly pale, often described as 'white as a sheet', falls down and becomes unconscious. They are due to excessive vagal tone, which causes temporary cardiac arrest and thus brain hypoxia/ischaemia. They last a few seconds only and the progronsis is very good. Both 'blue' and 'white' breath-holding attacks are benign, but frightening for parents and require full explanation.

Headaches

Headache is a very common symptom in children. Some 95% of school children are said to have had one or more headache within a year and 10% of these are tension headaches, and 6% migraine. Headaches tend to be classified as acute, occurring during an illness, and chronic, occurring for a longer period of time and not generally associated with febrile illness.

Acute headache Children from the age of 2–3 years are able to localize pain and will complain of headache, often during a febrile illness such as an URTI or sinusitis, but also with more serious illnesses, such as meningitis, both viral and bacterial. In the history, features such as headache, dislike of light, and signs such as neck stiffness and rash, will require urgent referral from the GP to hospital. Following full history and examination a cause may be found. Generally, treatment of the underlying problem, for example throat or ear infection, with antibiotics if indicated and analgesics such as paracetamol/ibuprofen, will be sufficient to resolve the headache.

Chronic tension headache These tend to occur in older children and are when they describe a band-like pain around the head. The headache is often present all day and resistant to normal medication. After a careful and full examination, which is normal in these cases, very full reassurance needs to be given and ongoing support is also vital in managing the condition.

Migraine Six per cent of children suffer from migraine and 75% have a positive family history. Children can have classic migraine when there is an aura or warning before the headache develops or a more common variety with no aura. Rarely, migraine is associated with neurological disturbance, such as numbness or weakness of a limb or face, which, in most cases, resolve spontaneously. The headache can be unilateral and associated with nausea and vomiting, but this is not always the case. In young children, episodes of nausea, vomiting, visual abnormalities, for example blurring/flashing, and recurrent abdominal pain may precede the development of recurrent headaches. Triggers include stress; relaxation after stress, for example weekends; certain foods, including cheese and chocolate; food additives; and, in girls, the onset of menstruation. Referral to the GP for further advice and often hospital referral for further tests may be part of the management plan.

A rare cause of headache is raised intracranial pressure, which may be due to a brain tumour. The headache is often present first thing in the morning, associated with vomiting and worse lying down. In older children, personality changes can occur and a decline in school performance may be noted. Early referral to hospital for further tests, which include MRI brain scan may be needed. Other causes of headache include refractive errors, in older children drug abuse and, rarely, high blood pressure.

Psychological symptoms

Sleep disturbances

These are common problems in young children and often impact on the whole family. They are discussed in Chapter 6.

Temper tantrums

Temper tantrums are a normal response of children to frustration (see Chapter 7) when they are not allowed to do something they wish to do. While, in the majority of cases, the children have no ongoing problems, a few are discovered to have hearing impairments, for example glue ear and others may have global or speech/language delay. An important factor if the tantrums become recurrent is to try and analyze what has led to the tantrum and then to avoid the triggers. If no trigger is apparent a caring and empathic approach by the parents is important, while being firm and consistent in their handling of the situation. A 'time out' approach may be used as a method of dealing with recurrent tantrums, where the child is put somewhere, such as another room, for a short period while they calm down.

Eating problems

In the pre-school child food refusal is a common problem. Mealtimes may become a battle between parent and child. The child is usually well nourished, growing well and doesn't see this as a problem. The parent feels the child is either not eating a sufficient amount or sometimes lacking an adequate diet. A full history and examination needs to be taken with the parents and the child together and plotting the child's growth on an appropriate growth chart will help to demonstrate that the diet is, indeed, adequate and he is growing normally. Further help from the Child Mental Health Service might be needed if the problem continues.

Anorexia nervosa This condition is found in approximately 1% of teenage girls and is related to a distorted body perception, such that they feel that they must lose weight. Initial dieting does not produce specific problems but, after a while, the preoccupation with food and weight and often excessive exercise tends to dominate their lives and severe weight loss intervenes. If post–pubertal, sexual functioning may cease. The peak age of onset is about 14 years and girls out-number boys by about 10:1. Initial management is recognition of the problem and then referral to the appropriate child mental health service. Prognosis is reasonably good, but about one-quarter develops a relapsing condition.

Bulimia This is the other side of the coin to anorexia nervosa where binge eating is followed by vomiting. It is thought to be about ten times more common than anorexia and, again, mainly affects girls. The young person often lacks self-esteem and becomes obsessed by their shape and size. Denial of the problem is common and the classic signs of bulimia include enlargement of the parotid gland and erosion of the dental enamel by stomach acid from self-induced vomiting. To manage this problem both the child and the family need to be involved, along with a psychotherapeutic approach. In both anorexia and bulimia there is a mortality associated of approximately 5%, hence the need for quick identification of the problem and early intervention.

Further reading

Bellman M, Kennedy N 2000 Paediatrics and Child Health. Churchill Livingstone, Edinburgh
David TJ 1995 Symptoms of Disease in Childhood. Blackwell, Oxford

Websites

www.bad.org.uk/public/leaflets (information on skin conditions)
www.yourchildshealth.nhs.uk (comprehensive information about common health issues)

14 Postscript: two case studies

M. Bellman, E. Peile

▼ OVERVIEW

In Chapter 11 (special senses) we made reference to 'Mother's sixth sense', and underlined the importance of listening to the parent. We conclude this book on the normal child with two case studies.

CASE STUDY 1

Molly

Molly was born to a mother who had a history of mental health disease and was a drug abuser. Labour and delivery went well, she was small for dates but bottle fed well and made satisfactory progress as an infant. Developmental milestones were at the slow limit of the normal range. Age 18 months she started to walk and babble and her health visitor advised mother to 'wait and see'.

Shortly afterwards, the mother was admitted to a psychiatric mother and baby unit for treatment of her drug addiction for 3 months. When Molly was 2 years old the mother consulted her GP because of behaviour problems as well as continuing slow development. She had about three single words, was walking slightly unsteadily and had poor play skills. Mother was reassured that Molly would make developmental progress in due course when the home situation was more stable. Molly was seen again by her GP age $2^1/_2$ when there was little change, but she was having more temper tantrums and had a short attention span. Mother reported that she had noticed episodes when Molly would go quiet and still for 1–2 minutes from about 6 months ago. The GP said he was not worried, but referred to a paediatrician.

When seen in the paediatric clinic 1 month later the mother asked if Molly had epilepsy. The paediatrician said it was unlikely and that Molly's episodes were signs of behavioural disorder. He requested an EEG, which was normal. The mother was reassured, but because she was anxious, Molly was followed up in the paediatric clinic 6–monthly.

Both the GP and the paediatrician considered the mother to be overanxious and unreliable and dismissed her observations and worries. Molly made slow developmental progress and had little interest in playing. The mother reported continuing 'vacant' episodes that had not been seen by anyone else. Age 3$\frac{1}{2}$ Molly started nursery and after a few weeks her key worker also noticed occasional 'absence' episodes. At the next paediatric appointment the mother insisted again that Molly had epilepsy. The paediatrician ordered another EEG that showed frequent runs of epileptic activity in the frontal lobes. Molly was started on anticonvulsant medication and the episodes stopped and she became more interested in her surroundings and her behaviour, attention and play skills improved.

CASE STUDY 2

Fawzul

Fawzul was a full–term normal delivery infant who made good neonatal progress and satisfactory developmental progress in the first year. He was a 'good' baby who slept well and seemed happy. He passed his routine 18-month check with the health visitor.

Just before his 2nd birthday the mother went back to the clinic and said that Fawzul's grandmother thought that something was wrong, as he was not speaking or playing properly. Developmentally he was in the normal range, but his speech had not progressed since he was last seen. His behaviour was good and he played contentedly with simple toys on his own. The health visitor reassured his mother that he would catch up.

When Fawzul was 2$\frac{1}{2}$ his mother went to her GP asking if he was autistic as that had been suggested by a friend who had looked it up on the Internet and the description fitted him. Fawzul had five siblings including a baby aged 9 months and the grandmother lived with the family, so the mother was very busy. The father worked long hours in a restaurant and took no part in child care. The GP said Fawzul's problems were environmental owing to the mother's preoccupation with her other family and he ignored her question and referred Fawzul to speech therapy. Fawzul had a speech and language assessment 6 months later followed by a course of therapy sessions. He made very little progress with his language and age 3$\frac{1}{2}$ the speech and language therapist made a referral to the child-development team because, in addition to the communication problem, she was worried about Fawzul's poor social and play skills.

By the time he was assessed by the multidisciplinary team Fawzul had a severe language disorder, no imaginative play, very poor interactive social skills and would not cooperate with adult-directed tasks. A report from his nursery confirmed that Fawzul showed no interest in playing with other children and his play was mechanical and repetitive. Autistic spectrum disorder was confirmed as the diagnosis.

In both these cases the mothers' anxieties and diagnostic questions were dismissed, for varying reasons. However, in both cases, mother eventually was proved right.

Appendix
Tables of normal
neurodevelopmental data

M. Bellman, E. Peile

All children are normal: whatever their circumstance, in respect of their health, development or environment, each child has his or her own norms.

If things are going awry, it is highly likely that a parent or carer who is sensitively tuned into the child will be able to pick up on the signs or symptoms, even if only by means of the 'sixth sense'. We hope that these chapters will have given some insight into the normal world of the child, and also of the vast array of professional expertise that exists to support parents bringing up children.

PRIMITIVE REFLEXES

Table 1 Neonatal primitive reflexes

Reflex	Method to elicit	Response	Appears	Disappears
Moro	Suddenly extend head or arms	Symmetrical extension, abduction and the flexion of arms	Birth	6 months
Placing	Bring dorsum of foot up to edge of table	Foot is lifted and placed on surface	4 weeks	6 months
Stepping	Support in standing position	Alternate legs flex at knees and hips and baby 'walks' forward	Birth	3 months
Grasp	Place finger in palm of baby's hand	Fingers close tightly round examiner's finger	Birth	4 months
Asymmetric tonic neck (ATNR)	Hold shoulders flat and turn head to either side	Limbs on face side extend and on occiput side flex	Birth	6 months
Head righting	In supine position turn head to either side	Pelvis and shoulders turn in same direction	4 months	2 years
Parachute	From ventral suspension suddenly lower the baby towards a surface	Arms and legs extend and abduct	6 months	Persists

DEVELOPMENTAL MILESTONES

Motor skills

Table 2 Prone position (adapted from Bellman M, Lingam S, Aukett A 1966 The Schedule of Growing Skills II NFER-Nelson, Windsor)

	Mean	Range
Lifts head momentarily	1 month	0.5–2 months
Lifts head about 45°	2 months	1–3 months
Head and upper chest up on forearms	3 months	2–5 months
Head and chest up on extended arms	6 months	4–8 months
Gets into crawling position	8 months	6–12 months

Table 3 Upright posture (adapted from Bellman M, Lingam S, Aukett A 1966 The Schedule of Growing Skills II NFER-Nelson, Windsor)

	Mean	Range
Bears some weight on feet	7 months	6–9 months
Takes full weight	8 months	6–12 months
Stands holding on	9 months	7–14 months
Pulls to stand	10 months	9–10 months
Stands alone	11 months	9–16 months

Table 4 Gross movements (adapted from Bellman M, Lingam S, Aukett A 1966 The Schedule of Growing Skills II NFER-Nelson, Windsor)

	Mean	Range
Rolls (or squirms) forwards or backwards	8½ months	6–11 months
Crawls	9½ months	7–13 months
Walks with support	10 months	8–12 months
Walks alone	13 months	11–18 months
Squats to pick up object	14½ months	12–19 months
Runs	16 months	15–20 months
Jumps	18 months	
Walks on tiptoe	20 months	
Runs on tiptoe	24 months	
Hops on one foot	3 years	

Table 5 Stairs (adapted from Bellman M, Lingam S, Aukett A 1966 The Schedule of Growing Skills II NFER-Nelson, Windsor)

	Mean	Range
Walks upstairs with hands held	16 months	12–24 months
Walks upstairs with two feet on each step	25 months	19–30 months
Walks upstairs, one foot per step and downstairs 2 feet per step	3 years	
Walks upstairs and downstairs one foot per step	4 years	

Manipulative skills

Table 6   Building with bricks (1 inch) (adapted from Bellman M, Lingam S, Aukett A 1966 The Schedule of Growing Skills II NFER-Nelson, Windsor)

Number of bricks	Mean	Range
2	15 months	11–19 months
4	18 months	15–24 months
8	24 months	21–23 months
Bridge	3 years	27–39 months
3 steps	4 years	

Table 7   Drawing skills (adapted from Bellman M, Lingam S, Aukett A 1966 The Schedule of Growing Skills II NFER-Nelson, Windsor)

Drawing skill	Mean
Scribbles	15 months
Imitates vertical line	2 years
Imitates horizontal line	$2\frac{1}{2}$ years
Imitates circle	3 years
Imitates cross	4 years

Language skills

Table 8   Speech (adapted from Bellman M, Lingam S, Aukett A 1966 The Schedule of Growing Skills II NFER-Nelson, Windsor)

Speech sounds	Mean	Range
Grunts	4 weeks	1–6 weeks
Vocalizes (coo)	$6\frac{1}{2}$ weeks	4–9 weeks
Laughs	$3\frac{1}{2}$ months	2–5 months
Babbles (monosyllabic)	$6\frac{1}{2}$ months	4–8 months
Imitates sounds	10 months	8–12 months
Jargon	12 months	10–15 months
One word	15 months	12–18 months
1–6 words	18 months	15–21 months
7–20 words	21 months	18–24 months
50 words	2 years	18–27 months
Joins 2 words	2 years	18–30 months
200 words	$2\frac{1}{2}$ years	24–36 months
Joins 3–4 words	$2\frac{1}{2}$ years	$2\frac{1}{4}$–3 years
Questions (why, what, where, who)	3 years	$2\frac{1}{2}$–$3\frac{1}{2}$ years
Pronouns (I, you, he, she)	$3\frac{1}{2}$ years	3–4 years
Conjunctions (and, but)	4 years	3–$4\frac{1}{2}$ years
Sentences of 5+ words	4 years	3–$4\frac{1}{2}$ years
Complex explanations and sequences	$4\frac{1}{2}$ years	4–$5\frac{1}{2}$ years

Table 9   Comprehension (adapted from Bellman M, Lingam S, Aukett A 1966 The Schedule of Growing Skills II NFER-Nelson, Windsor)

	Mean	Range
Understands 'no'/bye-bye'	7 months	6–9 months
Recognizes own name	8 months	6–10 months
Recognizes familiar names	12 months	10–15 months
Selects 3 out of 4 objects	15 months	12–18 months
Points to body parts on person	15 months	12–18 months
Points to body parts on doll	18 months	15–21 months
Follows a 2-step command	2 years	18–27 months
Understands prepositions (in, on, under)	$2\frac{1}{2}$ years	2–3 years
Understands simple negatives	3 years	$2\frac{1}{2}$–$3\frac{1}{2}$ years
Follows a command with 2 instructions	$3\frac{1}{2}$ years	3–4 years
Understands complex negatives (neither/nor)	4 years	$3\frac{1}{2}$–5years
Follows a command with 3 instructions	$4\frac{1}{2}$ years	4–$5\frac{1}{2}$ years

Social skills

Table 10   Feeding (adapted from Bellman M, Lingam S, Aukett A 1966 The Schedule of Growing Skills II NFER-Nelson, Windsor)

	Mean
Holds spoon but does not feed	12 months
Holds spoon, brings it to mouth but cannot prevent it turning over	15 months
Holds spoon and gets food safely to mouth	18 months
Eats skilfully with spoon	2–$2\frac{1}{2}$ years
Eats with fork and spoon	3 years
Eats skilfully with little help	$3\frac{1}{2}$–4 years
Copes with entire meal unaided	5 years

Table 11   Toileting (adapted from Bellman M, Lingam S, Aukett A 1966 The Schedule of Growing Skills II NFER-Nelson, Windsor)

	Range
Reflex emptying of bladder	Up to 6 months
Empties bladder less frequently (CNS inhibition of reflex)	6–12 months
Indicates or vocalizes toilet needs or wetness	1–2 years
Bowel control	$2\frac{1}{2}$–4 years
Dry during the day (occasional accident)	3–4 years
Dry at night (occasional accident)	$3\frac{1}{2}$–5 years
Able to control voiding, and micturate on command	4–5 years

Table 12   Play (Bellman M, Lingam S, Aukett A 1966 The Schedule of Growing Skills II NFER-Nelson, Windsor)

	Range
Shakes rattle	3–6 months
Transfers objects from hand to hand	6–9 months
Plays 'pat-a-cake' and 'peep-bo'	9–11 months
Casts	12–15 months
Imitates domestic activities	18 months–2 years
Isolated pretend play	2–3 years
Cooperate play with other children	3–4 years
Takes turns to play	4–5 years
Plays games to rules	$4\frac{1}{2}$–6 years

Appendix Immunization

M. Bellman, E. Peile

It is generally agreed that after education, clean water and sanitation (which are social actions), the most beneficial and cost-effective *health* intervention is immunization for the primary prevention of infectious diseases. For that reason all countries in the world have a childhood immunization programme supported by the World Health Organization. Despite this, infections remain the commonest cause of death in children across the globe. However, in Western countries, which have a universal childhood immunization programme, the incidence of severe morbidity and mortality from infectious diseases is low.

In the UK childhood immunization against diphtheria was introduced in 1940, followed in the next few years by immunization against pertussis (whooping cough) and then tetanus. The incidence of all three diseases plummeted with a concordant dramatic reduction in the number of deaths. The number of available vaccines has steadily increased and now protection is offered against 11 infectious diseases and deaths from these particular causes are now rare.

One of the primary aims of immunization is to provide a population with *herd immunity* so that the number of susceptible individuals is so small that the infectious organism cannot survive by chain transmission of infection. This is the best way of protecting people who are unimmunized for any reason, for example immunocompromised or not accessed immunization. Effective herd immunity can only be achieved by immunizing around 90% of the target population, which is why it is very important that every eligible child should have it as no vaccine is 100% effective.

Mothers are often worried about the safety of vaccines and are very aware of side effects, which often receive a lot of publicity. However, serious adverse reactions to immunization are extremely rare and the risks are vastly outweighed by the benefits. There are valid contraindications in a very a small number of children and these are listed in the 'Green Book' published by the Department of Health (HMSO 1996).

IMMUNIZATION SCHEDULE IN THE UK

Protection against tuberculosis (TB) is provided by offering BCG vaccine to a targeted population of individuals at increased risk, for instance because they live in an area with a high incidence or whose parents were born in a country with a high incidence of TB. It can be given to such infants age less than 3 months without any prior tests, but older children should first be assessed for previous infection with a Mantoux test (Table A2.1)

Table: Immunisation schedule in the UK		
Age	Vaccine	Method
2 months	Diphtheria/Tetanus/Pertussis/Poliomyelitis/ Haemophilus type B (DTaP/IPV/Hib)	1 injection
	Pneumococcal vaccine	1 injection
3 months	DTaP/IPV/Hib	1 injection
	Meningococcus group C (MenC)	1 injection
4 months	DTaP/IPV/Hib	1 injection
	MenC	1 injection
	Pneumococcal vaccine	1 injection
12 months	Hib/MenC	1 injection
13 months	Measles, Mumps and Rubella (MMR)	1 injection
	Pneumococcal vaccine	1 injection
3 yrs 4 mths-5 yrs	Diphtheria, Tetanus, Pertussis and Polio (D*TaP/IPV or d+TaP/IPV)	1 injection
	MMR	1 injection
13-18 years	Diphtheria, Tetanus and Polio (Td/IPV)	1 injection

*D – full dose diphtheria vaccine
+d – reduced dose diphtheria vaccine for children over 10 years and younger children who have completed a primary immunisation course in infancy

References

Department of Health 1996 Immunisation against infectious disease. Scottish Office, Welsh Office, DHSS (Northern Ireland). HMSO, London

Websites

www.immunisation.nhs.uk (up-to-date source of information on vaccines, disease and immunization in the UK)

3

Appendix
Sexualized behaviour

M. Bellman, E. Peile

Sexual behaviour is a normal part of children's play as they grow, change shape and become more social. While the stages and progress of physical sex development are fairly well mapped out (see Chapter 4), the process of cognitive and emotional development is relatively poorly understood and variable. Many factors influence the way in which children behave sexually, the most important perhaps being experience and peer pressure.

It is not uncommon for sexualized behaviour to be observed in a child and a decision must be made about whether or not it is normal, and therefore best ignored, or whether it is abnormal, and therefore to be acted on and possibly reported. The difficulty of the decision for a child care professional is compounded by the knowledge that reporting will possibly lead to a full child protection procedure, which is stressful for all concerned. Observers will have their own cultural and personal concept of acceptability which may determine their reactions. However, in all cases, the best interests of the child are paramount and cannot be compromised. Hence it is crucial that the professional knows about the range of normal sexual behaviour, so that when appropriate, no action is taken or 'non-invasive' management, such as gentle discouragement, distraction or stopping the child from being seen by peers can be carried out. Unfortunately, the boundary of normal sexual behaviour with abnormal is fuzzy and there may be no easy answer.

Child sexual abuse is distressingly common and the possibility must be borne in mind. The following guidelines in Tables 1–3 may help to distinguish 'normal' from potentially 'abnormal' activity, which requires further investigation:

Table 1 Typical sexual knowledge	
Age 2–6 years	**Age 7–12 years**
Knows that girls and boys have different private parts	Knows about physical aspects of puberty, especially after age 10
Knows words (usually slang) for genitalia	Knows correct terms for genitalia although often uses slang words in conversation
Has limited knowledge about pregnancy and childbirth	Has increased knowledge about pregnancy, intercourse and masturbation

Table 2 Common sexual behaviours	
Age 2–6 years	**Age 7-12 years**
No strong sense of modesty and enjoys own nudity	Sexual play with familiar friends
Uses 'elimination' words (wee/poo) for fun	Interested in sexual content in media
May explore body differences between boys and girls	Touches own genitalia in private
Curious about private parts	Looks at nude pictures with interest
May touch genitalia in public	Interested in the opposite sex
Some sex play with siblings and friends	Shy about undressing
Enjoys touching genitalia	Shy with opposite sex adults
Limited masturbation	More intense masturbation in private

Table 3 Uncommon (worrying) sexual behaviour age 2-12 years	
Puts mouth on private parts	Suggests sex acts with friends
Inserts objects into rectum or vagina	Imitates intercourse
Masturbates with objects	Undresses other people
Masturbates for attention or asks others to participate	Asks to watch sexually explicit material on television
Touches other people's private parts after being told not to	Makes sexual sounds

Index

Notes
    Page number in **bold** refer to tables
    Page number in *italics* refer to
        figures

A

abdomen, fetal 15–17
abdominal pain 187, 188
abortion 10, **20**
absolute poverty 158, **158**
abuse 157, 170
    see also neglect
acceptable behaviour 110, 114
accessory nerve development 13
acquired childhood aphasia (ACA)
    98
acute otitis media (AOM) 186
adaptive response 107
adenoids 65, 186
adenotonsillectomy 65
adolescents
    growth spurt, gender differences
        34
    health 165, 165–167
    play 111
        peer pressure 115
    pregnancy 165–167
        high risk groups 166
        impact **166**
        rates 166
    risk behaviour 165–167
    role imitation/rehearsal 112
    sleep-wake behaviour 65, 69
adrenaline (epinephrine) injectors
    58
adults
    play 115
    sleep **65**
    see also parents
AIDS, breast feeding
    51
air quality 168
alcohol, adolescent *165*
allantois 16
allergens 184
    avoidance during weaning 52
allergic (perennial) rhinitis 184
allergy 55–58, 183–184

definition 55
diagnosis 183–184
treatment 183–184
see also specific allergies
ambient noise 136–137, *137*
amblyopia 132
analgesia, endogenous 144
analgesic drugs 144
androgens
    boys 34, 41
    girls 41
aneuploidy 6
Angelmann syndrome 5–6
anorexia nervosa 191
antenatal time course 10, *10*
antibiotics
    intrapartum 22
    preterm baby 25
anus
    agenesis 15
    anal fissure 188
    fistula 15
anxiety 80
    maternal 147
    new environment 80
    separation 68, 80, 144–145
    sleep disturbances 65, 67
aorta 13
Apgar score **24**
    preterm baby 24
apnoea
    central 65
    of prematurity 25–26
appendicitis 143
appropriate for gestational age **20**
aqueous humour 131
arachidonic acid (AA) **48**
arm swing, reciprocal 125
arousal disorders 70
articulation disorders 99–100
artificial feeding 48, **48**, **49**
    developing countries 59
Aspergers syndrome (AS) 81, 109
asthma 185
asylum seekers 154
asymmetric tonic neck reflex (ATNR)
    106, **195**
atopic eczema 180
atopy 184
atrium, development 13
attachment 145

attention 76–77
    assessment 77
    definition 76
    development 76–77
    difficulties/disorders 77, 81, *81*
    motor development 123–124
    psychological tests **75**
attention deficit disorder (ADD) 81
attention deficit hyperactivity
        disorder (ADHD) 81, *81*
auditory association **139**
auditory attention **139**
auditory closure **139**
auditory discrimination **139**
auditory figure-ground **139**
auditory integration **139**
auditory memory **139**
aura 190
auricle (pinna) 135
authoritarian parenting style 157
autistic spectrum disorders (ASD)
        81
    case study 194
    co-ordination difficulties 128
    language impairment 98, 100
autonomic nervous system
        development 10
autonomy 78
autosomal inheritance 2–4
    disorders 3, 4
    dominance 3, *3*
    recession 3, 3–4
autosomes 2
auxologists 45

B

baby walker 123
balance (equilibrium) 140, *140*
balanced translocation 6
Barker hypothesis 172–173
BCG vaccine 199–200
bear walking 123
Beckwith–Wiederman syndrome 5
beclomethasone, antenatal 22
bedtime routine 67
behaviour
    acceptable 110, 114
    development 73–82

behaviour, cont'd
   environmental effects 159–167
   parental 159, *160*, 165
   risk behaviour in adolescents
         165–167
   sexualised 201
   sleep-wake *see under* sleep
behavioural problems 78–80
   British children 150
   case studies 193–194
   communication breakdown 92
   eating 58, 79
behavioural support, temper tantrums
      79
behaviourism, play theories 104
bilingualism 91, **178**
binge eating 191
biological programming 172–173
birth weight
   cognitive development 44
   definitions **20**
   environmental factors **173**
bladder
   control 66, 78, **198**
   development 16
blankets, self-soothing 68
blastocyte 9
blastocyte cavity 10
blastomere 9
blind spot *130*, 131
blocked ear 135
blocked nose 184
blue breath-holding attacks 190
body hair development 42, *43*
body mass index (BMI) 55
   boys *56*
   girls *57*
body temperature control
   preterm baby 24, 25
   sleep 65–66
bonding 144
bones 31, 34
bottom shuffling 122, **178**
bowel retraining methods 78
bow legs (genu varum) **118**, 124,
      177–178, *179*
brain development
   abnormal 12
   early life 173–174
   embryonic 12, *12*
   environmental factors 173–174
   fetal growth 12
   preterm baby 25, 27
   see also cognition
bran 54
bread **54**
breast, puberty and *41*, 41–42
breast feeding 47–48

advantages 48–50
allergic disease reduction 50
atopic eczema 180
breathing problems protection 50
caffeine intake 68
developing countries 59
ethnic groups 160
HIV/AIDS 51
hormones **48**
maternal benefits 50
preterm baby 50
problems 51–52
social class 160
social environment 160–161, *161*
special circumstances 50–51
special needs baby 50
breast milk
   composition 48–49, **49**
   infection protection 49–50
   preterm baby 24, 50
breast milk jaundice 26
breath-holding attacks 190
brick building **197**
Britain, children in 153, **153**
British Picture Vocabulary Scale
      (BPVS reference) 74
bronchodilators 185
bruxism (toothgrinding) 70
bug-busting 181
built environment 168
bulimia 191
buzzer alarms, enuresis 189

C

café-au-lait patches 181
Cambridge crowded letter test 134
camera phones 170
canal of Schlemm 131
capilliary haemangioma (strawberry
      naevi) 180
carbohydrates, in milks **49**
Cardiff 'count to ten' 21
cardinal veins 13
cardiotocography (CTG) 21
cardiovascular system
   abnormal development 14
   disease, preterm delivery risk **21**
   embryology 13–14
   sleep and 65
β-carotene **48**, **54**
catch-up-growth 30
celiac disease 58
central apnoeas 65
central auditory nervous system
      (CANS) 137–138

central auditory processing (CAP)
      138, **139**
central auditory processing disorder
      (CAPD) 138–139
central nervous system development
      12–13
   brain *see* brain development
   spinal cord 12
cerclage 22
cereals **54**
cerebral palsy 25, 26
cervical incompetence 22
cervical suture 22
chatrooms 170
chemical irritant dermatitis 179
chicken pox 181, **182**
child directed speech (CDS) 87
children in need **155**
Children's National Service
      Framework 169
Children's Trusts 169
child's rights 153
chin tucking 120
chlamydia 166
*Choosing health: making healthy choices
      easier* 162, 169
choroid 130
chromosome(s) 2, 6
   see also DNA; inheritance
chronic lung disease (CLD) 27
ciliary body 18, 130
circadian rhythms 62–63
cleft palate 17
clumsy children 126
cochlea 136, 137
   implants 93
cochlear duct 136
cochlear nucleus 137
cocooned baby 123
codon 2
coelom 10
cognition
   development 73–80
   early 73–74
   measurement 74–77
      cultural issues 74
      tests *75*
   play 108–109
   space and time awareness 77
   speech processing difficulties 99
cognitive theory, language acquisition
      86–87
cold receptors **141**
colic 51–52, 187–188
coloboma 18
colostrum 47–48
colour blindness 4, 133
colours, complementary 133

comforting rituals 81
commando crawling 122
commerce 170
commercial world 170–172
communication 83–102
  definition 83
  development 87–88, *98*
    birth-2 months **88**
    2 - 5 months **89**
    5 - 7 months **90**
    7 - 10 months **91**
    10 - 13 months **92**
    13 - 18 months **93**
    18 months - 2 years **94**
    2 - 2.5 years **95**
    2.5 - 3.5 years **96**
    3.5 - 5 years **97–98**
    factors affecting 88–92, *98*
  expressive *see* expressive
      communication
  infants 73
  media 170–172
  play 109–110
  problems
    primary difficulties 99–100
    secondary to other conditions
      93–98
  see also language
communities 152, 167
comprehension milestones **198**
concomitant squint 131
concrete operational period 111
conductive deafness 18
cones, eye 130
conflict, play 114–115
confusional arousals 70
congenital adrenal hyperplasia 17
consonant sounds 84
constipation 78, 188
convergent squint 131
conversation **84**
cooing sounds **89**
coordination 126–128
  definition 126
  language difficulties 126
  problems
    identification 126–128, 127f
    treatment approaches 127
corkscrewing 121
cornea 129
corneal light reflection 134
coryza 184
co-sleeping 66
cough 184–185
cough reflex 184–185
count by rote **95**
country of birth, birth weight **173**
cover test 134

cow's milk 48
  composition **49**
  intolerance 58, 184
  weaning 53
cradle cap (seborrhoeic dermatitis)
    179
cranial nerves development 13
crawling 122, *122*
cries/crying 182
  colic 51–52, 187–188
  reflexive **88**
crime, adolescents *165*
crista ampullaris 136, 140
crown-rump measurement 45
cruising 123
crying *see* cries/crying
cuddling 145
cultural environment, play 114–115
cupula 140
cutaneous receptors **141**, *141*, 141–143
cystic fibrosis 4

D

daytime sleeping 64
  adolescents 65
  children aged 1-5 years 64
  sleep-phase delay 68–69
deafness *see* hearing impairment
decibels 136
deciduous teeth 182–183, **183**
dehydration 31, 187
deletion, genetic material 5
delta waves **62**
dependence 145
depression 80
  maternal 71
dermatomes 141
Desmopressin 189
despair, post-separation 145
detachment, post-separation 145
development
  communication *see under*
      communication
  domains **117**
  embryonic 9–18
  emotional 80–82
  gait 124–125
  memory 76
  milestones **196–198**
  normal variation 177–191, **178**
  selected movements 120
  see also growth; *specific
      organs/systems*
developmental dyspraxia 100
developmental theories

motor skill 117–119
play 104
dexamethasone, antenatal 22
diabetes mellitus 189
  preterm delivery risk factor **21**
diarrhoea 187
diencephalon 12
diet 160–163
  income and **162**
  see also food; nutrition
digestive system development 15
diphtheria vaccine 199, **199**
diplopia (double vision) 131–132
disability 154–155
discipline 157
distraction test 139
DNA
  analysis 6–7
  sequencing/cloning 6–7
  structure 1–2, *2*
docosahexaenoic acid (DHA) **48**
domestic violence 156
dominant inheritance
  autosomal 3, *3*
  X-linked *4*, 4–5
Doppler ultrasound, fetal blood flow
    22
dorsal column, sensory pathway
    141–142, **143**
double vision (diplopia) 131–132
Down's syndrome 6
drawing skills **197**
drugs, adolescents *165*
ductus arteriosus 14
  preterm baby 25
ductus venosus 13, 14
dummies 183
duodenal stenosis 15
duodenum development 15
dynamic equilibrium 140
dysarthria 98
dysfluency **97**, 100–102, **101**
dyslexia *81*
dyspraxia *81*, 100
dysuria 189

E

ear *135*, 135–136
  development 18
  pain 186
  see also hearing
ear, nose and throat symptoms
    184–186
earache (otalgia) 186
early morning waking 69

Early Years Movement 152
eating problems 191
  behavioural 58, 79
echolalia **94, 101**
economic environment, child
      health/wellbeing 157–159
ectoderm 10, *11*
education 168–169
eggs **54**
egocentric speech **93**
ejaculation, spontaneous 34
elective Caesarean delivery, preterm
    baby 24
elective mutism 92
embryo 10
embryoblast 10
embryology 9–18
  see also fetus
embryonic arches 13
embryonic disc 10
emotional deprivation, growth 44
emotional development 80–82
emotional problems
  British children 151
  communication breakdown 92
  developmental 81–82
encephalin 144
encopresis 188
endoderm 10, *11*
endolymph 136
endorphins 144
enuresis 64, 66, 78, 189
  nocturnal 189
  secondary 78
environment
  birth weight and **173**
  built 167–168
  communication development
    89–92
  cultural 114–115
  developmental progress **178**
  diet 161–162, *162*
  enuresis 78
  exploration 107, *107*
  global 168
  linguistic 87
  new, anxiety in 80
  obesogenic 159
  physical 167–168
  play 112–115
  preterm baby 24
  restrictions to play 113
  sleep 66
  social *see* social environment
epiblastic cells 10
epilepsy 189, 193–194
epinephrine (adrenaline) injectors 58
epistaxes (nose bleeds) 186

equilibrium (balance) 140, *140*
erythema infectiosum (fifth disease)
    181, **182**
ethnicity
  birth weight and **173**
  developmental progress and **178**
  education issues 168–169
  health and 154
Eustachian tube 135
executive function 77
exercise 55, 163–164
  factors affecting *164*
  sleep problems 67
exons 7
experimental vocal play **90**
expressive communication 84, *84*, **84,**
    87
  birth - 2 months **88**
  2 - 5 months **89**
  5 - 7 months **90**
  7 - 10 months **91**
  10 - 13 months **92**
  13 - 18 months **93**
  18 months - 2 years **94**
  2 - 2.5 years **95**
  2.5 - 3.5 years **96**
  3.5 - 5 years **97–98**
external auditory canal 135
external (outer) ear 18, 135
extremely low birth weight **20**
extremely preterm babies 19, **20**
extrusion reflex, weaning 52
eye
  development 17–18
  movements 131
  muscles 131
  structure 129–131, 130f
  see also vision

F

face, development 17, *17*
facial nerve development 13
faints 189–190
fair trade movement 170
families/family environment
  breakdown 156
  composition 156
  health *155*, 156–157
  language development 90
  trends **156**
  see also parents
fathers, bonding with child 144
fats **49, 54**
fears/fear reaction 80
febrile convulsions 189

feeding 47–59
  artificial 48, **48, 49,** 59
  breast *see* breast feeding
  breast or bottle decision 47
  cycle, sleep-wake behaviour 63
  developmental milestones **198**
  early, problems in 51–52
  preterm baby 24
  problems 79
  weaning *see* weaning
  see also food
feet
  postural deformities 177–179
  touching 121
female genitalia development 16–17
'ferocious fours' 79
fertilization 9
fertilization age 9
fetal circulation 14, *14*
fetus
  blood flow assessment 22
  definition 19
  early development 10–13, *11*
  hearing 134
  heart rate 21
  movements 21
  sex 9
  wellbeing assessment 21–22
fifth disease (erythema infectiosum)
    181, **182**
finger foods 53
first words 92
fish **54**
FISH test 6
fits 189–190
'5 A Day' campaign 162
flat feet **118,** 177, *178*
flutter **143**
follicle-stimulating hormone (FSH)
    41, 43, 44
follow-on milks 53
food
  allergy 180, 184
  avoidance, emotional disorder 79
  as comfort 55
  costs 161
  environmental factors 161–162, *162*
  income and 162–163
  intolerance 55–58
  labelling 161
  refusal 58, 191
  school 161
  see also diet; feeding; nutrition
food poverty 162–163
food wars 58
foramen ovale 13, 14
foramen primum 13
foramen secundum 13

forebrain 12
foregut 15
foreign body inhalation 185
fore-milk 48–49
formula feeds, composition **48, 49**
four point crawling 122, *122*
fovea 131
fricative sound 84
frontal lobe development 173–174
fruit **54,** 162
funny turns 189–190

G

gag reflex, preterm baby 25
gait **118,** 124–128
  analysis 126
  development 124–125
    12-18 months 124
    18-24 months 124–125
  maturation 125
    2-3 years 125
    3-4 years 125
    4-7 years 125
    7-9 years 125
  parental concerns 125–126
  postural alignment 125
  referrals 125–126
gallop 125
'games with rules' 108
gametes 2
gastro-enteritis 186, 187
  bacterial causes 187
  breast feeding 50
gastro-intestinal tract
  function in sleep 65
  symptoms 186–188
gastro-oesophageal reflux 51, 187
  preterm baby 25
gastro-oesophageal reflux disorder
    (GORD) 65, 187
gastroschisis 15
gastrulation 10
gender
  adolescents growth spurt 34
  developmental progress **178**
  language development 90
general practitioners, sleep problems
    71
genetic code 2
genetics 1–7, **178**
genital system
  congenital abnormalities 17
  development 16–17
  pubertal changes 34, 41
genomic imprinting 5

genotype 2
genu valgum (knock knees) **118,** 125,
    178–179, *179*
genu varum (bow legs) **118,** 124,
    177–178, *179*
geography, health 154
germ layers 10, *11*
gestational age 9, 20
gestation length 30
gestures
  hearing loss 94–96
  multiple birth children 90
glandular fever (infectious
    mononucleosis) 185–186
glaucoma 131
global environment 168
globe, eye 129
glossopharyngeal nerve development
    13
glue ear 186
gluten intolerance 58
good-enough-mother 146
grasp reflex **195**
grass pollen allergy 184
Green book 199
Griffiths Developmental scales 74
gripe water 188
grommets 186
group B Streptococci (GBS)
    transmission prevention 22
growing pains 45, 179
growth 29–46
  birth, as interruption in 30–31
  differential 31, 34
  drivers of 44
  infant 31, *32–33*
  measurement 45
  obesity 30
  puberty 34–44
  toddler 31, *32–33*
  in uterus 29–30
  wellbeing marker 44
growth hormone
  bone age 34
  secretion 44, *45*
growth hormone-insulin-like growth
    factor (GH-IGF) 44

H

habitual polydypsia 189
haematuria 189
haemoglobinopathies 4
β haemolytic streptococcus 185
hair cells, ear 136
half-kneeling position 123, *123*

hands, moving to mid-line 120–121
haploid cells 2
hardwired brain 173
hayfever 184
head
  control 120
  growth 31
  size measurements 34, *35–36*
headaches 190
headbanging 70
head lag 120
head lice 181
head righting reflex **195**
head-rolling 70
head turning 120
health
  Britain's children 150–151
  determinants 150–151
  different circumstances 153–156
  factor influencing *151,* 151–174
  normal boundaries 177–191
health services 169
  neonatal 22–23, **23**
  perinatal 22–23, **23**
  sleep problems 71
health visitors, sleep problems and 71
Healthy Eating 53–54
Healthy School Programme 169
hearing 134–139
  acoustics 136–137
  auditory processing *137,* 137–139,
    138
  ear anatomy *135,* 135–136
  fetal 134
  infants 134
  speech production 99
  tests 27, 100, 139
hearing aids 93
hearing impairment
  communication difficulties 93–96
  congenital 18
  non-verbal communication 94–96
hearing threshold 139
heart development 13
height charts *32–33, 37–40*
herd immunity 199
Hertz 136
Heschl's gyrus 138
heterozygous characteristics 3
high dependency units **23**
high guard elbows 124
hillocks of His 18
hindbrain 12
hindgut 15
hind-milk 49
hip flexion 121
Hirschsprung's disease 15
HIV, breast feeding 51

holding 146
homozygous characteristics 3
homunculus 142, *142*
hopping 125
House of Commons Select Committee Report on Obesity 170
housing 168
human chorionic gonadotrophin (hGC) 10, 16
human genome 2
Human Genome Project 7
humanism theories, play 104–105
human papilloma virus 180
human rights 153
hyaloid artery 18
hydrocephalus 12
hyperactivity 82
hyperalgesia **141,** 143
hyperbilirubinaemia 26
hypermetropia 132, *132*
hypnagogic hallucinations 69
hypnic myoclonia ('sleep starts') **62,** 69
hypochloraemic alkalosis 52
hypoglossal nerve development 13
hypoglycaemia, preterm baby 25
hypothermia, preterm baby 25

I

imaginary characters/friends 109
imitation
    play 112
    speech 86
immunization 181, **199,** 199–200
imperforate anus 15
imprinting 145
impulsivity 82
inattention **81,** 82
in-care children, teenage pregnancy 166
independence 78
indeterminate sleep, newborn 63
Infacol 188
infantile colic (3-month colic) 51–52, 188
infants/infancy
    communication 73
    growth 31, *32–33*
    hearing 134
    later health 172–173
    mortality rate, ethnicity 154
    nutrition in developing countries 58–59
    rapid growth 30
    sleep-wake behaviour 63–64

infections
    preterm baby 25
    systemic 181–182
    see also specific infections
infectious mononucleosis (glandular fever) 185–186
infestations 181
inheritance 2–6
    Mendelian 2–5
    mitochondrial 6
    non-Mendelian 5, 5–6
inhibin B 43–44
innate capacity theory, language acquisition 86
inner ear 136
    development 18
insecure attachment 156–157
insulin resistance 30
intellectual ability, psychological tests **75**
intensive care units, premature babies **23**
interventricular septum 13
in-toeing 177, *178*
intolerance 55–58
intracranial pressure, raised 190
intrauterine growth restriction (IUGR) 20, *20*
inverse care law 169
IQ tests 74, **75**
iris 18, 130, 133
iron 54
    deficiency **178**
    vegetarian diet 53
irritation, sleep disturbances 67
isodopsin 130

J

jargon **92**
jaundice, preterm baby 26
joint attention **91**
joint laxity **118**
joint receptors 141
jumping 125

K

kangaroo mother care, preterm baby 25
karyotype 6
kick-count 21
kidney
    congenital abnormalities 16

development 15–16, 18
    disease, preterm birth risk factor **21**
knock knees (genu valgum) **118,** 125, 177–178, *179*

L

labyrinth, ear 136
lactase 187
lactose intolerance 58, 187
language 75–76, 83–85
    acquisition theories 86–87
    arbitrary 84
    components 85
    delayed 89
    development 75, 89–92, **197–198**
    disordered 89
    environmental factors affecting 89–92
    expressive *see* expressive communication
    input 87
    pragmatic impairment 100
    psychological tests **75**
    receptive *see* receptive language
    secret, multiple birth children 90
    semantic impairment 100
    symbolic 83
    see also communication
language acquisition device (LAD) 86
large for gestational age 19–20, **20**
large intestine development 15
laryngotracheal diverticulum 15
laxatives 78, 188
learning difficulties
    communication difficulties 96–98
    moderate 96
    severe 96–97
learning theory, language acquisition 86
legs, postural deformities 177–179
leisure time, adults 115
lens (crystalline) 18, 130
'let down' reflex **48**
life course approach, epidemiology 174
lifestyle choices, low-income families 158
light/dark adaptation 133
light (pupillary) reflex 133
lipase 50
listening, speech production 99
literacy, psychological tests **75**
liver development 15

local environment, child
health/wellbeing 167–172
localization, sound **139**
locomotion development **178**
locomotor screening markers **119**
logical thinking 111
long chain polyunsaturated fatty acids
(LCPs), formula feeds **48**
low birth weight **20**
luteinizing hormone (LH) 41, 43, 44
lymphocytes, chromosomal analysis 6
Lyon hypothesis 6

M

macrobiotic diet 53
macula 131, 140
malathion 181
male genitalia
fetal development 16
pubertal development 42, *42*
manipulative skills, developmental
milestones **197**
manner of articulation 84
marketing 170–172
mastitis 51
masturbation 201–202
measles 181, **182**
meat **54**
mebendazole 181
mechanoreceptors **141**
media 170–172, *171*
communication 170–172
play trends 114
meiosis 2
Meissner corpuscles *141*, **143**
melatonin 62
infants 64
manufactured 71
memory 76
menarche 34
Mendelian inheritance 2–5
mental health teams, sleep problem
referrals 71
Merkel cells *141*, **143**
mesencephalon 12
mesenchyme 10
mesoderm 10, *11*, 16
mesonephroi 15
metanephric diverticulum (ureteric
bud) 16
metanephric mesoderm 16
metanephroi 15–16
metatarsus varus 177
metencephalon 12
midbrain 12

middle ear 135
development 18
problems, communication
difficulties 93
midgut 15
midline
hands, moving to 120–121
inability to cross 127
moving out of 121
mid-parental centile charts 45
migraine 190
milia 180
milk 54, **54**
follow-on 53
minerals, in **49**
products **54**
see also breast milk; cow's milk
minerals, in milks **49**
Minister for Children 168
miscarriage 10, **20**
mitochondrial inheritance 6
mitosis 2
mobile phones 170
molluscum contagiosum 180
Mongolian blue spots 181
Montgomery's tubercles 47
mood 80
Moro reflex **195**
morphemes 85
morphine 144
morphology, language 85
morula 9
mosaicism 6
mother(s)
age-birth weight relationship **173**
anxieties 147
behaviour patterns recognition 147
bonding 144
as caretaker 145–146
as child 146
depression, sleep problems 71
early mother-baby relationship *156*,
156–157, 172
medication and breast feeding 51
sixth sense 144–147
as witness 147
motor development 119
early **118**
milestones **196**
sensory integration 119–120
motor skills 117–128
mouth development 17
movements
control development 106–107
developmental milestones **196**
normal 120–123
Mullerian inhibiting factor 16
multiple births

breast feeding 50
language development 90–91
mumps 181, **182**
muscle/joint problems 126
muscle receptors 141
muscles, of eye 131
mutations 2
myelencephalon 12
myopia 132, *132*

N

napkin rashes 179
National Teenage Pregnancy Strategy
166, 166–167
nausea 186
neck righting reaction 120
necrotizing enterocolitis
breast feeding 50
preterm baby 25
neglect
health 157
language development 91–92
neonatal services
levels of care **23**
regionalization 22–23
neonates **20**
blood in the stool 188
circulation 14
emotional responses 80
sleep-wake behaviour 63, 67
social world 172
weight loss 30–31
neonatology **20**
nervous system development 12–13
neural crest 10
neural folds 10, 12
neural plate 10, 12
neural tubes 10, 12
neuroectoderm 10, *11*
neurofibromatosis 181
neurological symptoms 189–190
neuromaturational theory 118
neuromuscular disorders,
communication problems 98
neuro-ophthalmology 133
neuropathic pain 144
newborn *see* neonates
NHS Direct 182
night blindness 130
night disturbances 64–65
nightmares 70
night terrors 70
night waking 69
children aged 1-5 years 64
infants 64

nit comb 181
nociceptors 141, **141**
non-concomitant (paralytic) squint
        131
non-fluency, normal **97**
non-Mendelian inheritance 5, 5–6
non rapid eye movement (NREM)
        sleep 61
    cardiovascular control 65
    children aged 5-10 64
    deprivation 63
    infants 64
    newborn 63
    parasomnias 70
    stages **62**
nose
    bleeds (epistaxes) 186
    blocked 184
    development 17
notochord 10
nucleotide bases 1–2, 2
nucleotides, formula feeds **48**
numeracy, psychological tests **75**
nutrition
    developmental progress **178**
    growth 44
    later childhood 161–162
    see also diet; food
nutrition programmes 59
nystagmus 131

O

obesity 55, 56–57, 150, 163, **163**
    coronary risk factors 30
    definition 55
    eating habits 55
    growth 30
    impacts **163**
    junk food marketing campaigns 170
obesogenic environment 159
object recognition **93**
obligate carriers 4
obsessions 81
obsessive compulsive disorder (OSD)
        81
obstructive sleep apnoea (OSA) 65
occipito-frontal head circumference
        34, 35–36
ocular albinism 4
oesophagus development 15
oestradiol 43, 44
oestrogen 41
oils **54**
olfactory nerve development 13
omphalocele 15

oocyte 9, 16
operant conditioning 86
opioid peptides 144
optic cup 17
optic disc 130–131
optic nerve 13, 17, 130, 133
optic sulci 17
optic vesicles 17
organ of Corti 136
oromotor dyspraxia 100
ossicles, middle ear 135
otalgia (earache) 186
otic vesicles 18
otitis externa 186
otitis media
    acute 186
    secretory 135
    speech acquisition 99
oto-acoustic emission (OAE) 139
otoliths 140
out-toeing (external rotation) 177
overwiring phenomenon 173
oxytocin 48, **48**

P

Pacinian corpuscles 141, **143**
paediatricians, sleep problem referrals
        71
paedophiles 170
pain 143–144
    receptors 143
    referred 143
    sleeplessness 66–67
    threshold 143
pain control 144
pain inhibition 144
palate development 17
palatine processes 17
panic reactions 80
parachute reflex **195**
parallel play **94**
parasomnias 69–70
    deep sleep related 70
    light sleep related 70
    REM sleep related 70
    sleep onset related 69–70
parenting style
    child health/wellbeing 157
    early childhood 172
parents
    behaviour 159, 160, 165
    bonding with child 144
    counselling, preterm birth
        24, 27
    separation from, sleep and 67–68

size/height, growth projections 31
    see also mother(s)
partners, birth weight **173**
'passing phases' 115
peanut allergy 58, 184
penis
    fetal development 16
    pubertal development 42, 42
perennial (allergic) rhinitis 184
perinatal services
    levels of care **23**
    regionalization 22–23
peripheral nervous system
        development 13
permanent teeth 183, **183**
permethrin 181
permissive parenting style 157
pertussis (whooping cough) vaccine
        199, **199**
phantom limb pain 144
pharyngeal pouches 15
pharyngitis 185
phenotype 2
phobias 80
phonemes 84
phonetic skills (PAT reference) 74
phonological development 85
phonological disorders 99
photoreceptor cells 130
phototherapy 26
physical activity 163–164
physical environment, child
        health/wellbeing 167–168
physiotherapists, gait analysis 126
Piaget, Jean 103–104
Pierre Robin syndrome 17
pineal gland 62
pinna (auricle) 135
piperazine 181
pituitary gland development 12
placenta
    function, fetal growth 30
    insufficiency, fetal blood flow 22
place of articulation 84
placing reflex **195**
play 103–116
    adults 115
    characteristics 105–106
    child development 105
    cognitive skills 108–109
    communication 109–110
    cultural environment 114–115
    definitions 103
    developmental milestones **198**
    environmental influences 112–115
    group 114
    imitative 112
    physical environment 113

risk-taking 105–106
role development 111–112
self-development 111
skills used 106–112
social development 109–110
social environment 114–115
stimulation 105
theories 103–105
play audiometry 139
playfulness, levels of 106
playfulness theories 104
plosive sound 84
policy environment 168
polydypsia, habitual 189
polymerase chain reaction (PCR) 7
polyunsaturated fats **54**
polyuria 189
poor neighbourhoods 168
port wine stains 180
positive feedback, play 111
possetting 51, 187
post-nasal drip 185
posture, developmental milestones
    196
poverty 157–159
    diet and 162–163
    eradication initiatives 159
    health inequalities 158–159
    impact 158–159
    material deprivation 159
    progress in the UK 159
    psychosocial effects 159
    rural 154
'practice play' 108
Prader–Willi syndrome 5–6
pragmatics 85
pre-babble vocalizations **90**
precocious puberty 43
pregnancy
    embryology 9–18
    smoking during 164
    testing 10
    see also fetus
premature baby see preterm baby
prenatal life, later health 172–173
prepubertal stage 43
pretend play 109
preterm baby
    breast milk 50
    definition **20**
    at delivery 23–24
    disability rates 26
    energy requirements 24
    feeding 24
    growth 30
    initial management 24
    intensive care 20
    motor development 119

outcomes 26
problems 24–26
transport 23
undescended testes 16
preterm birth 19–28
    causes 20
    complication prevention 22
    definition 19–20
    delivery decisions 22
    follow-up 26–27
    prevention interventions 22
    risk factors 21
primitive streak 10
primordial follicles 16
projectile vomiting, persistent 52
prolactin 48
promethazine, sleeplessness 68
prone position, developmental
    milestones **196**
proprioception **143**
protein, in different milks **49**
protest, post-separation 145
proto words **92**
pseudoephedrine, sleeplessness 68
psychodynamic theories, play 104
psychological symptoms 191
psychological theories, play 104–105
psychosomatic abdominal pain 187
puberty 34–44
    biological clock 43
    breast changes *41*, 41–42
    hair development 42, *43*
    hormonal regulation 43–44
    late onset 34
    male genital development 42, *42*
    precocious 43
    secondary sexual changes 34, 41
    skeletal growth 34, *37–38, 39–40*
    sleep-wake behaviour 65
    timings **41**
pubic hair 42, *43*
public services 168
public transport 170
pulses **54**
Punnett's square 2, *3*
pupil 130
pupillary (light) reflex 133
pure tone audiometry 139
pyloric stenosis 52, 186
pyloromyotomy (Ramstedt
    procedure) 52, 186

Q

Quetelet Index see body mass index
    (BMI)

R

Ramstedt procedure
    (pyloromyotomy) 52, 186
rapid eye movement (REM) sleep
    61–62, 63
    body temperature regulation
        65–66
    cardiovascular control 65
    children aged 5-10 64–65
    deprivation 63
    dreaming 62
    newborn 63
    parasomnias 70
rashes 179–181
    viral infections 181–182
Rastafarian diet 53
receptive language *84*, **84**, 84–85, 87
    birth - 2 months **88**
    2 - 5 months **89**
    5 - 7 months **90**
    7 - 10 months **91**
    10 - 13 months **92**
    13 - 18 months **93**
    18 months - 2 years **94**
    2 - 2.5 years **95**
    2.5 - 3.5 years **96**
    3.5 - 5 years **97**
receptor organs 140–143
recessive inheritance
    autosomal *3*, 3–4
    X-linked 4, *4*
red reflex 134
referred pain 143
reflex anoxic seizures 190
reflexes 120
    asymmetric tonic neck reflex
        (ATNR) 106, **195**
    cough reflex 184–185
    extrusion reflex, weaning
        52
    gag reflex, preterm baby
        25
    'let down' reflex **48**
    light (pupillary) reflex
        133
    primitive neonatal **195**
    reflexive cries/crying **88**
    see also *individual reflexes*
reflexive noises **88**
refraction 132, *132*
regression to the mean **178**
relative poverty 158, **158**
renal agenesis 16
renal disease, preterm birth risk factor
    21

respiratory disease, preterm birth risk factor **21**
respiratory distress syndrome (RDS) 25
restrictive eaters 79
resuscitation, preterm baby 24
retailing 170
retina 17, 130
retinol (vitamin A) deficiency 130
retinopathy of prematurity (ROP) 26
retrieval 145
reward system 124
rhodopsin (visual purple) 130, 133
rhythmic movement disorder 69–70
road-traffic accidents 170
rods, eye 130
rolling 121
rooming-in 144
roseola infantum 181, **182**
rotation 120
rubella 181, **182**
Ruffini endings *141*, **143**

S

saccades 131
salt, dietary 54
saturated fats **54**
scabies 181
school
  attendance 169
  exclusion, teenage pregnancy 166
  food 161, 162
  phobias 80
  physical education (PE) *164*
School Fruit and Vegetable Scheme 162
sclera 130
seborrhoeic dermatitis (cradle cap) 179
sedatives, sleep problems 71
selective eaters 79
selective mutism 92
selenium, formula feeds **48**
self-consciousness 111
self-development, play 111
self-evaluation ability 111, 114
self-soothing methods 64, 68
semantics 85
semicircular canals 136, 140
sensorimotor skill, play 106–108
sensorineural deafness 18

sensory development, motor integration 119–120
sensory motor stage, language acquisition 86–87
sensory nerves, development 13
sensory stimulation, play 112–115
separation anxiety 80, 144–145
  sleep problems 68
septum primum 13
septum secundum 13
sex chromosomes 2
sex cords, primary 16
sex-linked inheritance 4–5
sexual behaviour 201
sexually transmitted diseases 166
Sheridan-Gardener cards 134
short-term (working) memory 76
siblings, developmental progress **178**
sidesitting *121*, 121–122
significant others 147
single nucleotide polymorphisms (SNiPs) 7
sinus venosus 13
sitting 121–122
skin problems 179–181
skin-to-skin contact 144
skipping 125
sleep 61–71
  bladder function 66
  cardiovascular control 65
  characteristics 63–65
  child *vs.* adult **65**
  cycles 62, *62*
  daytime *see* daytime sleeping
  daytime routine 67
  deprivation 63
  function 63
  gastro-intestinal function 65
  intermediate 62
  interruptions during *see* parasomnias
  learning associations 67
  non-rapid eye movement *see* non rapid eye movement (NREM) sleep
  normal, at wrong time 69
  normal behaviour establishment 66–68
  normal variation 68–70
  parental separation 67–68
  physiology 61
  problematic 70–71, 78–79
    referral options 71
  rapid eye movement *see* rapid eye movement (REM) sleep
  reluctance 68–69
  respiration 65
  sleep-wake behaviour 63–65, *64*

  adolescents 65
  children aged 1-5 years 64
  children aged 5-10 64
  infants 63–64
  newborn 63
  stages 61–63, **62**
  sudden infant death syndrome 66, **66**
sleeplessness 68–69
sleep paralysis 69
sleep-phase delay 68–69
'sleep starts' (hypnic myoclonia) **62**, 69
sleep sweating 66
sleeptalking 70
sleep walking 70
slow-wave sleep *see* non rapid eye movement (NREM) sleep
small-for-date baby 30
small for gestational age **20**
small intestine development 15
smiles **88**
smoking 164–165
  adolescent *165*
  birth weight **173**
  fetal growth 30
  pregnancy 164
  preterm delivery risk factor **21**
smothering mother 146
Snellen chart 134
snuffles 184
social capital 167
social class
  birth weight **173**
  gradients 158
social development, play 109–110
social development theory 109
social environment 149–175, *151*
  behavioural effects 159–167
  birth weight **173**
  breast feeding 160–161, *161*
  growing child 172–174
  layers 151–167, **152**, *152*
  lifestyle 159–167
  play 114–115
social exclusion 167
social inclusion 167
social inequalities, health 154
social interaction 87
  birth - 2 months **88**
  2 - 5 months **89**
  5 - 7 months **90**
  7 - 10 months **91**
  10 - 13 months **92**
  13 - 18 months **93**
  18 months - 2 years **94**
  2 - 2.5 years **95**
  2.5 - 3.5 **96**
  3.5 - 5 years **97**

social organizations 152
social policy 168
social skills, developmental
        milestones **198**
socioeconomic status
    early life 172
    preterm delivery risk factor **21**
softwired brain 173
soiling 78, 188
somatic cells 2
somato-sensory system 140–144
somites 10
Sonksen Silver test 134
sore throat 185–186
sound frequency, speech 99
sound waves 136, *136*, 137
space perception 77, 107
spatial judgement ability 108
special care units **23**
special senses 129–147
specific language impairment (SLI)
        98–99
speech 84–85
    anatomy 84, *85*
    delayed production 99–100
    developmental milestones **197**
    disordered production 99–100
    see also communication; language
speech and language therapy 89
    referrals 100, **101**
speech articulators 84
sperm 9
spermarche 34
spina bifida 12
spinal cord
    development 12
    somato-sensory pathways
        141–143
spinothalamic tract 142
squint (strabismus) 131–132, 134
stairs
    developmental milestones **196**
    as 'toy' 113
stammer 100–102, **101**
standing *122*, 122–123
static equilibrium 140
stepfamilies 156
stepping reflex **195**
steroids
    antenatal 22
    inhaled 185
stillbirth **20**
stimulant substance avoidance, sleep
        68
stomach development 15
stools 188
stool softeners 188
stork marks 180

strabismus *see* squint (strabismus)
strangers, fear of 80
strawberry naevi (capilliary
        haemangioma) 180
stretch receptors 141
Sturge–Weber syndrome 180
stutter 100–102, **101**
STYCAR 134
sudden infant death syndrome
        66, **66**
suprachiasmatic nucleus (SCN) 62
surface ectoderm 10, *11*
susceptibility genes 7
sustainability 168
swaddling 123
'symbolic play' 108
synaptic pruning 173
syncope, vasovagal attack 190
syncytiotrophoblast 10
syntax 85
systems theory 118–119

T

talipes 178, *179*
tears 129
teenagers *see* adolescents
teeth
    deciduous 182–183, **183**
    permanent 183, **183**
    staining 183
teething 182–183
    night waking 64, 67
    pain relief 183
telegraphic speech **95**
telencephalon 12
television 170–172
    educational benefits 171
    watershed 171
temperature, sleep 66
temper tantrums 79–80, 191
tension headaches, chronic 190
term baby **20**, 30
'terrible twos' 79
testis
    descent 16
    fetal 16
    pubertal development 42, *42*
testis-determining factor 16
testosterone 41, 43
    fetal 16
tetanus vaccine 199, **199**
tetracycline 183
thelarche *41*, 41–42
    premature 43
thermoreceptors **141**

threadworms 181
thrifty phenotype 172–173
tics 82
time orientation 77
'time out' approach 191
tip-toe walking 124
toddler
    blood in the stool 188
    gait 124
    growth 31, *32–33*
    sleep-phase delay 68–69
    social world 172
toddler diarrhoea 187
toileting **198**
tonsillitis 185
tonsils
    enlarged, obstructive sleep apnoea
        65
    growth 31
too-good-mother 146
tooth *see* teeth
toothgrinding (bruxism) 70
touch, light **143**
Tourette's syndrome 82
toys 113
    self-soothing 68
    traditional 114
    trends in 114
    see also play
tracheo-oesophageal fistula 15
tracking, eye 131
transcutaneous electrical nerve
        stimulation (TENS) 144
transitional care units 23
transitional movements, absence of
        124
transport 170
travel, active *164*, 170
    physical environment 168
Treacher Collins syndrome 17
trigeminal nerve 13, 143
trigeminal tract 143
trisomy 21 6
trisomy rescue 5
trophoblast 10
tuberculosis 199–200
tuning fork tests **143**
turn taking 108, *109*, 110
twitches 82
tympanic membrane 135

U

ultradian rhythm 63
ultrasound
    fetal growth assessment 21–22, 30

ultrasound, *cont'd*
  gestational age estimation 20
umbilical arteries 13, 14
umbilical hernia 15
umbilical veins 13, 14
umbilication 180
uniparental disomy 5–6
United Nations Convention on the
    Rights of the Child 153, 168
upper respiratory tract infections
    (URTI) 184
urachus 16
ureteric bud (metanephric
    diverticulum) 16
urethra development 16
urinary tract
  development 15–16
  infections 189
    formula feeding 50
  symptoms 188–189
urine
  blood in 189
  fetal 15
urogenital system development 15–17
urticaria 184
uterus development 16
uveal tract 130

V

vaccines 199
vagus nerve development 13
valsalva manoeuvre 135
variegated babble **91**
vasovagal attack 190
vegetables **54**
vegetative noises **88**
ventricles, primitive 13–14
verbal behaviour theory 86

verbal dyspraxia 100
verruca 180
very low birth weight **20**
very preterm babies 19
vestibulitis 186
vestibulo-cochlear nerve development
    13
vibration **143**
Vineland screening scale 74
violence
  adolescents *165*
  imitation 112
viral infections 181–182
visceral receptors 141
visceral sensation **143**
visible light *132*, 133
vision 129–134
  monocular 131
  optics *132*, 132–133
  stereoscopic 131–132
  testing 133
visual acuity tests 134
visual organizational ability 77
visual pathway 133, *133*
visual persistence 133
visual purple (rhodopsin) 130, 133
visual reinforcement audiometry 139
visual sensation 133
visuospatial ability 77
vitamin(s)
  deficiency 130
  milks, varying content **49**
  supplementation 53
vitamin A **54,** 130
vitamin C **54**
vitelline veins 13
vitreous humour 131
vomiting 186
vowel sounds 84–85
vulnerable children 155, **155**

W

wakefulness 61
walking 123, *123*
warts 180
water, in different milks **49**
wax, ear 135
weaning 52–55
  dietary balance 53–55
  food composition 52–53
  purées to lumps progression 53
  signs that baby is ready **52**
  vegetarian 53
weight charts *32–33, 35–40*
wheezing 185
white breath-holding attacks 190
whooping cough (pertussis) vaccine
    199, **199**
wobbly teeth 183
working (short-term) memory 76
World Health Organization (WHO),
    breast feeding
    recommendations 47

X

X-linked inheritance *4,* 4–5

Z

zinc 54–55
zygote 9